The Science of
Leaky Gut Syndrome:
Intestinal Permeability
and Digestive Health

By Case Adams, Naturopath

The Science of Leaky Gut Syndrome: Intestinal Permeability and
    Digestive Health
Copyright © 2014 Case Adams
LOGICAL BOOKS
Wilmington, Delaware
http://www.logicalbooks.org
All rights reserved.
Printed in USA
Front cover image: © Sebastian Kaulitzki
Back cover image: © Garry DeLong

Publishers Cataloging in Publication Data
    Adams, Case
The Science of Leaky Gut Syndrome: Intestinal Permeability and
    Digestive Health
    First Edition

    1. Medicine. 2. Health.
    Bibliography and References; Index

    ISBN-13: 978-1-936251-42-1

Other Books by the Author:

ARTHRITIS - THE BOTANICAL SOLUTION: Nature's Answer to Rheumatoid Arthritis, Osteoarthritis, Gout and Other Forms of Arthritis

ASTHMA SOLVED NATURALLY: The Surprising Underlying Causes and Hundreds of Natural Strategies to Beat Asthma

BREATHING TO HEAL: The Science of Healthy Respiration

ELECTROMAGNETIC HEALTH: Making Sense of the Research and Practical Solutions for Electromagnetic Fields (EMF) and Radio Frequencies (RF)

HEALTHY SUN: Healing with Sunshine and the Myths about Skin Cancer

HEARTBURN SOLVED: The Real Causes and How to Reverse Acid Reflux and GERD Naturally

NATURAL SLEEP SOLUTIONS FOR INSOMNIA: The Science of Sleep, Dreaming, and Nature's Sleep Remedies

NATURAL SOLUTIONS FOR FOOD ALLERGIES AND FOOD INTOLERANCES: Scientifically Proven Remedies for Food Sensitivities

ORAL PROBIOTICS: The Newest Way to Prevent Infection, Boost the Immune System and Fight Disease

PROBIOTICS: Protection Against Infection

PURE WATER: The Science of Water, Waves, Water Pollution, Water Treatment, Water Therapy and Water Ecology

THE CONSCIOUS ANATOMY: Healing the Real You

THE LIVING CLEANSE: Detoxification and Cleansing Using Living Foods and Safe Natural Strategies

THE ANCESTORS DIET: Living and Cultured Foods to Extend Life, Prevent Disease and Lose Weight

TOTAL HARMONIC: The Healing Power of Nature's Elements

Table of Contents

Introduction

For many years, naturopaths and herbalists described a digestive disorder they called "leaky gut syndrome." This condition was largely dismissed by the medical establishment as anecdotal and non-existent.

Furthermore, many in the medical establishment labeled those who taught 'leaky gut' as heretics. These included such prominent physicians of their era as Benedict Lust, Jethro Kloss, John Harvey Kellogg, Allan Eustis, Herbert Shelton, Paavo Airola, Bernard Jensen and many others.

Over the past couple of decades, however, research on intestinal drug absorption by the pharmaceutical industry has consistently confirmed that the lining of the small intestine is subject to alteration. This, they found, dramatically affected the absorption of drugs through the intestines. They termed this "increased intestinal permeability."

As this research progressed, a number of protocols were developed by researchers to rate the level of altered—increased—permeability existing within the intestines. They soon discovered that drug absorption wasn't the only issue affected by increased permeability. They found that increased intestinal permeability increased the admission of macromolecules, toxins and microorganism endotoxins into the body's tissues and bloodstream. Increased intestinal permeability became a scientifically credible disorder.

While pharmaceutical researchers were the first to define the disorder in the research, soon the research took another turn: Into the issues of disease causation. International government, university and hospital research has since linked intestinal permeability syndrome to a host of inflammatory diseases, including allergies, asthma, arthritis, liver disorders and other issues.

Much of this research has been led by medical researchers from France, Canada, Germany, Switzerland, the Netherlands, the UK and elsewhere in the world.

However, U.S research into this area remained limited to drug research, while the international scientific community has embraced the condition.

We will also show the scientific evidence for the existence of leaky gut syndrome by examining the science of increased intestinal

1

permeability. We'll present the research connecting increased intestinal permeability to many inflammatory and degenerative diseases.

We will prove for once and for all that leaky gut syndrome in the name of increased intestinal permeability, is associated with a multitude of inflammatory diseases.

We will then go further, to prove the causes of the disorder, and its relationships with gluten sensitivities along with other food sensitivities and allergic conditions.

Then we will provide clear solutions for the disorder.

Because many in the health community have branded this syndrome as leaky gut, this text inherits the moniker, while at the same time clarifies the medical condition termed increased intestineal permeability or IIPS.

It is time to lay down the clear science about this disorder, and clearly understand those choices we can make which will prevent and even reverse the condition. This will cover which types of foods, beverages, herbs and other choices can prevent, reverse and/or significantly improve leaky gut or IIPS.

While this text is intended for both health professionals and lay persons, the reader is advised to consult with their health professional before engaging any significant dietary, herbal or lifestyle changes: Working with someone who understands our medical history and the relative risks of change can guarantee that these concepts are applied correctly and at the appropriate time.

Chapter One

Increased Intestinal Permeability

Is IIPS the Same as Leaky Gut Syndrome?

Yes and no. The reader might try a little experiment: Walk into a medical doctor's office and ask the doctor if he or she knows what leaky gut syndrome is, and if so, whether they believe that it is a real condition.

Then ask either the same doctor or another doctor if they know what increased intestinal permeability is and if so, whether that is a real condition.

Most likely the doctor will either not know what leaky gut syndrome is, or simply believe that it does not exist as an actual condition.

At the same time, the majority of doctors will certainly know what IIPS is. Why? Because IIPS has been the subject of medical and clinical research for the past three decades.

Most doctors will admit to IIPS as a medical condition because they have to. Medical doctors must recognize that some people assimilate pharmaceutical drugs faster than others. This is because some people have greater absorption rates through their intestinal walls. They have greater permeability, in other words.

Research scientists studying pharmaceutical drugs had to understand why some people reacted more strongly to their medications than others. In order to understand this, they ran tests on urine to measure the metabolites of the drugs that were absorbed and processed. This gave them the first hint that some people absorbed the drugs faster than others.

But to be sure of the effect, they had to remove the possibility that some people were just metabolizing (breaking down) the drugs faster than others. So they established protocols to test substances that the body did not readily break down. This way, they could isolate whether some were absorbing faster or simply metabolizing faster.

The researchers found out that people were absorbing compounds at different rates. Those who had greater effects from pharmaceuticals were also absorbing the non-metabolizing drugs faster. Their intestines, for some reason, were more porous: They had greater permeability. This resulted in the name: *Increased intestinal permeability*.

All of us have intestinal permeability. If we didn't we could not absorb any nutrients through our intestines. But some people absorb more than others. And some absorb much more than others—and absorb larger molecules for some reason. So they have larger pores in their intestinal walls..

To say that this is the same as leaky gut syndrome could be considered accurate, but then again not. Our intestines do not "leak." Even the intestines of someone with IIPS do not "leak." Our intestines are not like big balloons filled with air or water, and some of these have holes in them and others don't.

Rather, our intestinal walls have pores--better described as gaps. Our intestines are lined with porous, villous epithelial cells. They have junctions that tie them together and tiny pores or gaps between them that allow particular molecules through. And since they are cells, there are also pores in their cell walls. We'll discuss the physiology more specifically later, but an intestinal wall with increased permeability simply has wider gaps between them, allowing larger molecules to be absorbed into the bloodstream.

The word "absorbed" is important. It means that the intestines are set up in such a way that they *draw* nutrients through to the bloodstream. This means they pull certain nutrients through, using a combination of ions and magnetically charged pores. This also utilizes a mucous membrane lining filled with a complex combination of ions, enzymes, probiotics and other elements—which help breakdown and filter nutrients, and in many cases, escort them through the intestinal walls.

In other words, the moniker 'leaky gut syndrome' would be like calling our mouth a vacuum cleaner. It would be like describing the process of eating as vacuuming food in. Rather, the act of eating is much more delicate and complex. Food doesn't just get sucked into our mouths. Eating is a complex process involving precise feeding, chewing, initial digestion with enzymes and so on.

The process of intestinal absorption is also quite complex. So while 'leaky gut syndrome' is more accurately described as IIPS, here we will use it to clarify the condition from a scientific perspective, as we lay out the evidence.

Some History

Dr. Harvey Kellogg was one of the most well-known physicians of the late Nineteenth century through the second World War. Dr. Kellogg is most famous for his invention of a whole grain breakfast cereal called corn flakes. More importantly, his accomplishments and stature within the health and medical communities during that era rose to great heights, and also fell to great depths.

Dr. Kellogg was a native of Battle Creek, Michigan, which became the eventual home for his medical center and his brother's breakfast cereal factory. Dr. Kellogg graduated from what is now Eastern Michigan University and then graduated from the New York University Medical College in 1875 with a medical doctor's degree.

Dr. Kellogg's specialty was digestive health. He was a surgeon who performed thousands of surgeries on the intestines and colon, removing cancers, polyps and even sectioning intestines when necessary. At one point, he said:

> *"Of the 22,000 operations that I have personally performed, I have never found a single normal colon, and of the 100,000 that were performed under my jurisdiction, not over 6% were normal."*

Dr. Kellogg also cared for many more thousands of patients in the hospitals he worked at, and at his medical center in Battle Creek. Here he promoted natural healing methods, but at the same time was conversant with all of the most modern medical treatments. He became renowned across the country for healing people that were pronounced untreatable by conventional medicine. Dr. Kellogg was a maverick, but his theories proved to be accurate.

For example, decades before modern medical research found that fiber reduces colon cancer, cholesterol and many other conditions, Dr. Kellogg was teaching and recommending high fiber whole foods. Through his abundant clinical experience, he saw that a fibrous diet with plenty of plant-based foods prevented colon cancer, constipation and many other intestinal disorders.

His dry cereal recipes promoted the concept of fiber for breakfast, as breakfast for most Americans of his day was eggs and bacon—in recent years shown to increase cholesterol and induce hardening of the arteries. Dr. Kellogg was a big proponent of nuts and beans as a protein source, and became one of the first producers of heart-healthy soy products. He was a proponent of yogurt for intestinal health before anyone had ever heard of yogurt.

Dr. Kellogg wasn't only focused on diet. His therapies ranged from breathing exercises to hydrotherapy to massage and water therapy. Dr. Kellogg also promoted massage and water therapy, both of which were rejected by western conventional medicine until after World War II, when army veteran hospitals discovered that massage and water therapy speeded up rehabilitation from war wounds.

Dr. Kellogg also recognized, long before western medical researchers discovered the need for vitamin D, that sunlight was critical to maintaining health and preventing disease. Now, almost a century after Dr. Kellogg's ideas about sunbathing for health and disease prevention were ridiculed by conventional western medicine, conventional western medical research has proven in double-blind placebo-controlled and randomized research that a deficiency of vitamin D (which is produced by sunlight) is associated with the cause or worsening of more than 70 different diseases.

In all these respects, Dr. Kellogg and other "natural doctors" of his time such as Dr. Benedict Lust, Dr. Jethro Kloss, Dr. Allan Eustis, Dr. Herbert Shelton, and later Dr. Paavo Airola and Dr. Bernard Jensen, shared a vision of natural health that was rejected by the conventional western medical institutions of the early-to-mid twentieth century.

This vision of health was based upon prevention. They used their medical degrees and clinical experience to determine that particular activities prevented disease, and other activities tended to cause disease. They also found that many of these same preventative therapies were also powerful healing therapies for diseased conditions.

Today, practically every one of these natural strategies, from high fiber to probiotics to vitamin D to alternative protein sources has proven to prevent disease in conventional western medical research.

These weren't the only theories that Dr. Kellogg and his colleagues held that have proven out. They also held the understanding that should the intestines become diseased through poor diet and the consumption of other toxins, the intestines could allow toxins access to the bloodstream and the body's tissues.

This internal exposure to toxins, they held, caused many inflammatory disease conditions. The condition was eventually described inaccurately as leaky gut. As we'll find, this theory, long disputed by western conventional medicine, has—like many other concepts by Kellogg and his colleagues—proven out to be true in modern randomized, double-blind placebo-controlled research.

Determining Intestinal Permeability

So how do scientists and physicians test for increased intestinal permeability? Many of the studies we'll discuss in this book utilize one or more of these procedures, so we ought to clarify them early on. Intestinal permeability is typically measured by giving the patient a compound that is not readily metabolized—or broken down—in the body.

Intestinal absorption is gauged using difficult-to-metabolize compounds of varying molecular sizes. Those compounds consisting of larger molecules will gauge the intestinal wall's ability to absorb larger molecules. Those with smaller molecule sizes will gauge levels of less permeability. Substances scientists have used for testing absorption through the intestines include:

- Horseradish peroxidase
- Ethylenediaminetetraacetic acid (CrEDTA or EDTA)
- Mannitol
- L-rhamnose
- Lactulose
- Cellobiose
- Polyethylene glycols of various molecular weights (such as Polyethyleneglycol 400)

These substances are not readily metabolized (broken down) in the body—particularly in the intestines, bloodstream and liver. So if they are absorbed into the bloodstream through the intestines, they can readily be measured in the urine. This will show the level of permeability within the walls of the intestines. They also have varying molecular sizes, allowing them to be used to measure gut permeability.

Absorption testing is controlled by giving the test subject two different substances of different molecular sizes at the same time. Increased permeability will allow larger molecules through at a higher rate. This allows the tests to accurately gauge permeability independent of the person's variations in metabolism.

For example, sugars and sugar alcohols such as lactulose and mannitol are often used. These indicate intestinal permeability because of their different molecular sizes and the fact that they are not readily metabolized after ingestion. After ingestion, the patient's urine is tested to measure the quantities that these two molecules were absorbed through the intestinal walls.

Because lactulose is a larger molecule than mannitol, it will thus be more present in the urine compared to mannitol when there is greater permeability of the intestinal wall. Intestines with normal permeability will have less lactulose absorption. This creates a ratio between lactulose and mannitol, which scientists call the L/M ratio. The L/M ratio has become an international standard to quantify intestinal permeability. When the lactulose-to-mannitol ratio is higher, more permeability exists. When it is lower, less (and normal) intestinal permeability exists. Higher levels are graduated using what many researchers call the *Intestinal Permeability Index*.

The procedure is simple. The researcher feeds a mixture of the two compounds, or the two separate compounds to the subject at the same time. After several hours—typically five or more—the subject's urine is tested. The urine is then analyzed for its contents of the two substances of relatively different sizes.

Over years of testing with these same substances, levels of the smaller and larger compounds have become standardized. This allows researchers or doctors the ability to immediately gauge the level of intestinal permeability in the patient or subject.

The standardized ratio becomes the ruler to measure by, associated with the period of time from ingestion to urination test. For example, the standardized L/M ratio is the proportion of lactulose to mannitol found in the urine after five hours of feeding to a patient.

Newer methods of determining permeability by international researchers include transepithelial electrical resistance testing. This methodology measures the ion resistance across the intestinal wall. This is a similar method used by electricians to determine the conductivity and electrical potential of circuits. The reasoning is that the intestinal wall is a conducting medium. The intestines draw nutrients or other molecules through epithelial gaps via ion conductance.

Diseases Related to IIPS

In the last two decades, increased intestinal permeability has been associated with a number of disorders. The list can be very long, depending upon our sources. Here we will focus on add associations made in modern clinical research with clinical findings of peer-reviewed health professionals and their respective organizations.

We'll be presenting numerous studies showing a myriad of diseases associated with IIPS. Let's start with a short sampling of some of the clinical human research that has found IIPS associated with disorders affecting millions of people around the world:

Asthma

Researchers from the Immunity and Allergy Department at France's Calmette Hospital (Benard *et al.* 1996) studied the potential of intestinal permeability among 37 asthma patients using chromium 51-labeled ethylenediaminetetraacetatic acid (CrEDTA) urinary recovery. They compared the test results with 13 COPD patients without asthma and 26 healthy people. They found that CrEDTA recovery among the asthma group was 2.5%, versus 1.16% in the COPD group and 1.36% in the healthy group—about double the levels of the non-asthma groups.

Furthermore, the asthma patients with allergic asthma had higher levels (2.94%) than the non-allergic (no IgE sensitivity) group (1.92%).

The researchers proceeded to continue the testing over a period ranging from two to 13 months to confirm the results. The results stayed consistent. The researchers concluded: "Our results support the hypothesis that a general defect of the whole mucosal system is present as a cause or a consequence of bronchial asthma."

Researchers from Sweden's University Hospital in Uppsala (Knutson *et al.* 1996) studied 12 patients with allergic asthma who were sensitive to birch pollen—along with 12 healthy controls. They found that exposure to the birch pollen allergen increased the intestinal permeability of the allergic group, but not the healthy group. They concluded: "This would suggest less organ specificity and more general allergic recognition shared by several immunocompetent tissues in the body, probably mediated by circulating IgE antibodies."

Medical researchers from Kuwait University (Hijazi *et al.* 2004) studied 32 asthmatic children together with 32 matched healthy children. They conducted a lactulose/mannitol test to determine intestinal permeability among both groups. They found that the asthmatic group exhibited more than three times the levels of intestinal permeability than did the control group. They also eliminated other possible relationships, such as eczema and inhaled steroid use.

Food Allergy

Oslo researchers (Kovács et al. 1996) found that higher antibody levels to food allergens was associated with increased intestinal permeability. They found that IgA and IgG antibodies against eight common food antigens among 35 allergy patients and 12 healthy controls were tested for IgA levels and 28 allergy patients and 20 controls were tested for intestinal permeability using the Cr-EDTA test. The two tests were performed among 17 patients, and 21 of the entire group permitted a repeat of the tests five years after.

The tested found that higher IgA antibody titers were associated with increased intestinal permeability among the allergic patients.

Medical researchers from Italy's University of Bari (Polimeno et al. 2010) studied the relationship between anisakiasis—an infection of the *Anisakis simplex* parasite—and intestinal permeability in 540 persons. They found that an anisakiasis infection significantly increased intestinal permeability. They also found that those who ate raw fish were most exposed to the parasite. Those with more intestinal permeability were also exposed to other pathogens, and when their parasitic infections were resolved, many showed improved permeability.

We'll show more of this research later as we discuss IIPS physiology, its causes, and its solutions.

Eczema

Eczema is characterized by rashes, itching, swelling and inflammation on the skin. Research has found eczema associated with allergies and toxic exposures.

Medical researchers (Jackson *et al*. 1982) gave polyethylene glycol to eight eczema patients with food allergies and 10 patients with supposed non-allergic eczema in order to investigate intestinal permeability. Both groups absorbed macromolecules in excess of the normal subjects. They concluded that eczema with and without food allergy was associated with "intestinal mucosal defects" (increased intestinal permeability).

Other Allergies

Medical researchers at Norway's University of Bergen (Lillestøl *et al*. 2010) found that irritable bowel syndrome was associated with intestinal permeability. Of the 71 adult subjects, 93% had irritable bowel syndrome and increased intestinal permeability, while 61% had other allergic conditions—primarily rhinoconjunctivitis. All the allergic sufferers also had respiratory allergies, and 41% had food allergies.

Hepatitis

Researchers from China's People's Hospital of Guangxi (Song, et al. 2009) studied 60 chronic severe hepatitis B patients and 30 healthy volunteers. They tested intestinal permeability using the urine lactulose/mannitol ratio (L/M), as well as serum diamine oxidase testing. They found that the hepatitis B patients had significantly more intestinal permeability than the healthy controls.

Irritable Bowel Syndrome

Researchers from Ohio State University's Medical School Zhou *et al*. 2009) studied 54 patients with irritable bowel syndrome along with 22 controls. They found that those patients with higher pain

11

intensity and higher levels of diarrhea also had greater levels of increased intestinal permeability.

Researchers from China's Qilu Hospital and Shandong University found that increased intestinal permeability is associated with irritable bowel syndrome. They also found that IIPS decreased significantly after the supplementation with probiotic fermented milk with *Streptococcus thermophilus, Lactobacillus bulgaricus, Lactobacillus acidophilus* and *Bifidobacterium longum.*

Anemia

A study from the Cochin St Vincent de Paul Hospital in Paris (Kalach *et al.* 2001) studied 64 children with milk allergy symptoms, and found that higher intestinal permeability levels were associated with anemia.

Bacteria Infections

Researchers from South Korea's Sungkyunkwan University Kangbuk and Samsung Hospital (Kim et al. 2011) studied 113 patients with advanced liver cirrhosis and gastrointestinal bleeding. Those patients with higher levels of increased intestinal permeability were higher among those patients with bacterial infections.

HIV Infection

Researchers from the Human Immunology Section of the U.S. National Institutes of Health's Vaccine Research Center (Sandler et al. 2011) stated in their background information of a study that associated HIV death with lipopolysaccharides and CD14, that: "Chronic human immunodeficiency virus (HIV) infection is associated with intestinal permeability and microbial translocation that contributes to systemic immune activation, which is an independent predictor of HIV disease progression. The association of microbial translocation with clinical outcome remains unknown."

Researchers from the University of Natal in Durban, South Africa (Rollins et al. 2001) found among 272 infants with HIV that HIV infections were associated with significantly increased intestinal permeability. They utilized the lactulose/mannitol test. They found that the level of permeability increased with more severe HIV infections.

Researchers from London's Centre for International Child Health (Filteau et al. 2001) studied 238 infants with HIV-infections. They found that HIV was associated with significantly increased levels of intestinal permeability. Their controlled study found that daily supplementation with antioxidants vitamin A (retinyl palmitate) and beta-carotene resulted in significantly lower levels of intestinal permeability among the infected children. Vitamin A supplementation did not make a difference in permeability levels among the healthy children.

Pancreatitis

Researchers from China's Third Affiliated Hospital of Nanchang University (Zhang et al. 2010) studied 63 patients with severe pancreatitis, along with healthy controls. They found that those with severe pancreatitis had significantly increased levels of intestinal permeability. Several measures, including levels of serum diamine oxidase, endotoxins, transepithelial electrical resistance and F-actin rearrangement of the epithelial monolayer were all used to identify what they concluded was "gut mucosal dysfunction."

Rheumatoid Arthritis

Scandinavian researchers (Sundqvist et al. 1982) found that intestinal permeability was increased among patients with rheumatoid arthritis. They used the PEG 400 test to determine permeability. They also found that intestinal permeability in the subjects decreased after a period of fasting.

Depression

It might seem odd that intestinal permeability can be linked with a mood disorder, but considerable research from other studies has connected bacterial endotoxins with moods.

Belgium researchers (Maes et al. 2008) found that major depression was associated with IIPS. They found that depression was related to an inflammatory response system triggered by pro-inflammatory cytokines and an increased translocation (movement from one part of the body to another) of lipopolysaccharides (LPS) from gram negative bacteria.

The researchers examined serum concentrations of IgM and IgA against LPS taken from several species of gram-negative enterobacteria including *Hafnia Alvei, Pseudomonas Aeruginosa, Morganella Morganii, Pseudomonas Putida, Citrobacter Koseri,* and *Klebsielle Pneumoniae.* They tested normal and depressed patients, and found that IgM and IgA antibodies to LPS was significantly higher in the depressed patients than the healthy patients. The researchers concluded:

"The results show that intestinal mucosal dysfunction characterized by an increased translocation of gram-negative bacteria (leaky gut) plays a role in the inflammatory pathophysiology of depression. It is suggested that the increased LPS translocation may mount an immune response and thus IRS [inflammatory response system] activation in some patients with MDD [major depression] and may induce specific "sickness behaviour" symptoms. It is suggested that patients with MDD should be checked for leaky gut by means of the IgM and IgA panel used in the present study and accordingly should be treated for leaky gut."

Celiac Disease

Researchers from Sweden's Orebro University Hospital (Ludvigsson et al. 2008) studied 15,325 people with celiac disease along with 14,494 in-patient control subjects. They found that those celiac disease patients diagnosed during adulthood had a significantly greater risk of sepsis. Sepsis is a systemic—whole body—infective state, often associated with bacterial infections.

The researchers stated: "Potential explanations include hyposplenism, increased mucosal permeability and an altered composition of the intestinal glycocalyx in individuals with celiac disease."

Sepsis

Medical researchers from the University of Copenhagen (Jørgensen et al. 2006) studied nine patients with septic shock, seven patients with severe sepsis along with eight healthy persons. They found that colorectal permeability, gauged by testing with DTPA within the blood and after application to the walls of the rectum, along with urinary clearance of CrEDTA. They found that permeability was significantly increased among the sepsis patients as compared to the healthy control patients. They concluded that, "metabolic dysfunction of the mucosa contributes to increased permeability of the large bowel in patients with severe sepsis and septic shock."

Researchers from Rush University's Division of Gastroenterology and Nutrition and the Rush-Presbyterian-St. Luke's Medical Center in Chicago (DeMeo *et al.* 2002) found that damage to the intestinal wall (which creates increased permeability as we'll discuss later) was associated with immune dysfunction and sepsis.

Diarrhea

Researchers from the Centre Health and Population Research in Bangladesh (Rabbani et al. 2004) found that small intestine intestinal permeability was significantly higher among diarrhea patients using lactulose-mannitol testing. They also found that green banana and pectin (a fiber found in apples and other fruits) dramatically decreased levels of diarrhea and intestinal permeability among the patients.

Multiple Organ Dysfunction

Researchers from China's Chong Qing Medical University (Zhang et al. 2010) studied 22 patients with multiple organ dysfunction and found that they also suffered from damage to the walls of the intestines. They also determined the patients had increased intestinal permeability, increased levels of serum diamine oxidase and endotoxins, as measured by transepithelial electrical resistance testing.

Other Conditions

In addition to these, other conditions have been associated with IIPS in animal and *in vitro* studies. Also, European and Asian doctors, along with many alternative practitioners have associated IIPS (or leaky gut in their syntax) with an even longer list of conditions. Here is a longer list, which also includes most of those mentioned above:

➢ Rheumatoid arthritis
➢ Colitis

- Irritable bowel syndrome
- Sinusitis
- Asthma
- Crohn's disease
- Migraines
- COPD
- Constipation
- Fibromyalgia
- Ulcers
- Urinary disorders
- Cardiovascular disease
- Cirrhosis
- Hepatitis
- Mental conditions
- Food allergies
- Diabetes
- Immunosuppression
- Depression
- HIV/AIDS
- Sepsis
- Celiac Disease
- Infections
- Pancreatitis

In some cases, the association with the conditions listed above is considered causative. In others, it may be the other way around. Many of these conditions are classified as autoimmune diseases. As a matter of association then, IIPS might be considered autoimmune. This is supported by the fact that autoimmunity is defined as a condition where the immune system or physiology begins to attack its own cells. In the case of IIPS, the immune system is simply responding to the damage and resulting greater permeability amongst the intestinal wall cells.

Other Signs of Intestinal Permeability

In addition to gauging the level of absorption through the intestines, there are a variety of other ways to confirm that the wrong molecules have gotten through the intestinal barrier and entered the bloodstream. Typically, when the wrong molecules get into the bloodstream, the body's immune system finds them and memorizes them using antibodies. This memory becomes expressed by different types of immunoglobulins. As our immunoglobulins are measured and analyzed, doctors can establish what we have been exposed to and how long we have been exposed.

The following tests have been used conclusively to confirm, after the fact, that certain macromolecules have been memorized by the immune system for inflammatory response. This is based on the fact that the immune system will launch an inflammatory attack when it registers contact with a substance that has wrongly gotten into the bloodstream. This inflammatory attack is typical of allergies, eczema and other allergic inflammatory episodes, which typically launch histamine. We'll discuss this process more in the next chapter. For now, here is a brief summary of the tests that determine what our bloodstream has been exposed to:

Immunoassays

Blood may be drawn and submitted to what some refer to as a *radioallergosorbent test* (or RAST). This is more accurately called the *immunoassay for allergen-specific IgE,* however. This test will measure the content of allergen-specific immunoglobulin Es in the bloodstream.

When we say allergen-specific IgEs, know that an IgE responsive to wheat protein will not be the same as an IgE that is responsive to milk proteins. This means that the immunoassay may determine whether an allergy exists, and if so, what the allergen might be.

A well-respected immunoassay test for accuracy is the CAP-RAST test. Because CAP-RAST immunoassay tests determine the level of an allergen-specific IgE in the blood, they are considered more accurate. Typically the test comes with a level on a 1-to-100 scale, with 100 being the highest level and one being the lowest. A score of 75 will typically produce an allergy diagnosis. On the other hand, a level that is, say, 10 or 15, might be problematic to diagnose. At this level, there may be tolerance to a molecule that was previously considered an allergen to the body.

Indeed, one of the problems of immunoassay testing is the fact that different people have different levels of tolerance at the same IgE levels. The immunoassay test also does little to indicate the severity or type of allergic reaction a person might have. A person, for example, might have a high immunoassay IgE number but have a strong immune system that manages the response quite well. On the other hand, an immunosuppressed person with a lower IgE level might have severe reactions to the molecule.

On the other hand, one of the benefits of obtaining such a clear number is that from successive tests, a person can find out whether their sensitivity is dropping or increasing with time. A higher number can indicate increasing sensitivity, while a lowering number can indicate increased tolerance. This can be truly helpful with some of the strategies we'll discuss later on.

Skin Prick Tests

In skin prick testing (often referred to as SPT), a small amount of a substance that the allergist thinks we are sensitive to is inserted underneath the top layer of skin by a pricking of the skin. The skin is then monitored for response. If the skin responds with a *weal* (a small circular mark or welt), this indicates the existence of a sensitivity to that substance.

There are typically three methods used to apply this skin prick test. A skin prick instrument may be soaked in the substance before the skin is pricked with it. The diagnostician may also place a drop of the substance onto the skin before pricking the skin underneath the drop with a needle or probe.

The diagnostician may also inject the allergen underneath the skin with a needle. This is rarely employed for food allergies.

Once the prick is done, it usually takes about 10-15 minutes for the weal to come up. It will often look like a small pimple. It is the histamine response that makes this happen. A salt water prick test is often deployed to test for skin sensitivity to the pricking alone.

Skin prick testing has proven to be one of the least accurate forms of testing, however. While a negative response (no weal) usually confirms no allergy to that substance, a positive response may not indicate an actual allergy. Research has revealed that up to 60% of positive results can be false *(false positives)*.

Double Blind Challenges

If there is a strong suspicion of an allergy, the allergist may invoke a challenge by feeding the patient with first a tiny amount, and then increasingly larger doses of a substance while they watch for reactions. This can be a painstaking and extensive test. And for someone who is showing signs of allergies, this test should only be performed by or in the presence of a trained health professional prepared to react with medical care should anaphylaxis result.

There are a number of different types of challenge tests, but the most employed method is giving the patient a capsule of the allergen (or a placebo). When a placebo is employed, it is called a *double-blind, placebo-controlled challenge*. In other words, neither the diagnostician nor the patient will know whether the capsule contains the allergen or the placebo. This can eliminate results produced through the inclinations of either the health professional or patient.

As mentioned earlier, the double-blind, placebo-controlled challenge is considered the gold standard among diagnostic tests for allergies and most sensitivities.

Enzyme-linked Immunosorbent Assays (ELISA)

This test and its relative, the ALCAT test, have been met with significant resistance and criticism from conventional Western physicians. The complaint of some physicians is that ELISA testing has not been proven to be reliable for allergy diagnosis.

This was illustrated by researchers from India's Post Graduate Institute of Medical Education and Research (Sharnan *et al.* 2001). The scientists gave skin prick tests and ELISA tests to 64 children with food allergies previously confirmed through food challenges, along with 32 control subjects. They found that the ELISA tests had greater specificity than the skin prick tests (88% versus 64%). But while they found that ELISA provided reliability for a lack of allergy, the ELISA testing generally did not provide a reliable basis for determining an allergy was present. They concluded that ELISA provided no useful advantage over skin prick testing.

One of the issues with ELISA testing (and some say its advantage) is that it yields levels of other immunoglobulins such as IgG, IgG4 and IgA. Some research has indicated that IgG4 is indicative of a hidden food allergy (Shakib *et al.* 1986), but other research has shown that allergen-specific IgG4s can also simply indicate a recovery from a prior food allergy (Savilahti *et al.* 2010).

The advantage of ELISA testing for intestinal permeability is that it gauges the exposure of the immune system to particular types of proteins or other allergens. If the IgG immunoglobulin is sensitive to a particular molecule of a particular size, it can provide confirmation of increased intestinal permeability that allowed the particle to get through the intestinal walls.

Chapter Two

The Physiology of Increased Intestinal Permeability

The Intestinal Brush Barrier

Lining our intestines are barriers that let only selected parts from the contents of our intestines into our bloodstreams. This barrier is very complex. It has various layers, made of different materials and densities. This is called the intestinal brush barrier.

In total, the brush barrier is a triple-filter that screens for molecule size, ionic nature and nutrition quality. Much of this is performed via four mechanisms existing between the intestinal microvilli: tight junctions, adherens junctions, desmosomes, and colonies of probiotics. The tight junctions form a bilayer interface between cells, controlling permeability. Desmosomes are points of interface between the tight junctions, and adherens junctions keep the cell membranes adhesive enough to stabilize the junctions. These junction mechanisms together regulate permeability at the intestinal wall.

The top layer of the intestinal brush barrier is a complex mucosal layer of mucin, enzymes, probiotics and ionic fluid. It forms a protective surface medium over the intestinal epithelium. It also provides an active nutrient transport mechanism.

This mucosal layer is stabilized by the grooves of the intestinal microvilli. It contains glycoproteins, mucopolysaccharides and other ionic transporters, which attach to amino acids, minerals, vitamins, glucose and fatty acids—carrying them across intestinal membranes. Meanwhile the transport medium requires a delicately pH-balanced mix of ionic chemistry able to facilitate this transport of useable nutrient.

Furthermore, the mucosal layer is policed by billions of probiotic colonies, which help process incoming food molecules, excrete various nutrients, and control pathogens.

One of the key regulating factors that regulate the tight junctions between the intestinal cells is a protein called zonulin.

Zonulin governs the junctions between the intestinal cells. Research has determined that increased zonulin levels increases permeability, while decreased zonulin decreases permeability.

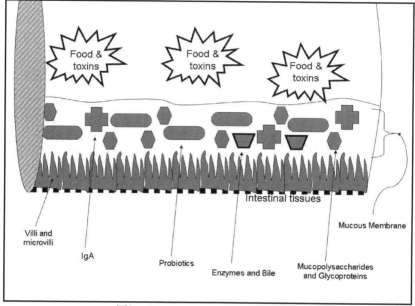

The Healthy Intestinal Wall

This mucosal brush barrier creates the boundary between intestinal contents and our intestinal cells. Should the chemistry of the mucosal layer become altered, its protective abilities become compromised. Its ionic transport mechanisms become weakened, allowing toxic or larger molecules to be presented to the intestinal wall—the microvilli junctions.

This contact of elements not normally presented to the intestinal wall can irritate the microvilli, causing a subsequent inflammatory response. This is now considered a contributing cause of IBS.

Accompanying this inflammatory response as mentioned is an increase in zonulin production.

The breakdown of the mucosal membrane causes it to thin. This depletes the protection rendered by the mucopolysaccharides and glycoproteins, probiotics, immune IgA cells, enzymes and bile. This thinning allows toxins and macromolecules that would have been screened out by the mucosal membrane to be presented to the intestinal cells.

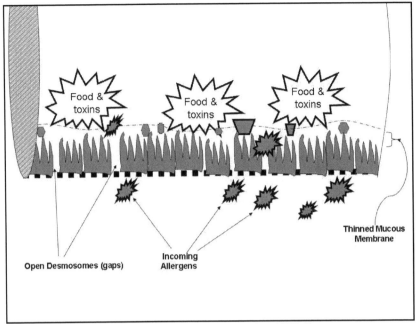

The Unhealthy Intestinal Wall

This mucous membrane thinning, intestinal cell irritation and inflammatory immune response cause desmosomes and tight junctions to open. These gaps now allow larger macromolecules to enter the tissues and bloodstream. These can include large food proteins, endotoxins from pathogenic yeasts and bacteria, and many other substances that have no business in the body.

Intestinal Permeability and Immunity

The consensus of the research is that the gastrointestinal tract, from the mouth to the anus, is the primary defense mechanism against antigens as they enter the body. The mucous membrane integrity, the probiotic system, digestive enzymes, and the various immune cells and their mediators work together to orchestrate a "total defense" structure within the mucosal membrane. However, should this barrier be weakened or become imbalanced, hypersensitivity can result. The weaknesses in the barrier can be influenced by a number of factors, including toxins, diet, genetics, and environmental factors (Chahine and Bahna 2010).

In other words, poor dietary choices, toxin exposures and environmental forces related to lifestyle and living conditions can wear down and thin this mucosal membrane. Once the membrane is damaged, the intestinal cells become exposed to the foods and toxins we consume.

The intestines also have a microscopic barrier function. The tiny spaces between the intestinal epithelial cells—composed of villi and microvilli—are sealed from the general intestinal contents with the tight junctions. As we discussed earlier, should the tight junctions open up, this barrier or seal will be broken.

This results in increased intestinal permeability.

When tight junctions are open—as they are normally in the bladder or the colon—the wrong molecules can cross the epithelium through a transcellular pathway. Researchers have found more than 50-odd protein species among the tight junction. Should any of these proteins fail due to exposure to toxins, the barrier can break down, giving access to what are called macromolecules—molecules that are larger than nutrients than the intestinal cells, liver and bloodstream are accustomed to. Once these macromolecules access the intestinal tissues, they can stimulate an immune response: an inflammatory reaction.

The epithelial mucosal immune system has two anti-inflammatory strategies: The first is to block invaders using antibodies, probiotics and acids. This controls microorganism colonies and inhibits new invasions. The body's immune response counteracts local and peripheral hypersensitivity by attempting to remove them before a full inflammation attack is launched. This is referred to as oral tolerance when it is stimulated in the intestines.

The biochemical constituents of the mucosal membrane (glycoproteins, mucopolysaccharides and so on) also attach and escort nutrients across the intestinal barrier, while resisting the penetration of unrecognized and potentially harmful agents. Intestinal permeability allows molecules that are normally not able to cross the intestines' epithelial barrier access to the bloodstream.

When the intricate balance between the intestinal epithelial layer is destroyed by exposure and inflammation, abnormal protein antigens gain access to the intestinal subepithelial compartment. Here they stimulate the release of immune cells and degranulation (Yu

2009). This produces what is commonly known as an allergic response.

Let's examine the research supporting these conclusions:

Louisiana State University researchers (Chahine and Bahna 2010) found that the intestinal wall uses specific immunologic factors to defend the body against antigens. They showed that integrity of the mucous membrane lining of the intestine is critical. A defective lining, on the other hand, leads to allergic responses and hypersensitivity reactions, according to their research. They named the cause of these *"defects in the gut barrier."*

Hungarian researchers (Kovács *et al.* 1996) tested intestinal permeability among 35 food allergic patients and 20 healthy controls. Intestinal permeability was determined using EDTA. Of the 35, increased intestinal permeability was determined in 29 of the food allergy patients. Of these 29, 21 volunteers were tested for intestinal permeability five years later. IgA antibody titers were increased, among wheat, soy and oat antigens. Significant correlations between intestinal permeability and IgA antibody titers was found, especially against soy and oat proteins.

French researchers (Bodinier *et al.* 2007) studied wheat proteins with patients with intestinal permeability syndrome. They compared the translocation of native wheat proteins with those in a pepsin-hydrolyzed state. They found that the native wheat proteins were crossing the intestinal cell layer, and were able to associate this with their allergic responses.

Hospital Saint Vincent de Paul researchers (Dupont *et al.* 1991) pointed out in their research that the extent of intestinal permeability depends upon the molecule size and the state of the intestinal mucosa. Some intestinal *"porosity,"* as the researchers put it, is normal. However, when macromolecules that were normally not allowed to enter the bloodstream gained entry—primarily protein macromolecules—this stimulated the immune system according to their research.

Increased Intestinal Permeability Immune Mechanisms

Once permeability is increased in the intestinal tract, there is no telling what the immune system will begin responding to. At this point it is likely that the immune system is greatly burdened by the many strange and different molecular structures now gaining entry into internal tissues and the bloodstream. What is known is that once permeability is increased, a self-perpetuating cycle of increased permeability and immune response produces more intestinal dysfunction and more immune response (Heyman 2005).

Researchers from Ontario's McMaster University (Berin *et al.* 1999) studied the role of cytokines in intestinal permeability. They found that interleukin-4 (IL-4) increased intestinal permeability and increased horseradish peroxidase (HRP) transport through intestinal walls. They found that IL-4 was inhibited by the soy nutrient genistein, and anti-IL-4 antibodies also reduced the HRP transport. The researchers concluded that: "We speculate that enhanced production of IL-4 in allergic conditions may be a predisposing factor to inflammation by allowing uptake of luminal antigens that gain access to the mucosal immune system."

Research has indicated that CD23 encourages the transport of intestinal IgE and allergens across intestinal epithelium. This opens a gateway for antigen-bound IgE to move across (transcytose) the intestinal cells. This sets up the immune response of histamine and atopic environmental conditions (Yu 2009).

Researchers from the University of Cincinnati College of Medicine (Groschwitz *et al.* 2009) determined that mast cells are critical to the regulation of the intestinal barrier function. The type and condition of the mast cells seems to affect the epithelial migration through intestinal cells.

Researchers from the Cincinnati Children's Hospital Medical Center (Forbes *et al.* 2008) found that interleukin-9 appears to help stimulate, along with mast cells, increased intestinal permeability. The researchers found that this *"IL-9- and mast cell-mediated intestinal permeability"* activated conditions for food allergen sensitization.

French INSERM researchers (Desjeux and Heyman 1994) concluded that increased protein permeability in milk allergies follows what they called *abnormal immunological response*. This abnormal immune response, they observed, leads to general mucosal and systemic inflammation.

Stimulating Inflammation

French researchers (Heyman and Desjeux 2000) found that not only can intestinal permeability cause various disorders, but disorders can worsen intestinal permeability. They pointed out that as undigested food antigens are transported through the intestinal wall, the immune system launches an inflammatory response. Intact proteins and large peptides, they pointed out, stimulate inflammation among the mucosa of the intestinal wall. IFN gamma and TNF alpha are cytokines that are often part of this inflammatory response. These two—IFN gamma and TNF alpha—also so happen to increase the further opening of the tight junctions.

Researchers from Brazil's Federal Fluminense Medical School (Soares *et al.* 2004) studied the associations between IBS and food intolerance. The researchers used 43 volunteers divided into three groups: an IBS group, a dyspepsia group, and a group without gastrointestinal difficulties. All test subjects were given skin prick tests for nine food allergens. The IBS group presented the highest level of positive allergen responses. The researchers concluded that, "The higher reactivity to food antigens in group I compared to groups II and III suggests that intestinal permeability may be increased in patients with IBS."

Researchers (Forget *et al.* 1985) tested intestinal permeability using EDTA in ten normal adults, eleven healthy children, seven children with acute gastroenteritis, and eight infants with eczema. They found significantly greater intestinal permeability among those with either gastroenteritis or eczema.

Researchers from Paris' Cochin-St Vincent de Paul Hospital (Kalach *et al.* 2001) studied 64 children with cow's milk allergy symptoms, and found that higher intestinal permeability levels were also associated with anemia.

Researchers from London's Middlesex Medical School tested intestinal permeability among eight patients with food-intolerance using EDTA testing. While fasting levels were normal, after they ate the sensitive foods, permeability levels changed some, but not that significantly.

Researchers from Paris' Saint-Vincent de Paul Hospital (Barau and Dupont 1990) tested intestinal permeability using the lactulose and mannitol test with 17 children with irritable bowel syndrome

(IBS). Of the 17, nine tested positive to IgE food allergies. Among these, permeability levels increased when the children were given foods they were sensitive to, illustrating the link between IBS, food allergies and intestinal permeability among many IBS sufferers.

Russian researchers (Sazanova *et al.* 1992) studied 122 children, four months old to six years old with food intolerances. Symptoms included atopic dermatitis among 52 children, and chronic diarrhea among 70 children. They found antibodies to food antigens among all the children. They also found chronic gastroduodenitis (duodenum and stomach inflammation) among every child with atopic dermatitis and among 95% of those with chronic diarrhea. They observed that lactase deficiencies and microorganism growth in the duodenum increased the levels of intestinal permeability and subsequent allergy response.

Inflammation coordinates the various immune players into a frenzy of healing response. This is a good thing. Imagine for a moment cutting your finger pretty badly. First you would feel pain—letting you know the body is hurt. Second, you will probably notice that the area has become swollen and red. Blood starts to clot around the area. Soon the cut stops bleeding. The blood dries and a scab forms. It remains red, maybe a little hot, and hurts for a while. After the healing proceeds, soon the cut is closed up and there is a scab left with a little redness around it. The pain soon stops. The scab falls off and the finger returns to normal—almost like new and ready for action.

Without this inflammatory process, we might not even know we cut our finger in the first place. We might keep working, only to find out that we had bled out a quart of blood on the floor. Without clotting, it would be hard to stop the bleeding. And without some continuing pain, we would be more likely to keep injuring the same spot, preventing it from healing.

Were it not for our immune system and inflammatory process slowing blood flow, clotting the blood, scabbing and cleaning up the site, our bodies would simply be full of holes and wounds. Our bodies simply could not survive injury.

The probiotic system and immunoglobulin immune system work together to deter and kill particular invaders—hopefully before they gain access to the body's tissues. Should these defenses fail, they can stimulate the humoral immune system in a strategic attack that includes identifying antigens and recognizing their weaknesses. B-cells and probiotics coordinate through the stimulation of immunoglobulins and CDs.

This progression also stimulates an activation of neutrophils, phagocytes, immunoglobulins, leukotrienes and prostaglandins. Should cells become infected, they will signal the immune system from paracrines located on their cell membranes. Once the intrusion and strategy is determined, B-cells will surround the pathogens while T-cells attack any infected cells. Natural killer T-cells may secrete chemicals into infected cells, initiating the death of the cell.

Leukotrienes immediately gather in the region of injury or infection, and signal to T-cells to coordinate efforts in the process of repair. Prostaglandins initiate the widening of blood vessels to bring more T-cells and other repair factors (such as plasminogen and fibrin) to the infected or injured site. Histamine opens the blood vessel walls to allow all these healing agents access to the injury site to clean it up.

Prostaglandins also stimulate substance P within the nerve cells, initiating the sensation of pain. At the same time, thromboxanes, along with fibrin, drive the process of clotting and coagulation in the blood, while constricting certain blood vessels to decrease the risk of bleeding.

In the case where the pathogen is an allergen, the inflammation response will also accompany an H1-histamine response. As mentioned earlier, histamine is primarily produced by the mast cells, basophils and neutrophils after being stimulated by IgE antibodies. This opens blood vessels to tissues, which stimulates the processes of sneezing, watering of the eyes and coughing. These measures, though sometimes considered irritating, are all stimulated in an effort to remove the toxin and prevent its re-entry into the body. As histamine binds with receptors, one of the resulting physiological responses is alertness (also why antihistamines cause drowsiness). These are natural responses to help the body and mind remain vigilant in order to avoid further toxin intake.

At the height of the repair process, swelling, redness and pain are at their peak. The T-cells, macrophages, neutrophils, fibrin and plasmin all work together to purge the allergen from the body and repair the damage.

As macrophages continue the clean up, the other immune cells begin to retreat. Antioxidants like glutathione will attach to and transport the byproducts—broken down toxins and cell parts—out of the body. As this proceeds, prostaglandins, histamines and leukotrienes begin to signal a reversal of the inflammation and pain process.

One of the central features of the normalization process is the production of bradykinin. Bradykinin slows clotting and opens blood vessels, allowing the cleanup process to accelerate. A key signalling factor is the production of nitric oxide (NO). NO slows inflammation by promoting the detachment of lymphocytes to the site of infection or toxification, and reduces tissue swelling. NO also accelerates the clearing out of debris with its interaction with the superoxide anion. NO was originally described as endothelium-derived relaxing factor (or EDRF)—because of its role in relaxing blood vessel walls.

The body produces more nitric oxide in the presence of good nutrition and lower stress. Probiotics also play a big role in nitric oxide production in a healthy body. Lactobacilli such as *L. plantarum* have in fact been shown to remove the harmful nitrate molecule and use it to produce nitric oxide (Bengmark *et al.* 1998). This is beneficial to not only reducing inflammation: NO production also creates a balanced environment for increased tolerance.

Low nitric oxide levels also happen to be associated with a plethora of diseases, including diabetes, heart failure, high cholesterol, ulcerative colitis, premature aging, cancers and many others. Low or abnormal NO production is also seen among lifestyle habits such as smoking, obesity, and living around air pollution.

The intestinal cells are often damaged first by other toxins, resulting in an inflammatory cascade. Once the intestine's cells are damaged, macromolecules/allergens can enter the system through the damaged intestinal wall.

Thus IIPS is usually the result of three events: The first being a thinning of the mucosal membranes that line the wall of the intestines. The second is injury to the cells of the intestinal wall, as invaders penetrate the normally protective mucosal membranes of our intestines. The mucosal lining can be thinned and damaged by an assortment of toxins, poor dietary choices, microorganism pathogens, stress, smoking, alcohol, pharmaceuticals and toxins. Once the membrane is damaged, food macromolecules or allergens can also damage and irritate the cells of the intestinal walls.

Once the cells of the intestinal wall are damaged, the immune system will launch an inflammatory injury response through the T-cell system as described earlier. The T-cells will "repair" the problem by killing off these intestinal cells. This is often described as an autoimmune issue, but in reality, the T-cells are responding to real damage to these cells. They are not confusing "self" with "nonself" as theorized by many.

While this damage and response is active, the intestinal cell wall barrier is altered. This alteration creates further increased intestinal permeability. Now large molecules (macromolecules) and/or allergens may readily enter the tissues and bloodstream, stimulating the IgE-histamine allergic immune response and/or other physiological and immune responses that produce the various conditions that IIPS causes, as outlined in the previous chapter.

The Hypersensitivity Response

There are four kinds of hypersensitivity responses within the body once an intruder leaks through the intestines and gains access to the blood and tissues: Type I, Type II, Type III and Type IV. These might sound very similar but they are actually quite different. Let's review these:

Type I: Immediate Hypersensitivity

This response occurs when IgE antibodies bind to antigens. Antigens include proteins, fatty acids, lipopolysaccharides and polysaccharides among others. When this binding between an antigen and IgE takes place, the bound IgE will typically set off the release of inflammatory mediators from mast/basophil/neutrophil white blood cells. These mediators include histamine, prostaglandins and leukotrienes. Depending upon the location and type of mast/basophil/ neutrophil cells, these mediators will spark an allergic response within the airways, sinuses, skin, joints and other locations. This kind of response will typically be immediate, within about two hours of ingestion of the offending allergen.

Type II: Cytotoxic Response

In this type of immune response, antigens have penetrated the tissues, and the body responds to kill these cells. This typically takes place through an antigen binding to IgG or IgM immunoglobulins in a delayed immune response. This response can happen concurrently to other allergic responses; though it is still most often a delayed response.

Should the red blood cells be involved in the antigen absorption, hemolysis (the destruction of red blood cells) and anemia (a lack of red blood cells) may result.

Type III: Immune-Complex Response

Here the allergen-bound antibody complex actually penetrates cell tissues and injures them. This can occur within the intestinal cells, liver, or virtually anywhere around the body. In some instances these immune complexes can increase vascular permeability or intestinal permeability, as we've discussed.

This type of response is also often a delayed response, occurring hours or even a day or two after exposure.

Sometimes the immune complexes will stimulate mast/basophil/neutrophil cell degranulation of histamine, prostaglandins and leukotrienes, and stimulate inflammation within the tissue system. This can result in a variety of conditions, which are sometimes attributed to autoimmunity.

Type IV: T-Cell Responses

This type of response is independent of other types of sensitivity. For example, the Type III may generate a T-cell response once the cell and tissue damage begins. But this Type IV occurs without the binding of an antigen by an antibody. In this response, a cell is directly affected by the allergen or constituent. Conditions of colitis are typical of this type of response, because the antigen directly stimulates toxicity within the intestinal cells. Once the intestinal cells are damaged, T-cells launch an immune response to clear out the invaded cells. As mentioned, this response is also often attributed to autoimmunity. Rather it is an immune response to cellular toxicity.

This type of response will typically take from two to four days from exposure to response.

Sensitization

The type I hypersensitivity response can be broken down into two stages: sensitization and elicitation.

The molecule sensitization process takes place when a potential protein antigen happens to come into contact with a type of immune cell called a progenitor B-cell. As part of their immune system responsibilities, these B-cells will break apart the protein into smaller peptides. These will be attached to hystocompatibility complex class II complex molecules.

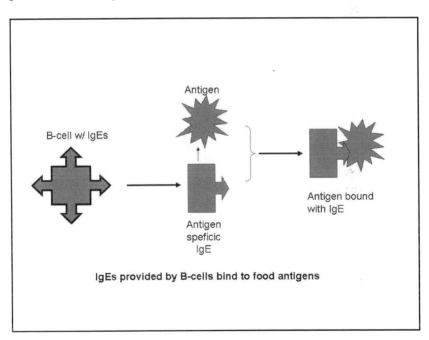

IgEs provided by B-cells bind to food antigens

The T-cell hystocompatibility complex is transferred onto the surface of the B-cell, which binds to a particular allergen. Once upon the B-cell surface, T-helper cells take notice of this foreign particle stuck to the B-cell. The T-helper cell cytokine CD4 receptors trigger a response, and this stimulates the production of the IgE immunoglobulins. These particular IgE immunoglobulins are now sensitized to the particular epitope of the antigen in the future.

Elicitation

Once sensitized, the IgE associates with the specific IgE receptors that lie on the surface of the neutrophil, basophil or mast cells. Within these cells are packages called granules.

The granules are stock full of a variety of inflammatory mediators. The most notorious of these in allergies is histamine as we've been discussing. As the allergen-specific IgEs connect with the IgE receptors on these immune cells, the immune cells will release the inflammatory mediators such as histamine and leukotrienes into the bloodstream and lymph. This is what drives much of the symptoms of an allergic attack, including but not limited to hives, asthma, uritica, sinusitis and others.

The below diagram illustrates elicitation:

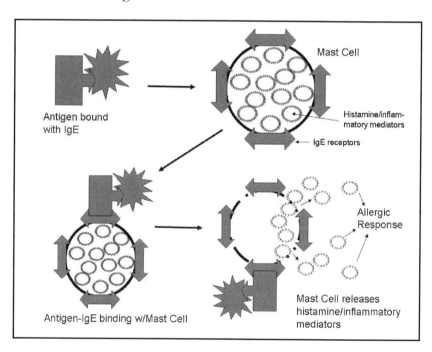

IIPS and The Liver

The liver is the key organ involved in detoxification and the production of a variety of enzymes and biochemicals. The liver produces over a thousand biochemicals the body requires for healthy functioning. The liver maintains blood sugar balance by monitoring glucose levels and producing glucose metabolites. It manufactures albumin to maintain plasma pressure. It produces cholesterol, urea, inflammatory biochemicals, blood-clotting molecules, and many others.

These functions are major reasons that the liver is significantly exposed to those intruders that can access the bloodstream through the intestines in an IIPS situation.

The liver sits just below the lungs on the right side under the diaphragm. Partially protected by the ribs, it attaches to the abdominal wall with the falciform ligament. The *ligamentum teres* within the falciform is the remnant of the umbilical cord that once brought us blood from mama's placenta. As the body develops, the liver continues to filter, purify and enrich our blood. Should the liver shut down, the body can die within hours.

Interspersed within the liver are functional fat factories called stellates. These cells store and process lipids, fat-soluble vitamins such as vitamin A, and secrete structural biomolecules like collagen, laminin and glycans. These are used to build some of the body's toughest tissue systems.

Into the liver drains nutrition-rich venous blood through the hepatic portal vein, together with some oxygenated blood through the hepatic artery. A healthy liver will process almost a half-gallon of blood per minute. The blood is commingled within cavities called sinusoids, where blood is staged through stacked sheets of the liver's primary cells—called hepatocytes. Here blood is also met by interspersed immune cells called kupffers. These kupffer cells attack and break apart bacteria and toxins. Nutrients coming in from the digestive tract are filtered and converted to molecules the body's cells can utilize. The liver also converts old red blood cells to bilirubin to be shipped out of the body. Filtered and purified blood is jettisoned through hepatic veins out the inferior vena cava and back into circulation.

The liver's filtration/purification mechanisms protect our body from various infectious diseases and chemical toxins. After hepatocytes and kuppfer cells break down toxins, the waste is disposed through the gall bladder and kidneys. The gall bladder channels bile from the liver to the intestines. Recycled bile acids combine with bilirubin, phospholipids, calcium and cholesterol to make bile. Bile is concentrated and pumped through the bile duct to the intestines. Here bile acids help digest fats, and broken-down toxins are (hopefully) excreted through our feces. This is assuming that we have healthy intestines containing healthy mucous membranes, barrier mechanisms and probiotic colonies.

The liver's filtration and breakdown process means that anything that leaks through the intestinal wall will be presented quickly to the liver. Endotoxins, infective agents, ethanol (alcohol), toxins and other intruders will damage the liver's cells quickly. If an allergen gets through the intestines, the liver gets a crack at removing it.

If the liver is not able to metabolize and neutralize the molecule, the body must rely upon the inflammatory immune response to rid the body of the molecule. Often this process is concurrent, but a strong liver will reduce the body's dependence upon the inflammatory processes for removing macromolecules. If the hepatocytes and kuppfer cells are abundant and resilient, they can remove many toxins. Should those cells be damaged or overwhelmed by too many toxins at once, their ability to break down and remove problematic macromolecules becomes diminished.

Research and a wealth of clinical evidence shows that the liver is damaged by pharmaceuticals, alcohol, infective agents, toxins and other intruders. This is the very reason that alcohol (ethanol) causes liver disease: ethanol damages the liver's hepatocytes and kuppfers.

Today our diets, water and air are full of many other chemicals that can damage the liver if they get through the intestinal walls. These include plasticizers, formaldehyde, heavy metals, hydrocarbons, DDT, dioxin, VOCs, asbestos, preservatives, artificial flavors, food dyes, propellants, synthetic fragrances and more. With every additional chemical comes a requirement for the liver to work harder to break down these synthesized chemicals. How do these chemicals get into the body? They typically come in via our lungs, our skin, or through our intestines.

Frankly, most modern livers—especially those in urban areas of industrialized countries—are now overloaded and beyond their natural capacity. What happens then? Generally, two things. First, the hepatocytes collapse from toxicity, causing an overactive immune system due to the additional burdens placed upon it. Second, liver exhaustion leads to increased susceptibility to infectious diseases such as viral hepatitis. The combined result is a downward spiraling of hypersensitivity.

Liver disease—where one or more lobes begin to malfunction due to the death or dysfunction of hepatocytes—can result in a life-threatening emergency. Cirrhosis is a common diagnosis for liver disease, often caused by years of drinking alcohol or taking prescription medications combined with other toxin exposure. During this progression towards cirrhosis the sub-functioning liver can also produce symptoms such as jaundice, high cholesterol, gallstones, encephalopathy, kidney disease, clotting problems, heart conditions, hormone imbalances and many others. As cirrhosis proceeds, it results in the massive die-off of liver cells, and the subsequent scarring of remaining tissues, causing the liver to begin to shutdown.

While most of us have heard about the damage alcohol can have on the liver, many do not realize that pharmaceuticals and so many other synthetic chemicals can also be extremely toxic to the liver. The liver must find a way to break down these foreign chemicals. The liver's various purification processes can become overwhelmed by these synthetic molecules. As liver cells weaken and die, their enzymes leak into the bloodstream. Blood tests for AST and ALT enzymes reveal this weakening of the liver.

A strong intestinal barrier will help protect the liver; while increased intestinal permeability will significantly weaken the liver (and the rest of the body) by exposing it to numerous foreigners.

Chapter Three

The Causes of Leaky Gut

The causative forces of increased permeability are a bit compli-cated. Infections, toxins, pharmaceuticals, probiotic deficiencies, breast milk deficiencies, metabolic stress and others have been iden-tified as potential causes of increased intestinal permeability.

Accordingly, French INSERM researchers (Desjeux and Hey-man 1994) concluded that increased protein permeability in milk allergies follows what they called *abnormal immunological response*. This abnormal immune response, they observed, leads to mucosal in-flammation and a dysfunction of intestinal cellular endocytic proc-esses (endocytosis is the process the cells undertake when they engulf or absorb amino acids and polypeptides). The researchers based this conclusion on the observation that the milk protein beta-lactoglobulin stimulated lymphocytes that released increased levels of cytokines tumor necrosis factor-alpha (TNF alpha) and gamma interferon. The cytokines stimulated an inflammatory response that in turn disturbed the intestinal cell wall barrier.

In other words, first an irritating toxin, abnormal macromole-cule or other stressor disrupts the intestinal mucous membrane. This exposes the intestinal cells, allowing intestinal cells to be dam-aged by the toxin. This in turn produces inflammation and opens gaps in the intestinal barrier.

On a biochemical level, electrogenic chloride secretion is in-volved in an ion transport chain that stimulates the inflammatory prostaglandin E2 (PGE2) response within the intestinal mucosa. This secretion is balanced by the chloride channel blocker diphenyl-amine-2-carboxylate in healthy persons. In unhealthy persons, in-flammatory cytokines alter the balance among intestinal barrier cells, with the effect of increasing permeability.

Medical researchers from the University Hospital in Groningen of The Netherlands (van Elburg *et al.* 1992) pointed out that the intestinal immunity mechanisms, which include IgA immunoglobu-lin and cell-mediated immune factors—and the brush barrier in general—do not completely mature until after about two years of age. Until this time, the barrier is sensitive to toxins and feeding problems.

Researchers from the Medical University of South Carolina (Walle and Walle 1999) found that mutagens formed when frying meat are associated with damaging the mucosal membranes and producing increased intestinal permeability. These mutagens, such as phenylimidazo-pyridine, were studied for their possible transport across human Caco-2 intestinal cells. The absorption was characterized as *"extensive and linear."* Equilibrium exchange tests showed that the mutagens form substrates with intestinal transporters. This indicates that these fried meat byproducts directly increase intestinal permeability.

A biochemistry researcher from Germany's Otto-von-Guericke University (Schönfeld 2004) discovered that dietary phytanic acid increases intestinal permeability through a function of ionic exchange and disruption of mitochondrial energy production. Damage to mitochondria may also explain the production of the inflammatory cytokine IL-4 within intestinal cells.

Researchers from the Department of Pediatrics at Italy's University of Federico II (Raimondi *et al.* 2008) found that bilirubin modifies the intestinal barrier. They also found among infants that cow's milk protein intolerance had higher levels of bilirubin and higher stool excretion. Those infants that had higher levels of bilirubin in the first year also had a greater risk of contracting cow's milk allergy.

To this, the French INSERM researchers added that stomach and upper intestinal infections with microorganisms such as *Helicobacter pylori* also increase intestinal permeability. Their observations led them to conclude that this was caused by an increased burden upon the immune system, and the resulting increase in inflammatory cytokines.

Medical researchers from Finland's University of Helsinki (Kuitunen *et al.* 1994) studied permeability using beta-lactoglobulin from cow's milk with 20 infants through eight months old or until they began weaning from breast milk. In one week after they weaned from breast milk, bovine beta-lactoglobulin levels were found in the bloodstream among 38% of the infants. After two weeks, 21% retained beta-lactoglobulin in the bloodstream. The researchers concluded that: "The gut may often be transiently permeable to BLG when cow's-milk-based formula is started."

INSERM researchers from the Hospital Saint-Lazare (Heyman *et al.* 1988) studied intestinal permeability with milk allergy among infants. They tested 33 children ages one month to 24 months, which included 18 healthy infants and 15 with milk allergies, using the protein marker horseradish peroxidase and jejunal biopsies. No absorption permeability was seen in the control children over two months of age, illustrating that "gut closure probably occurred earlier in life." However, milk allergy children had about eight times the permeability levels than the control children.

The connection may lie in the health condition of the mother. French doctors (de Boissieu *et al.* 1994) reported that in one case, a 1-month-old breast-fed boy who had regurgitation, diarrhea, feeding difficulties, and malaise—typical of food sensitivities. They conducted intestinal permeability tests on mother and baby. These illustrated that the mother's breast milk induced intestinal permeability in the baby. The child's symptoms continued without improvement after the mother eliminated dairy products from her own diet. Then the mother withdrew egg and pork from her diet. This resulted in an almost immediate disappearance of allergy symptoms in the child. The doctors tested the child again for intestinal permeability after provocation with mother's milk (the same test done previously). Intestinal permeability levels were normal. The doctors concluded that allergens can be transferred from mother to baby through breast milk.

Researchers from Rush University's Division of Gastroenterology and Nutrition and the Rush-Presbyterian-St. Luke's Medical Center in Chicago (DeMeo *et al.* 2002) found that nonsteroidal anti-inflammatory drugs, free radical oxidation, adenosine triphosphate depletion (metabolic stress) and damage to the epithelial cell cytoskeletons that regulate tight junctions were associated with IIPS.

Medical researchers from the University of Southampton School of Medicine (Macdonald and Monteleone 2005) have suggested that this epidemic of intestinal permeability among industrialized nations has been creating genetic mutations that produce greater levels of permeability among successive generations. This of course, provides the link between greater levels of allergies among those with allergic parents.

Thus we can conclude that intestinal permeability comes as a result of certain exposures and poor dietary choices, which include certain pharmaceuticals, fried meats, egg, pork and milk for some, as well as others. Let's dive more a bit further into some of these associations.

The Link between Intestinal Permeability and Early Milk Allergies

Researchers from the Department of Pediatrics of the Cochin St Vincent de Paul Hospital in Paris (Kalach *et al.* 2001) studied intestinal permeability and cow's milk allergy among children as they aged. The research included 200 children who exhibited symptoms of cow's milk allergies. Of this 200, 95 were determined as allergic using challenge testing. This left 105 children as control subjects. The researchers measured intestinal permeability using the L/M ratio. They found that the L/M ratio was significantly greater among the milk-allergic children. Abnormal intestinal permeability levels were present among 80% of the milk-allergic children who had digestive symptoms, and 40% of children who exhibited anaphylactic symptoms. Furthermore, L/M ratios improved among older children who became more tolerant to milk.

Medical researchers from Italy's University of Naples (Troncone *et al.* 1994) tested intestinal permeability among 32 children aged from three months old to 84 months old. They utilized a ratio related to L/M called the cellobiose/mannitol (C/M) ratio. Of those who had allergy symptoms after a challenge with milk, 90% had significantly increased C/M ratios, indicating increased intestinal permeability.

Researchers from France's St. Vincent de Paul Hospital (Dupont *et al.* 1989) measured intestinal permeability using mannitol and lactulose among 12 milk-allergic children; 28 children with atopic dermatitis; and 39 healthy children. L/M ratios indicated that intestinal permeability in the milk-allergic group was three times higher than the healthy group when they drank milk.

French INSERM researchers from the Hospital Saint-Lazare (Heyman *et al.* 1988) studied intestinal permeability with milk allergy among infants. They tested 33 children ages one month to 24 months, which included 18 healthy infants and 15 with milk allergies, using the protein marker horseradish peroxidase together with jejunal biopsies. No absorption permeability was seen in the control children over two months of age, illustrating that *"gut closure probably occurred earlier in life."* However, milk allergy children had about eight times the permeability levels than the healthy children.

Mucosal Damage and Diet

The consensus of the research is that the gastrointestinal tract, from the mouth to the anus, is the primary defense mechanism against antigens as they enter the body. The mucous membrane integrity, the probiotic system, digestive enzymes, and the various immune cells and their mediators work together to orchestrate a "total defense" structure within the mucosal membrane. However, should this barrier be weakened or become imbalanced, hypersensitivity can result. The weaknesses in the barrier can be influenced by a number of factors, including toxins, diet, genetics, and environmental factors (Chahine and Bahna 2010).

In other words, poor dietary choices, toxin exposures and environmental forces related to lifestyle and living conditions can wear down and thin this mucosal membrane. Once the membrane is damaged, the intestinal cells become exposed to the foods and toxins we consume.

The intestines also have a microscopic barrier function. The tiny spaces between the intestinal epithelial cells—composed of villi and microvilli—are sealed from the general intestinal contents with what are called tight junctions. As we discussed earlier, should the tight junctions open up, this barrier or seal will be broken.

This results in increased intestinal permeability, as we've mentioned before.

When tight junctions are open—as they are normally in the bladder or the colon—the wrong molecules can cross the epithelium through a transcellular pathway. Researchers have found more than 50-odd protein species among the tight junction. Should any of these proteins fail due to exposure to toxins, the barrier can break down, giving access to what are called macromolecules—molecules that are larger than nutrients that the intestinal cells, liver and bloodstream are accustomed to. Once these macromolecules access the intestinal tissues, they can stimulate an immune response: an inflammatory reaction.

The epithelial mucosal immune system has two anti-inflammatory strategies: The first is to block invaders using antibodies, probiotics and acids. This controls microorganism colonies and inhibits new invasions. The body's immune response counteracts local and peripheral hypersensitivity by attempting to remove them before a full inflammation attack is launched. This is referred to as oral tolerance when it is stimulated in the intestines.

The biochemical constituents of the mucosal membrane (glycoproteins, mucopolysaccharides and so on) also attach and escort nutrients across the intestinal barrier, while resisting the penetration of unrecognized and potentially harmful agents. Intestinal permeability allows molecules that are normally not able to cross the intestines' epithelial barrier access to the bloodstream.

When the intricate balance between the intestinal epithelial layer is destroyed by exposure and inflammation, abnormal protein antigens gain access to the intestinal subepithelial compartment. Here they stimulate the release of immune cells and degranulation (Yu 2009).

Let's examine the research supporting these conclusions:

Medical researchers at Norway's University of Bergen (Lillestøl *et al.* 2010) found that self-reported food hypersensitivity was highly associated with irritable bowel syndrome and intestinal permeability. Of the 71 adult subjects, 93% had irritable bowel syndrome and increased intestinal permeability, while 61% had atopic disease—primarily rhinoconjunctivitis. All the atopic sufferers had respiratory allergies, and 41% had food allergens.

Louisiana State University researchers (Chahine and Bahna 2010) found that the intestinal wall uses specific immunologic factors to defend the body against antigens. They showed that integrity of the mucous membrane lining of the intestine is critical. A defective lining, on the other hand, leads to allergic responses and hypersensitivity reactions, according to their research. They named the cause of these *"defects in the gut barrier."*

Medical researchers (Jackson *et al.* 1982) gave polyethylene glycol to eight eczema patients with food allergies and 10 patients with supposed non-allergic eczema in order to investigate intestinal permeability. Both groups absorbed macromolecules in excess of the normal subjects. They concluded that eczema with and without food allergy was associated with *"intestinal mucosal defects"* (increased intestinal permeability).

Hungarian researchers (Kovács *et al.* 1996) tested intestinal permeability among 35 food allergic patients and 20 healthy controls. Intestinal permeability was determined using EDTA. Of the 35, increased intestinal permeability was determined in 29 of the food allergy patients. Of these 29, 21 volunteers were tested for intestinal permeability five years later. IgA antibody titers were increased, among wheat, soy and oat antigens. Significant correlations between intestinal permeability and IgA antibody titers was found, especially against soy and oat proteins.

French researchers (Bodinier *et al.* 2007) studied wheat proteins with patients with intestinal permeability syndrome. They compared the translocation of native wheat proteins with those in a pepsin-hydrolyzed state. They found that the native wheat proteins were crossing the intestinal cell layer, and were able to associate this with their allergic responses.

Hospital Saint Vincent de Paul researchers (Dupont *et al.* 1991) pointed out in their research that the extent of intestinal permeability depends upon the molecule size and the state of the intestinal mucosa. Some intestinal *"porosity,"* as the researchers put it, is normal. However, when macromolecules that were normally not allowed to enter the bloodstream gained entry—primarily protein macromolecules—this stimulated the immune system, according to their research.

As we will read in the studies below, our diet, our childhood diet, and the diet of our mother during pregnancy and breastfeeding plays a significant role in the progression of increased intestinal permeability. The mechanisms relate directly to the immune system and the health of our intestines. As macromolecules and endotoxins enter our bloodstream via pores in the intestines, they can overwhelm the liver and immune system as they attempt to remove these intruders.

An exhausted immune system will inevitably react differently than a strong immune system to a perceived foreigner. The weakened immune system will typically over-react to these intruders, even if they have been part of foods eaten throughout our life-times. This immune response, as we discussed earlier, produces the inflammatory allergic response.

To tie this together, we can show that certain diets reduce the tendency for food allergies. This is because these diets reduce increased intestinal permeability syndrome.

Researchers from the University of Western Australia and the Princess Margaret Hospital (Jennings and Prescott 2010) reviewed the clinical data regarding diet and environmental changes with respect to autoimmunity. They concluded that dietary factors such as omega-3 fatty acids, oligosaccharides, probiotics, vitamin D, retinoic acid and various antioxidants in foods stimulate and assist immune function and the development of the immune system; and inherently decrease the risk of food allergies.

In a study of 460 children and mothers on Menorca—a Mediterranean island in Spain—medical researchers from Greece's Department of Social Medicine and the University of Crete (Chatzi *et al.* 2008) found that children of mothers eating primarily a Mediterranean diet (a predominantly plant-based diet) had significantly fewer food and other allergies. In fact, the higher the adherence to the Mediterranean diet during pregnancy, the fewer the allergies among the children.

The same researchers (Chatzi *et al.* 2007) surveyed the parents of 690 children from ages seven through 18 years old in the rural areas of Crete. The children also were tested with skin prick tests for 10 common allergens. They found that consuming a Mediterranean diet reduced the risk of allergic rhinitis by over 65%. The risk of skin allergies and respiratory conditions (such as wheezing) also reduced, but by smaller amounts. They also found that a greater consumption of nuts among the children cut wheezing rates in half, while consuming margarine more than doubled the prevalence of both wheezing and allergic rhinitis.

Remember the research showing that food sensitivities directly relate to asthma occurrence. Asthmatic parents increase the risk of food sensitivities among their children. Children who outgrow their milk allergy are more likely to contract asthma a few years later. Those with early allergies have a greater likelihood of later food sensitivities than those who don't.

An international group of researchers from around the world (Nagel *et al.* 2010) reported in the International Study on Allergies and Asthma in Childhood (ISAAC) that asthma occurrence is related to diet. The group conducted cross-sectional studies between 1995 and 2005 in 29 locations within 20 different countries. In all, 50,004 children ages eight through twelve years old were analyzed.

This study revealed that those with diets containing large fruit portions had lower incidence of asthma. This link occurred among both affluent and non-affluent countries. Fish consumption in affluent countries (where vegetable intake is less) and cooked green vegetables among non-affluent countries were also associated with a lower asthma rates. In general, the consumption of fruit, vegetables and fish was linked with reduced rates of asthma throughout life. At the same time, frequent consumption of meat burgers was linked with higher rates of lifetime asthma.

Consuming the Mediterranean diet (a predominantly plant-based diet), has clear results: It is linked with lower allergy and asthma rates.

The implication of this research is that diets weighted too far towards animal proteins increase the likelihood of IIPS. We can also see this connection in some of the research connecting IIPS with allergies.

Because a diet rich in antioxidants—and plant-based foods have more antioxidants—also typically contains more fiber and other nutrients that are helpful to our mucosal membranes, these diets help us retain healthy intestinal permeability.

Processed Foods

Processing robs our foods of important micro-nutrients and fiber that assist in the health of our intestinal walls. These micro-nutrients and fiber also feed our probiotics.

Food processing typically consists of chopping or pulverizing the food, heating it to high temperatures, distilling or extracting its contents, or otherwise isolating some parts of the food by straining off, clarifying or refining. Food processing is typically considered by humans as a good thing, because humans like to focus on one or two constituents or nutrients of a food as making up that food's intrinsic value.

In the end it is a value proposition, because all the energy and work required to produce the final food product must equal or be greater than the increase in the processed food's value.

Typically this increase in value is due to the food being sweeter, smoother or simply easier to eat or mix with other foods. In the case of oils or flours, the food extract is used for baking purposes, for example. In the case of sugar, which is extracted from a number of whole plants, including cane and beets, it is added to nearly every processed food.

Ironically, what is left out in this value proposition is the food's real value. The fiber and nutrients are typically stripped away during food processing. Plant fiber is a necessary element of our diet, because it renders sterols that aid digestion and reduce LDL cholesterol. Many nutrients are attached to food fiber. Once the fiber is stripped away, the food's nutrients can be easily damaged by the heat of processing.

What is being missed in the value proposition of food processing is that nature's whole foods have their greatest value, nutritionally, prior to processing. When a food is broken down, many of the molecular bonds that hold the food's fibers and polysaccharides are lost. As these bonds are lost, the remaining components can become unstable in the body. When they become unstable, they can form free radicals, requiring our bodies to neutralize them. This produces instability elsewhere in the body, and places a burden upon our immune system.

In other words, *whole foods* provide the nutrients our bodies need, in the combinations already provided by nature. In some cases, we might need to physically peel a food to get to its edible part. In other cases, such as in the case of grains, we may need to heat or cook the whole grains to soften the fibers to enable chewing and digestion. In the case of wheats, milling the whole grain (including the bran) will render a healthy flour.

Eating a food with its plant fibers intact will yield a more molecularly-balanced food. This is because the fibers deliver molecules the body recognizes. Our digestive enzymes and probiotics have evolved to break down (or not) certain types of molecules. Imbalanced or broken-down molecules are considered foreign.

We can also see how processing increases diseases when we compare the disease statistics of developing countries with developed countries.

For example, like many developing countries, India has more heart disease because of increased consumption of processed and fried foods. These processed foods damage intestinal health and promote free radicals. They are nutrient-poor. They burden and starve our probiotics. Frying foods also produces a carcinogen called acrylamide (Ehling *et al.* 2005).

Glycation

Researchers from France's University of Burgundy (Rapin and Wiernsperger 2010) have confirmed that protein or lipid glycation produced by modern food manufacturers is linked to intestinal issues and increased permeability.

Glycation is produced during the manufacturing of food products, specifically when sugars and protein-foods are heated to extremely high temperatures during cooking or filling. During glycation, sugars bind to protein molecules. This produces a glycated protein and glycation end products, both of which have been implicated in cardiovascular disease, diabetes, some cancers, peripheral neuropathy and Alzheimer's disease (Miranda and Outeiro 2010).

In Alzheimer's disease, one of the products of a glycation reaction is the amyloid protein. Glycation end products introduced to the cerebrospinal fluid have been directly implicated in the process of amyloid plaque build up among brain cells.

Glycation also takes place within the body. This occurs especially in diets containing high levels of refined sugars combined with considerable amounts of cooked or caramelized proteins.

The Western diet contains an incredible amount of processed protein compared to traditional diets. Americans eat far beyond the amount of protein required for health. Studies indicate that Americans eat an average of 80-150 grams of protein a day. This is significantly higher than the 25-50 grams of protein consumed in most healthy traditional diets around the world (Campbell and Campbell 2006; McDougall 1999).

This amount of protein in the American diet is also significantly higher than even U.S. RDA levels. The U.S. recommended daily allowance for protein is 0.8 grams per 2.2 lbs of body weight. This converts to 54 grams for a person weighing 150 pounds. Americans eat on average nearly double that amount.

To this we can add the sugar-laden Western diet. Today, nearly every pre-cooked recipe found in the mass market grocery stores contains refined sugar. Even processed organic foods contain organic cane syrup—a form of sugar that may not be as refined as white sugar, but is definitely refined, and stripped of the natural plant fibers in cane or beets.

Today, many brands are trying to white-wash the massive sugar content of their products by calling their sugar content "all natural." This is a deception, because nature in the form of fiber has been unnaturally stripped away from their refined sugar. This is hardly a "natural" proposition. Nature attaches sugars to complex fibers and nutrients in such a way that prevents them from easily attaching to proteins. Sugars that are cooked and stripped of their fibers become immediate glycation candidates within the body.

As our digestive system combines these sugars with proteins, many of the glycated proteins are identified as foreign by IgA, or IgE antibodies in immune-burdened or inflammatory intestines. Why are they considered foreign? Because, as we've mentioned, glycated proteins and their AGE end products damage blood vessels, tissues, brain cells and also stimulate cancerous cells. So the immune system is simply trying to protect us from our own diet!

There is no surprise that glycation among foods—and the glycation that occurs within the body as a result of the heavy consumption of refined proteins and sugars—is connected with the increase of allergies among Western societies over the past few decades. This has occurred with the increased consumption of overly-processed foods and manufacturing processes that pulverize and strip foods of their fiber; and blend denatured proteins and sugars using heating processes.

We should note that a healthy type of natural glycation also takes place in the body to produce certain nutrient combinations. Unlike the glycation produced by food manufacturers, this type of glycation is driven by the body's enzyme processes, resulting in molecules and end products the body uses and recognizes. When glycation is driven by the body's own enzyme processes, it is technically called *glycosylation.*

Hydrolyzation

Proteins are composed of very long chains of amino acids. Sometimes hundreds and even thousands of amino acids can make up a protein. A healthy digestive tract typically breaks apart these chains through an enzyme reaction called *proteolysis.*

Proteolysis breaks down proteins into amino acids and small groups of amino acids called polypeptides. This is also called *cleaving.* As enzymes break off these polypeptides or individual amino acids from proteins, they replace the protein chain linkages with water molecules to stabilize the peptide or amino acid. This process is called *enzymatic hydrolysis.* Breaking away the peptides or amino acids allows the body to utilize the amino acid or polypeptide to make new proteins within the body.

The body then assembles its own proteins from these amino acids and polypeptides. The body's protein assemblies are programmed by DNA and RNA. For this reason, the body must recognize the polypeptide combinations. Strange polypeptide combinations can burden the body, especially if the body does not have the enzymes to break those peptides apart. While some enzymes can break apart multiple proteins and polypeptides, some proteins, such as gliadins, require special enzymes to be properly broken down into body-friendly peptides and aminos. Protein-cleaving enzymes are called *proteases.*

Food manufacturers can synthetically break down proteins by extrusion, heating and blending with a variety of processing aids, including enzymes. These processes synthetically break apart the proteins in the food. As water is integrated into the process, synthetic hydrolysis results. This produces hydrolyzed protein foods. These synthetically hydrolyzed protein foods may not be recognized by the body's immune system.

French laboratory researchers (Bouchez-Mahiout *et al.* 2010) found by using immunoblot testing that hydrolyzed wheat proteins from skin conditioners produced hypersensitivity, which eventually crossed over to wheat proteins in foods. In other words, hydrolyzed wheat proteins in skin treatments are not necessarily recognized by the immune system. Once the body becomes sensitized to these hydrolyzed wheat proteins from skin absorption, this sensitivity can cross over to sensitivity to similar wheat proteins in foods.

Researchers from France's Center for Research in Grignon (Laurière *et al.* 2006) tested nine women who had skin contact sensitivity to cosmetics containing hydrolyzed wheat proteins (HWP). Six were found to react with either skin hives or anaphylaxis to different products (including foods) containing HWP. The whole group also had IgE sensitivity to wheat flour or gluten-type proteins. The tests showed that they had become sensitive not only to HWP, but also to unmodified grain proteins. As they tested further, they found that reactions often occurred among larger wheat protein peptide aggregates. The researchers concluded that the use of HWP in skin products can produce hypersensitivity not only to HWP, but this sensitivity can crossover to sensitivities to seemingly unrelated wheat proteins in foods.

Spanish researchers (Cabanillas *et al.* 2010) found that enzymatic hydrolysis of lentils and chickpeas produced allergens for four out of five allergic patients in their research.

The commercial enzymes used by many food manufacturers may also stimulate allergic responses. Danish researchers (Bindslev-Jensen *et al.* 2006) tested 19 commercially available enzymes typically used in the food industry on 400 adults with allergies. It was found that many of the enzymes produced histamine responses among the patients.

This means that these larger peptides are accessing our intestinal tissues and our bloodstream. How did they get there? Through increased intestinal permeability. And once they get there, they irritate the cells, producing greater porosity and further increases in permeability.

Food Additives

Many processed foods are chock full of many different artificial additives. These include hundreds of artificial food colors, preservatives, stabilizers, flavorings and a variety of food processing aids. A number of these additives have been found to cause irritable bowels and increased permeability in some people.

Illustrating the effects that food additives can have, Australian researchers (Dengate and Ruben 2002) studied 27 children with irritability, restlessness, inattention and sleep difficulties. The researchers saw many of these symptoms subside after putting the children on the Royal Prince Alfred Hospital Diet, which is absent of food additives, natural salicylates, amines and glutamates.

Using preservative challenges, the researchers were also able to determine that the preservatives significantly affected the children's behavior and physiology adversely.

Researchers from Britain's University of Southampton (Bateman *et al.* 2004) screened 1,873 three-year old children for hyperactivity and the consumption of artificial food colors and preservatives. They gave the children 20 mg daily of artificial colors and 45 mg daily of sodium benzoate, or a placebo mixture. The additive group showed significantly higher levels of hyperactivity than the group that did not consume the artificial colors and preservative.

While these studies are not proving these food additives increase permeability, we can say with confidence that they are somehow accessing the bloodstream through the intestines and affecting the release of neurotransmitters. We know they are also causing mood changes, and mood changes have been associated with IIPS as we've discussed. The logical conclusion that connects food additives with moods is IIPS. We'll discuss this further later.

Sulfites

Sulfites provide a classic case. The sulfite ion will aggressively preserve a food. Sulfites can also produce wheezing, tightness of the throat and other symptoms almost immediately after eating foods preserved with them. However, the effects of sulfites may not be as significant as often portrayed. It may well be that many sulfite-sensitivities seen among wine drinkers are actually the product of the alcohol rather than the sulfites.

Illustrating this, researchers from Australia's Centre for Asthma (Vally *et al.* 2007) tested eight wine-sensitive subjects with sulfite wine and non-sulfite wine. The researchers found that the wine sensitivities were unlikely caused by the sulfites in the wine.

Today, sulfites are used to preserve many wines, dehydrated potatoes and numerous dried fruits. Sulfites include potassium bisulfite, sulfur dioxide, potassium matabisulfite and others. Often labels do not disclose the use of sulfites, because the preservative may have been used early in the processing of the raw ingredients instead of added into the finished product. In addition, under current U.S. labeling laws, if an ingredient such as sulfite is less than 10 parts per million, there is no requirement for putting the ingredient on the panel.

Sulfite sensitivity may be the result of B12 deficiency. In a study presented to the American Academy of Allergy and Immunology, 18 sulfite-sensitive persons were given sublingual B12. The B12 effectively blocked adverse reactions to sulfites in 17 of the 18 (Werbach 1996). This illustrates a connection between the alcohol and/or sulfites and nutrient absorption.

Intestine-damaging Enzymes

The research clearly indicates that diets heavy in animal foods weaken the intestinal barrier. How does this happen? Animal foods deliver pathogenic bacteria, which produce enzymes that damage our intestinal barrier, and in turn harm our intestinal cells.

We can see this clearly as research has confirmed that the enzymes from red meat-rich foods increase the risk of colon cancer. Cancer, as we'll discuss, is the product of mutated cells, which is typically caused by those cells being damaged and altered. The enzymes that have been associated with this mechanism by the research include urease, beta-glucuronidase, beta-glucosidase and cholylglycine hydrolase.

In 1980, Dr. Barry Goldin, a professor at the Tufts University School of Medicine, led a series of studies that found that certain diets promoted a group of cancer-causing enzymes, including beta-glucuronidase, nitroreductase, azoreductase, and steroid 7-alpha-dehydroxylase. These enzymes had been linked with colon cancer in previous studies.

Furthermore, studies on vegetarians found lower levels of these enzymes, while those eating animal-based diets had greater levels. Apparently, these cancer-related enzymes originate from a group of pathogenic bacteria that tend to occupy the intestines of those with animal-based diets. It was discovered that the cancer-producing enzymes are actually the endotoxins (waste products) of these pathogenic bacteria.

Dr. Goldin and his research teams studied the difference between these enzyme levels in omnivores and vegetarians. In one study, the researchers removed meat from the diets of a group of omnivores for 30 days. A reduction of steroid 7-alpha-dehydroxylase was found. When the probiotic *L. acidophilus* was supplemented to their diets, this group also showed a significant reduction in beta-glucuronidase and nitroreductase. So there were now two dietary connections with these disease-causing enzymes: animal-based diets and a lack of intestinal probiotics. The two are actually related, because probiotics thrive in prebiotic-rich plant-based diets and suffer in animal-rich diets.

Two years later, Dr. Goldin and associates (Goldin *et al.* 1982) studied 10 vegetarian and 10 omnivore women. He found that the vegetarian women maintained significantly lower levels of beta-glucuronidase than the omnivorous women.

The association between colon cancer and red meat has been shown conclusively in a variety of studies over the years by the way. An American Cancer Society cohort study (Chao *et al.* 2005) examined 148,610 adults between the ages of 50 and 74 living in 21 states of the U.S. They found that higher intakes of red and processed meats were associated with higher levels of rectal and colon cancer after other cancer variables were eliminated.

Other studies have confirmed that vegetarian diets result in a reduction of these carcinogenic enzymes produced by pathogenic bacteria. Researchers from Finland's University of Kuopio (Ling and Hanninen 1992) tested 18 volunteers who were randomly divided into either a conventional animal products diet or an extreme vegan diet for one month. The vegan group followed the month with a return to the original omnivore diet. After only one week on the vegan diet, the researchers found that fecal urease levels decreased by 66%, cholylglycine hydrolase levels decreased by 55%, beta-glucuronidase levels decreased by 33% and beta-glucosidase levels decreased by 40% in the vegan group. These reduced levels continued through the month of consuming the vegan diet. Serum levels of phenol and p-cresol—also endotoxins of pathogenic bacteria—also significantly decreased in the vegan group.

After two weeks of returning to the animal diet, the formerly-vegan group's pathogenic enzyme levels returned to the higher levels they had before converting to the vegan diet. After one month of returning to the omnivore diet, the serum levels of toxins phenol and p-cresol returned to their previously higher levels prior to the vegan diet. Meanwhile, no changes in any of these enzymes or toxin levels occurred among the conventional omnivore diet (control) group.

A study published two years earlier by Huddinge University researchers (Johansson *et al.* 1990) also confirmed the same results. The conversion of an omnivore diet to a lacto-vegetarian diet significantly reduced levels of beta-glucuronidase, beta-glucosidase, and sulphatase (two other tumor-implicated enzymes) from fecal samples.

Another study illustrating this link between vegetarianism, pathogenic bacterial enzymes and cancer was conducted at Sweden's Huddinge University and the University Hospital (Johansson *et al.* 1998) almost a decade later. Dr. Johansson and associates measured the effect of switching from an omnivore diet to a lacto-vegetarian diet and back to an omnivore diet with respect to mutagenicity: testing the body's fluid biochemistry to determine the tendency for tumor formation.

In this extensive study, 20 non-smoking and normal weight volunteers switched to a lacto-vegetarian diet for one year. Urine and feces were examined for mutagenicity (cancer-causing bacteria and their endotoxins) at the start of the study, at three months, at six months and at twelve months after beginning the vegetarian diet. Following the switch to the lacto-vegetarian diet, all mutagenic parameters significantly decreased among the urine and feces of the subjects. The subjects were then tested once more, three years after converting back to an omnivore diet. The mutagenic biochemistry levels returned to their previously higher levels.

One might wonder what the connection is between cancer-causing enzymes and food sensitivities. The connection is found examining intestinal permeability and intestinal health in general. When intestinal cells are damaged, their likelihood of mutation increases. Intestinal cell damage and cancer-causing mutation stimulates the immune system to begin the inflammatory immune response, in this case, against the intestinal cells.

If the intestinal cells are becoming damaged by these enzymes, we know the intestinal barrier is being corrupted, and the intestinal cells are being exposed to the enzymes. The immune system launches a response to remove those damaged cells. This would typically consist of a cytotoxic T-cell attack against those damaged cells—the same mechanism observed in much of the intestinal permeability research.

Arachidonic Acid

Arachidonic acid is an essential fatty acid important to our diet, but only to a degree. Too much pushes our system towards inflammation. This has been shown by research from Wake Forest University School of Medicine, led by Professor Floyd Chilton, Ph.D.

Dr. Chilton has published a wealth of research data that have uncovered that foods high in arachidonic acid can produce a pro-inflammatory metabolism, especially among adults. As we've discussed, a pro-inflammatory metabolism is basically trigger-happy and hypersensitive: producing fertile ground for intestinal inflammation and subsequent IIPS.

In research headed up by Dr. Darshan Kelley from the Western Human Research Center in California, diets high in arachidonic acid stimulated four times more inflammatory cells than diets low in arachidonic acid content. And this problem increases with age. In other words, the same amount of arachidonic acid-forming foods will cause more inflammation as we get older (Chilton 2006).

According to the USDA's Standard 13 and 16 databases, animal meats and fish produce the highest amounts of arachidonic acid in the body. Diary, fruits and vegetables produce little or no arachidonic acid. Grains, beans and nuts produce none or very small amounts. Processed bakery goods produce a moderate amount of arachidonic acid.

Inflammation within the tissues and cells of the intestinal wall results in increased intestinal permeability, which in turn admits macromolecules into the intestinal tissues and bloodstream. This in turn invokes the IgE immune response.

Phytanic Acid

Another association we can make between intestinal wall health and primarily animal-based diets relates to phytanic acid. Phytanic acid (tetramethylhexadecanoic acid) is a byproduct of plant-food digestion inside the intestinal tracts of bovine (cows and bulls). Phytanic acid is thus present in the meat of these animals. When this branched-chain fatty acid degrades, mammalian peroxisomes are generated. Thus phytanic acid is deposited in tissues, and accumulated around the body.

Otto-von-Guericke University (Germany) professor Dr. Peter Schönfeld has shown that nonesterified phytanic acid directly alters inner mitochondrial membrane permeability though the conductance of hydrogen ions (H+). These open the cell's permeability transition pores, and causes the release of magnesium ions through the cell membrane (Schönfeld 2004).

This mechanism damages the cell, stimulating an inflammatory response. Among intestinal cells, this scenario contributes to intestinal permeability and autoimmunity—consistent with the observations from the research among primarily animal-based diets.

Microparticles

Some researchers have suggested that substances with microparticles can lead to increased intestinal permeability and food sensitivities (Korzenik 2005).

Microparticles are particles smaller than 100 μm, but larger than 0.1 μm. (Smaller molecules, in the nanometer range, are called nanoparticles.) Products that are produced with microparticles include toothpaste and mouthwashes. Food products that contain microparticles include powdered sugars and some refined flours.

We might better classify microparticles in the same category as overly processed foods. The bottom line is that the body can become sensitive to unnaturally-processed constituents should they be exposed to intestinal tissues and the bloodstream. These may not be recognized by the immune system, and thus provoke an inflammatory response.

Pharmaceuticals

After extensive research, medical scientists from the Department of Internal Medicine at France's University Hospital (Moneret-Vautrin and Morisset 2005) found that increased intestinal permeability is associated with the use of alcohol, aspirin, beta-blockers and angiotensin-converting enzyme (ACE) inhibitors.

Researchers from Rush University's Division of Gastroenterology and Nutrition and the Rush-Presbyterian-St. Luke's Medical Center in Chicago (DeMeo *et al.* 2002) has proposed that the gastrointestinal tract maintains one of the body's largest areas offering exposure to the outside environment. This is because everything we eat ends up facing the intestinal walls.

The Rush University researchers illustrated in their research that disruptions to the gut barrier follow inputs including nonsteroidal anti-inflammatory drugs, free radical peroxidation, adenosine triphosphate depletion (metabolic stress) and damage to the epithelial cell cytoskeletons that regulate tight junctions. They also pointed out evidence that associates gut barrier damage to immune dysfunction and sepsis—infection from microorganisms. This of course also alludes to the defenses provided by our probiotic microorganisms, which keep populations of infective microorganisms minimized—as we'll discuss in more detail later.

Medical researchers from the University of Southampton School of Medicine (Macdonald and Monteleone 2005) have suggested that this epidemic of intestinal permeability among industrialized nations has been creating genetic mutations that produce greater levels of permeability among successive generations. This of course provides the link between greater susceptibility for asthma and allergies among those with parents with those disorders. The asthma and allergies aren't necessarily being inherited, but the greater intestinal permeability is.

Alcohol

In a study also mentioned earlier, researchers from France's University Hospital (Moneret-Vautrin and Morisset 2005) found that the consumption of alcohol is implicated in increased intestinal permeability.

Alcohol is the same as ethanol, and ethanol damages cell membranes. Alcohol is very destructive to the cells, and this is evidenced in its damaging effects upon liver cells in alcoholic cirrhosis.

The research has revealed a link between intestinal permeability and liver damage (Bode and Bode 2003), and other research has found alcohol consumption linked to intestinal permeability (Ferrier *et al.* 2006).

When ethanol comes into contact with the cell membrane, it disrupts the ion channels that pump water, nutrients and waste products in and out of the cell. This disrupts the cell's ability to hydrate and manage its health. An increased level of osmosis within the cell membrane also allows not only ethanol, but also other damaging elements—such as free radicals into the cells, which damage them.

Ethanol disrupts the ionic balance within fluids. It disrupts the ability of water to balancing hydrogen bond exchange among the other elements of the fluid. This leads to greater levels of free radicals within the intestinal mucosal membranes, exposing our intestinal cells. These free radicals then damage intestinal cell membranes and the components of the gut barrier that protect our bloodstream.

The bottom line is that ethanol not only damages liver cells—it also damages the intestinal cells, producing increased intestinal permeability.

Genetically Engineered Foods

A genetically engineered food is a food whose genes have been modified in a laboratory. A gene from one species is synthetically inserted into the DNA of another species. More technically, genes from one seed are inserted into another seed utilizing a virus as the vehicle. This seed is then reproduced and sold to farmers.

Today about 70% of the packaged foods in a conventional supermarket contain ingredients grown from genetically modified seeds. Much of the U.S. supply of corn, soybeans, canola and cotton are now genetically modified. (Organic versions of these foods are not genetically modified.) A few other foods now are sometimes grown from GMO seed, such as squash and zucchini.

The main purpose of genetic modification in many cases is to yield plants that are tolerant to more pesticides. A few have been designed to produce their own pesticides.

This is because proteins are determined by the DNA of the plant. In other words, change the DNA, and you change some of the proteins.

Curiously, shortly after GMO soy was introduced to the U.K., soy allergies in England skyrocketed by 50%. GMO soy contains larger levels of a recognized allergen called trypsin inhibitor. It also contains a number of new proteins. In mice, GMO soy slowed down the production of pancreatic enzymes, which altered the breakdown of all foods. Mice also showed intestinal damage, organ damage, sperm damage and embryo damage after consuming GMO soy (Dona and Arvanitoyannis 2009).

In another study, when rats were given GMO soy, they suffered increased intestinal damage and damage amongst many organs, had greater levels of many diseases, and about 50% of the mice' offspring died within three weeks of feeding (Smith 2007).

It should also be noted that this topic is currently the subject of significant debate among scientists. Many believe that the risk of increased allergies is minimal. For example, a study of a GM soybean variety by Spanish researchers (Batista *et al.* 2007) found that there were two potential new allergens within the protein samples analyzed. But when they gave the GM soy to volunteers, none had an allergic response.

While this study illustrated that new potential allergens were produced in the new soy species, it did not prove allergic response. However, when we consider that the rate of allergies to soy is less than 1% of the entire population, the rate of allergenicity to these new allergens might even be less—perhaps .1%. This would mean that they would have needed to feed the soy to 1,000 people before they should see one allergic response.

It should also be noted that based on the science, many governments have banned the use of genetically modified crops and foods.

The critical issue here is to what extent we really understand the consequences related to genetic modification. This concern typically lands people in one of two camps: Do we trust that humans have the inherent wisdom to be able to modify nature in such a way that will ultimately benefit humanity and the planet, and not result in disaster?

To this point we could consider the rise of petroleum use and synthetic plastics, which have transformed society in many ways. These have certainly led to monumental environmental and health disasters: Ones that have not only destroyed or endangered many species, but could actually destroy the earth's ability to support the human race altogether.

Many scientists have proposed that GM crops should be banned simply for their possible allergenicity. In addition, many scientists argue that GM crops may introduce new allergens into the environment (Bachas-Daunert and Deo 2009).

There are also other issues with GM crops: One is the fact that growers must keep going back to the GM seed producers every year because the GM producers designed most seeds to not allow the plant to reproduce. This means that new seeds cannot be naturally produced by farmers—as they have for thousands of years.

Enzyme Deficiencies

If we are deficient in a particular enzyme, our foods will not be properly broken down. This can create a macromolecule that may be exposed to the cells and tissues of the intestines. If the intestinal barrier is already weakened, the immunoglobulins within the intestines can mark the macromolecule as an invader. Once within the intestinal tissues and bloodstream, an overloaded immune system may launch an inflammatory allergic attack against it, producing more intestinal permeability because of the increased histamine and other inflammatory factors.

The point is that the digestive tract has a very exacting way it breaks down proteins. As we discussed earlier, this requires specific protease enzymes and the process of natural enzymatic hydrolysis. This of course means that the body also needs to have plenty of water on hand as well.

Confirming the relationship between food allergies and digestive enzymes, researchers from the Medical University of Vienna (Untersmayr *et al.* 2007) studied the effects that incomplete digestion of fish proteins has on fish allergies. Healthy volunteers and those with diagnosed codfish allergies were challenged with codfish. They were also tested with fish proteins incubated with varying degrees of digestive enzymes. The subjects were tested for histamine release from fish allergen sensitivity with each type.

The researchers found that the inadequate breakdown of fish proteins produced more allergic responses, while a more complete breakdown by enzymes produced fewer allergic responses among both groups. Inadequate digestion produced macromolecules that the body became sensitized to.

Here is a short list of the body's major digestive enzymes:

Major Digestive Enzymes

Enzyme	Foods it Breaks Down
Amylase	Starches
Bromelain	Proteins
Carboxypeptidase	Proteins (terminal)
Cellulase	Plant fiber (cellulose)
Chymotrypsin	Proteins
Elastase	Proteins and elastins
Glucoamylase	Starches
Isomaltase	Isomaltose and Maltose
Lactase	Lactose
Lipase	Fats
Maltase	Maltose
Nuclease	Protein nucleotides
Pepsin	Proteins
Peptidase	Proteins
Rennin	Milk
Steapsin	Triglycerides
Sucrase	Sucrose
Tributyrase	Butter Fat
Trypsin	Proteins
Xylanase	Hemicellulose (plant fiber)

We can see from this list that there are many different protein enzymes. This is because there are so many different types of protein molecules to break down. There are numerous enzyme subtypes and others that break down specific food constituents and particular foods. The body makes some of these, but some are also obtained from our foods. Others are produced by our colonies of intestinal probiotics.

Breastfeeding

Research is increasingly illustrating that breastfeeding is critical to the health of the baby's intestines. Plenty of research on breast-feeding has found that babies breast-fed from healthy mothers have a lower incidence of disease, higher rates of growth, and stronger immune systems. The reasons for these include that breast milk contains a variety of proteins, fatty acids, vitamins, nucleotides and colostrum (a special immune system-stimulator). These all work to help mature the intestines by nourishing and strengthening the mucosal brush barrier that protects our intestinal cells from exposure, thus preventing macromolecules from entering the blood.

Breast milk from a healthy mother also contains a variety of important probiotics. Thus it is critical for establishing our resident intestinal probiotics—leading to a lifetime of intestinal protection.

We can see this effect among many studies. Here are a few:

Researchers from Japan's Shiga Medical Center for Children (Kusunoki *et al.* 2010) surveyed 13,215 parents of children aged from seven to 15 years old. The study compared allergic rates among three types of infant feeding histories: exclusive breastfeeding; mixed formula and breastfeeding; and exclusive formula feeding. The results showed conclusively that exclusive breastfeeding produced significantly fewer cases of bronchial asthma.

Researchers from University of Cincinnati's Department of Internal Medicine (Codispoti *et al.* 2010) studied 361 children, 116 who had allergic rhinitis. They found that prolonged breast-feeding among African American children decreased the allergy risk by 20%.

Researchers from Spain's University of Granada (Martínez-Augustin *et al.* 1997) studied intestinal permeability during the first month of life, along with antibody production to milk proteins. The study fed either cow's milk formula for low-birth weight or the same formula supplemented with nucleotides matching human breast milk. Blood and urine samples were obtained at one, seven and 30 days of age. They found that (low allergy risk) blood IgG antibodies to cow milk protein beta-lactoglobulin were higher among the babies that were fed the formula with the breast milk nucleotides.

Researchers from Sweden's Institute of Environmental Medicine (Kull *et al.* 2010) studied 3,825 children over a period of eight years to determine the role of breast feeding and food allergies. They determined that children who were exclusively breast-fed for four months or more experienced a significantly lower risk of asthma for the first eight years of their lives—as compared to those breast-fed for less than four months. The exclusively breast-fed group also were observed to have significantly better lung function.

Newborns and infants have under-developed intestinal epithelial barriers, and their immune system is still developing. For this reason, it is a sensitive time for the intestinal tract. Breast milk has been shown to stimulate greater levels of IgA within the intestinal tract—thereby reducing the risk of allergies (Brandtzaeg 2010).

However, this association between breast feeding and milk allergies is more complicated. University of Helsinki researchers (Saarinen *et al.* 2000) studied breast-fed and formula infants. From a sampling of 6,209 infants, 824 were found to be exclusively breast-fed. They found that the cumulative incidence of cow's milk allergies was higher in the cow's milk formula group than among the exclusively breast-fed group (2.4% versus 2.1%). This also illustrated that exclusive breast-feeding does not necessarily eliminate the potential for becoming allergic to milk. We would postulate that this rate of milk allergies was due to the mother's own IgE sensitivities to milk and passing these along, as we've discussed.

It also appears that some early exposure to cow's milk may reduce sensitivity. Israeli researchers (Katz *et al.* 2010) from the Assaf-Harofeh Medical Center studied 13,019 infants. The rate of IgE-mediated cow's milk allergy among the population was 0.5%. The average age that cow's milk feeding was introduced was significantly different between the allergic children and those not allergic. The healthy infants were started on milk an average of 62 days after birth. Those infants with cow's milk allergies were started on milk an average of 116 days after birth. Only 0.05% of those infants who were given cow milk formula within the first two weeks of life contracted milk allergies. This is compared to 1.75% of those children who took cow's milk formula between 105 and 194 days after birth contracting allergy to cow's milk.

No breast milk can result in other issues. Researchers from Italy's Siena University (Garzi *et al.* 2002) found that of the about-20% of infants given formula (not fed with breast-milk) suffered from gastroesophageal reflux (GERD), about a third also suffered from milk allergies.

Scientists from the Center for Infant Nutrition at the University of Milan (Arslanoglu *et al.* 2008) found that short-chain galactooligosaccharides (scGOS) and long-chain fructooligosaccharides (lcFOS) (both present in healthy breast milk) can reduce the incidence of atopic dermatitis (AD) and infections through six months of age. They fed 134 infants either a prebiotic-supplemented formula or a placebo-supplemented formula. Follow-ups continued until age two. Atopic dermatitis, asthma, and allergic urticaria rates were significantly higher among the infants given the placebo formula. Formula with oligosaccharide prebiotics lowers the risk of allergies. This of course relates to the fact that prebiotics increase probiotic populations within the intestines.

As we have discussed, the relationship between IIPS and allergies, asthma and eczema relates to the health of the intestinal brush barrier. If the brush barrier has not been given the nutrients, probiotics and immune factors, it will be more porous, allowing larger proteins or endotoxins into the intestinal tissues and bloodstream.

Anxiety, Stress and Depression

Mood and stress are critical to the intestinal barrier function. French researchers (Ducrotté 2009) have illustrated that irritable bowels and food sensitization can occur from a dysfunction of afferent neurons, which can produce disturbances among the *"brain-gut axis."*

In other words, the interplay between stress and digestive responsiveness can stimulate immune response and increased intestinal permeability. Research has found that chronic stress also plays a primary role in the occurrence and continuance of irritable bowel syndrome. This of course involves various neural and sensory relationships, as well as neurotransmitters and their receptors (Buret 2006).

Researchers from Norway's University of Bergen Medical School (Lillestøl *et al.* 2010) found that anxiety and depression are often associated in food intolerance. They studied 130 food sensitive patients with 75 healthy volunteers. They found that 57% of the food sensitive patients had at least one psychiatric disorder. Anxiety disorders were seen among 34% and depression disorders were seen among 16%. Meanwhile, 89% of the patients had irritable bowel syndrome. The researchers concluded that, *"anxiety and depression are common in patients with IBS-like complaints self-attributed to food hypersensitivity. Anxiety disorders predominate."*

The conclusion is that stress and anxiety induces intestinal hypersensitivity, and a higher risk of food sensitivities.

Sun Exposure

How can sun exposure affect the health of our intestines? We can find this association in food allergies, which again relate to macromolecules getting into the bloodstream. Multiple studies have found that allergies are significantly greater among regions further from the equator and those with less sunlight exposure. In both Europe and the U.S., those living in Southern regions have shown significantly lower incidence of food sensitivities and far fewer hospital visits for food allergies. As we've shown the connection between food allergies and IIPS, this also associates IIPS with sunlight.

One study followed 17,280 adults from different countries by researchers from Australia's Monash Medical School (Woods *et al.* 2001). Among developed countries, 12% reported either having food allergies or food intolerances. Food allergy rates were higher among those living in Northern Europe as compared with Southern European countries.

Researchers from the Children's Hospital Boston (Rudders *et al.* 2010) studied allergic emergency room visits throughout the United States. They found that those living in Southern regions had significantly lower incidence of food allergies and far fewer hospital visits for food allergies. The Northeast region had 5.5 visits per thousand, while the South had 4.9 visits per thousand. This difference was even greater when the analysis was restricted to food sensitivities. The risk of food sensitivities was 33% higher for those living in the Northeast than those living in the sun-drenched South. The researchers concluded that: *"These observational data are consistent with the hypothesis that vitamin D may play an etiologic role in anaphylaxis, especially food-induced anaphylaxis."*

Researchers from Massachusetts General Hospital (Vassallo *et al.* 2010) researched the connection between the season of birth and the contraction of food allergies. The records of three Boston food allergy clinics were reviewed. In all, 1,002 patients with food allergies were studied. Forty-one percent of children with food allergies were born in the spring or the summer. Fifty-nine percent were born in the fall or the winter time. Children born in the fall or winter had a significantly higher risk of food allergies. The researchers proposed that the findings indicate that greater levels of UV-B exposure and subsequent vitamin D production might explain this occurrence.

Vitamin D is now linked with over 70 inflammatory disorders. We can now associate vitamin D with intestinal permeability. (See the author's book, *Healthy Sun* for mechanisms involved in sunlight exposure.)

Tobacco

Tobacco smoke contains carbon monoxide, nicotine, aldehydes, ketones and other toxins. These can easily burden the immune system with toxin overload. While we might only think tobacco is inhaled, we should know that tobacco residues become ingested into the digestive tract, and are thus presented to the intestinal walls, where they can damage and irritate the intestinal cells, contributing to increased permeability.

Illustrating this, researchers from the Respiratory Diseases Department of France's Hospital of Haut-Lévèque in Bordeaux (Raherison *et al.* 2008), studied 7,798 children from six cities in France. The research found that children from parents (especially mothers) who smoked, had a significantly greater likelihood of having food allergies than children from families that did not smoke.

Yeast Infections

Overgrowths of yeasts like *Candida albicans* can also contribute to or be a primary cause for intestinal permeability issues. *Candida albicans* can also grow conjunctively with *Staphylococcus aureus*, resulting in the accelerated growth of both microorganisms. This can result in a tremendous burden for our intestinal probiotics as they try to defend against the incursion of the combined yeast and bacteria infections. We see this lethal combination involved in many of the fatalities from swine flu and other influenza contagions. The deaths typically occur in immunosuppressed patients with concurrent bacteria infections. Immunosuppression is also related to IIPS as we've discussed.

The immune system can easily become overloaded with the waste products produced by these microorganisms. These can damage mucosal membranes and seep into the bloodstream through permeable intestines. This produces a number of inflammatory-type symptoms as the immune system responds. This was illustrated from research from Australia's Ninewells Hospital and Medical School (McKenzie *et al*. 1990).

C-Sections

At birth, the baby travels through the birthing canal, picking up critical probiotics from mama. These make their way to the intestines of the baby, helping to form the baby's intestinal barrier. Without this barrier, the baby is more susceptible to allergies.

Researchers from the Netherlands' National Institute for Public Health and the Environment (Roduit et al 2009) studied the allergic status of 2,917 children with respect to whether they were born with a cesarean section. They tested 1,454 of the children for IgE antibodies for inhalants and food allergens at age eight. They found conclusively that babies born with cesarean section had a significantly increased risk of asthma and food sensitivities, both related to the lack of development of the infant's intestinal mucosa.

Researchers from Finland's National Institute for Health and Welfare (Metsälä *et al*. 2010) studied all children born in Finland between 1996 and 2004 that were diagnosed with cow's milk allergies. In all, 16,237 allergic children were found. Children born of cesarean section had a 18% greater risk of contracting milk allergies.

Researchers from the Germany's National Research Centre for Environment and Health and the Institute of Epidemiology (Laubereau *et al*. 2004) studied 865 healthy infants whose parents had allergies. They tested the babies at one, four, eight and twelve months old. They found that babies (147) born with cesarean section had over double the risk of sensitivities to allergens than their peers without C-section birth.

Toxins and Immunosuppression

Clinical research by Professor John G Ionescu, Ph.D. has concluded that environmental pollution is clearly associated with the development of allergic sensitivities—and so associating IIPS. Dr. Ionescu's research indicated that environmental noxious agents, including many chemicals, contribute to the total immune burden, producing increased susceptibility for intolerances.

Environmental toxins are also sensitizing in themselves, producing new trigger allergens. Professor Ionescu draws this conclusion from studying more than 18,000 atopic eczema patients:

> *"Beside classic allergic-triggering factors (allergen potency, intermittent exposure to different allergen concentrations, presence of microbial bodies dyand sensitizing phenols), the adjuvant role of environmental pollutants gains increasing importance in allergy induction."*

According to Dr. Ionescu, toxic inputs such as formaldehyde, smog, industrial waste, wood preservatives, microbial toxins, alcohol, pesticides, processed foods, nicotine, solvents and amalgam-heavy metals have been observed to be mediating toxins for new sensitization of a variety of atopic allergies.

Research has concluded that allergen responses are accelerated by pharmaceutical use because they stimulate histamine and/or acetylcholine. These provoke smooth muscle neuromediators, which stimulate rapid nutrient absorption within the intestines (Liu *et al.* 1977).

This is also consistent with findings of other scientists—as discussed earlier—that pharmaceuticals can increase intestinal permeability.

Immunosuppression may be a big word, but its meaning is very simple: The immune system has been overburdened and compromised by the combination of unnatural, synthetic or deranged foods or toxins. The chart on the next page itemizes a few of these toxins that theoretically produce inflammation and thus promote IIPS:

Major Modern Toxins

Source	Toxin
Antacids	Heavy Metals
Antiperspirant	Aluminum
Carpets, rugs	Molds, dander, lice, PC-4, latex
Cigarette Smoke	Carbon monoxide, nicotine, aldehydes, ketones
Cosmetics	Aluminum, phosphates and chemicals
Dental Fillings	Mercury, alloys, various chemicals
Dish soap	Perfumes, dyes, phosphates
Electric Blankets	EMFs, PC-4, various toxins
Food	Food colors, preservatives, trans-fats, pesticides, arachidonic acids, acrylamide, phytanic acid, artificial flavors
Soaps and Shampoos	Fragrances, chemicals, phosphates
House	Radon, formaldehyde, pollen, dust, mold, dander
Household cleaners	Chlorine, various phosphates
Indoor Light	Blinking fluorescent lights
Industrial Plant or Freeway	Lead, mercury, carbon monoxide
IUDs	Copper
Laundry soaps	Perfumes, dyes, phosphates
Old pillows	Lice eggs, dander, molds
Paints	Lead, arsenic, cadmium, various toxins
Pesticides	Neurotoxins, poisons
Pets	240 infectious diseases & parasites (65 from dogs/39 from cats)
Pipes	Lead, copper, deposits
Plastics	Plasticizers (see also tap water)
Pools and spas	Chlorine, various carbonates
Appliances	Electromagnetic frequencies

Restaurants	Parasites, pesticides, trans-fats
Pans	Aluminum, copper, lead
Shampoo	Chemical fragrances, phosphates
Stoves, Fireplaces	Carbon monoxide, arsenic, soot
Tap Water	Chlorine, microorganisms, pesticides, nitrates, pharmaceuticals
Toothpaste	Propylene glycol, microparticles, synthetic sweeteners
Work environment	Various toxins
Microorganisms	Various species

We might compare this to moving dirt. A small handful of dirt can be carried around easily, and dispersed without much effort. However, a truckload of dirt is another matter completely. If we dumped it on our lawn, we'd have a hill of dirt that would bury the front of our house, preventing us from getting in or out of the house.

This is a useful comparison because while our bodies can handle a small amount of toxins quite easily, modern society is increasingly dumping toxic 'dirt' into our atmosphere, water and foods, effectively inundating our bodies by the 'truckload.'

With this increased burden, the research shows that the body's defenses are lowered. The secretions of our mucosal membrane are reduced. The immune system is put on alert. In this less-protected immunosuppressed state, the intestinal cells are exposed to the wrong molecules (including those toxins). This contact serves to damage those cells, opening up gaps that increase permeability and allow the wrong molecules into our bloodstream.

Chapter Four

Leaky Gut and Dysbiosis

Our probiotics line the walls of our intestines and populate the mucosal membranes of our intestines. Probiotics police the intestinal walls and excrete acids that help manage the pH of the intestines. Should these critical probiotic colonies be damaged by toxins, infection, antibiotics or poor dietary choices, their symbiotic relationship with our intestines can come to an end or become severely limited. This is called dysbiosis. Dybiosis effectively thins the mucosal membrane and leaves the intestinal walls more exposed to macromolecules and toxins.

Should our probiotic colonies become scarce and our intestinal mucosal membranes thin, larger peptides, toxins and even invading microorganisms are allowed to have contact with the intestinal cells. This irritates the intestinal cells, producing an inflammatory immune response. This immune response creates pain and cramping within the intestines, known for such conditions as Crohn's and irritable bowel syndrome.

Again, the intestinal brush barrier as a whole includes the mucosal layer of enzymes, probiotics and ionic fluid. This forms a protective surface medium over the intestinal epithelium. It also provides an active nutrient transport mechanism. It contains glycoproteins and other ionic transporters, which attach to nutrient molecules, carrying them across intestinal membranes. However, this mucosal membrane is supported and stabilized by the grooves between the intestinal microvilli.

This support is provided by four mechanisms existing between the intestinal microvilli: tight junctions, adherens junctions, desmosomes and probiotics. The tight junctions form a bilayer interface between cells, controlling permeability. Desmosomes are points of interface between the tight junctions. The adherens junctions keep the cell membranes adhesive enough to stabilize the junctions. These junction mechanisms together with the zonulin protein regulate permeability at the intestinal wall.

In healthy intestines, the microvilli gaps are policed by billions of probiotic colonies. These perform a variety of maintenance tasks. They help process and break down incoming food molecules. They excrete acids to manage the environment. They secrete various nutrients. They control pathogenic bacteria that can threaten the region. They also communicate closely with the immune system to help signal invasions.

This symbiotic relationship gives the brush barrier its triple-filter mechanism that essentially screens for molecule size, ionic nature and nutrition quality. Before a molecule can come into contact with the intestines, tissues or bloodstream, it must pass through these filter mechanisms.

Should the probiotics become damaged, the entire mucosal brush barrier begins to break down. Zonulin levels also go up during a condition of dysbiosis.

The health of our probiotics and the health of the brush barrier can be threatened by many of the same factors mentioned in the last chapter.. Alcohol is one of the most irritating substances to our probiotics and the mucosal brush barrier in general (Bongaerts and Severijnen 2005).

In addition, many pharmaceutical drugs, notably NSAIDs, have been identified as damaging to probiotics and the mucosal brush barrier integrity. Foods with high arachidonic fatty acid capability (such as trans-fats and animal meats); low-fiber, high-glucose foods; and high nitrite-forming foods have been suspected for their ability to inhibit growth of our probiotics. They also can compromise the mucosal chemistry. Toxic substances such as plasticizers, pesticides, herbicides, chlorinated water and food dyes are also suspected. Substances that increase PGE-2 response also negatively affect permeability (Martin-Venegas et al. 2006).

In addition, the overuse of antibiotics can cause a die-off of our resident probiotic colonies. When intestinal probiotic colonies are reduced, pathogenic bacteria and yeasts can outgrow the remaining probiotic colonies. Pathogenic bacteria growth invades the brush barrier, introducing an influx of endotoxins (the waste matter of these microorganisms) into the bloodstream together with some of the microorganisms themselves.

Many distinguished scientists around the world have now attributed the breakdown of the mucosal brush barrier and the influx of macromolecules as the major cause for the increasing occurrence of food sensitivities in Western society. Healthy intestinal barriers prevent allergic response because they limit the entry of large food molecules into the body's tissues and bloodstream.

A food that has been a source of nutrition for many years can suddenly be identified by the immune system as a threat if its proteins get into the body's tissues before being properly broken down to size. This unfortunate circumstance results not only in the possibility of allergic response to some foods: Nutritional deficiencies can also result. Research is finally confirming these mechanisms (Laitinen and Isolauri 2005; Fasano and Shea-Donohue 2005).

Inflammatory responses resulting from increased intestinal permeability have now been linked to sinusitis, allergies, psoriasis, asthma, arthritis and other inflammatory conditions. These and food sensitivities are all related to dysbiosis.

Let's take a look at some of the research proving this:

In a study by scientists from China's Qilu Hospital and Shandong University (Zeng *et al.* 2008), 30 irritable bowel syndrome patients with intestinal wall permeability were given either a placebo or a fermented milk beverage with *Streptococcus thermophilus*, *Lactobacillus bulgaricus*, *Lactobacillus acidophilus* and *Bifidobacterium longum*. After four weeks, intestinal permeability reduced significantly among the probiotic group.

Researchers from Greece's Alexandra Regional General Hospital (Stratiki *et al.* 2007) gave 41 preterm infants of 27-36 weeks gestation a formula supplemented with *Bifidobacterium lactis* or a placebo. After seven days, bifidobacteria counts were significantly higher, head growth was greater. After 30 days, the lactulose/mannitol ratio (marker for intestinal permeability) was significantly lower in the probiotic group as compared to the placebo group. The researchers concluded that, "bifidobacteria supplemented infant formula decreases intestinal permeability of preterm infants and leads to increased head growth."

Granada medical researchers (Lara-Villoslada *et al.* 2007) gave *Lactobacillus coryniformis* CECT5711 and *Lactobacillus gasseri* CECT5714 or a placebo to 30 healthy children after having received conventional yogurt containing *Lactobacillus bulgaricus* and *Streptococcus thermophilus* for three weeks. The supplemented yogurt significantly inhibited *Salmonella cholerasuis* adhesion to intestinal mucins compared to before probiotic supplementation. The probiotic supplementation also increased IgA concentration in feces and saliva.

German scientists (Rosenfeldt *et al.* 2004) gave *Lactobacillus rhamnosus* 19070-2 and *L. reuteri* DSM 12246 or a placebo to 41 children. After six weeks of treatment, the frequency of GI symptoms were significantly lower (10% versus 39%) among the probiotic group as compared to the placebo group. In addition, the lactulose-to-mannitol ratio was lower in the probiotic group, indicating to the researchers that, *"probiotic supplementation may stabilize the intestinal barrier function and decrease gastrointestinal symptoms in children with atopic dermatitis."*

Researchers from the People's Hospital and the Jiao Tong University in Shangha (Qin *et al.* 2008) gave *Lactobacillus plantarum* or placebo to 76 patients with acute pancreatitis. Intestinal permeability was determined using the lactulose/rhamnose ratio. Organ failure, septic complications and death were also monitored. After seven days of treatment, microbial infections averaged 38.9% in the probiotic group and 73.7% in the placebo group. Furthermore, only 30.6% of the probiotic group colonized potentially pathogenic organisms, as compared to 50% of patients in the control group. The probiotic group also had significantly better clinical outcomes compared to the control group. The researchers concluded that: "Lactobacillus plantarum can attenuate disease severity, improve the intestinal permeability and clinical outcomes."

Researchers from the Department of Medical Microbiology at the Radboud University Nijmegen Medical Centre in The Netherlands (Bongaerts and Severijnen 2005) studied the intestinal permeability connection in food allergies with great focus. They came to the conclusion that:

> "Adequate probiotics can (i) prevent the increased characteristic intestinal permeability of children with atopic eczema and food allergy, (ii) can thus prevent the uptake of allergens, and (iii) finally can prevent the expression of the atopic constitution. The use of adequate probiotic lactobacilli, i.e., homolactic and/or facultatively heterolactic l-lactic acid-producing lactobacilli, reduces the intestinal amounts of the bacterial, toxic metabolites, d-lactic

acid and ethanol by fermentative production of merely the non-toxic l-lactic acid from glucose. Thus, it is thought that beneficial probiotic micro-organisms promote gut barrier function and both undo and prevent unfavorable intestinal micro-ecological alterations in allergic individuals."

Dysbiosis and Early Health

Our first major encounter with large populations of bacteria comes when our baby body descends the cervix and emerges from the vagina. During this birthing journey—assuming a healthy mother—we are exposed to numerous species of future resident probiotics. This first inoculation provides an advanced immune shield to keep populations of pathobiotics at bay. The inoculation process does not end here, however.

Because we get much of our bacteria as we pass through the vagina, cesarean section babies have significantly lower colonies of healthy bacteria. *Bifidobacterium infantis* is considered the healthiest probiotic colonizing infants. Some research has indicated that while 60% of vagina-birth babies have *B. infantis* colonies, only 9% of C-section babies are colonized with probiotics, and only 9% of those are colonized with *B. infantis*. This means that less than one percent of C-section babies are properly colonized with *B. infantis*, while 60% of vagina births are colonized with *B. infantis*. (The remaining 40% would indicate an unhealthy vagina.)

Our body establishes its resident strains during the first year to eighteen months. Following the inoculation from the vagina, these are accomplished from a combination of breast-feeding and putting everything in our mouth, from our parent's fingers to anything we find as we are crawling around the ground. These activities can provide a host of different bacteria—both pathobiotic and probiotic.

Mother's colostrum (early milk) can contain up to 40% probiotics. This will be abundant in bifidobacteria, assuming the mother is not taking antibiotics. Healthy strains of bifidobacteria typically colonize our body first and set up an environment for other groups of bacteria, such as the lactobacilli, to more easily become established.

Picking up a good mix of cooperative probiotic species is a crucial part of the establishment of our body's immune system. Some of the probiotic strains we ingest as infants may become permanent residents. They will continue to line the digestive tract to protect against infection while learning to collaborate with our immune system.

As our digestive tracts begin to become fully functional, interstitial and intercellular lymphocytes build up around our intestinal walls and mucosal membranes. However, these immune defenses only become functional when they are stimulated by the colonizing bacteria we gained from mother and the world around us. This probiotic stimulation renders the production of regulatory cytokines and immunoglobulins such as IgA.

These work together with our probiotics to seal up and defend our intestinal tissues from macromolecules and other potential allergens. IgA coats our intestinal cells and quietly removes allergens before they can invade our intestinal cells.

In other words, oral tolerance is established early in life as the body begins to respond to probiotic bacteria. This is called *down regulation of systemic immunity*. Oral tolerance marks the beginning of the maturity of the digestive tract. In other words, in order to become independent of mother, the baby body's immune system must recognize the good guys from the bad guys. Probiotics are the mediators for this discernment.

Imagine moving to a new location among the U.S. territories during the 1800s in the United States. The territories were full of different threats of various kinds. As we build our new log home and begin to settle in, we begin to try to distinguish between the creatures that will hurt us and those that won't. Say we are lucky enough to meet up with a frontiersman before we start building. The frontiersman has lived in 'these parts' for several decades. He begins telling us about what to 'watch out for' among the region. He also shows us how to prevent the bears from coming around and how to defend ourselves from the bears should they invade our new home. With his assistance, we can go about building our home and prepare for those threats.

Without his assistance, it would become difficult to determine what we should defend ourselves from. As a result, we might just shoot some very harmless (and even helpful) creatures, while allowing some dangerous creatures (such as bears) too much proximity.

Oral tolerance is like being able to distinguish between the good creatures and the bad ones. Our probiotics "show" our bodies what molecules are nutritious and what molecules should be blocked and destroyed by the immune system. How and why does this take place? Our probiotic bacteria are living beings. For millions of generations, these species have been living among our ancestors. Therefore, they have learned by experience what makes us healthy and what can make us sick. This information has been handed down through their generations through genetic evolution. In fact, it is more practical than that: What makes us sick likely also makes them sick.

Therefore, our probiotics can properly guide our immune system in terms of what is good for us and what is bad for us. Our immune system will then "mark" those "bad guys" for future responses when it comes into contact with them.

Of course, this does not exist in a vacuum, as our body's own DNA and immune system cells also will help our bodies recognize the good guys and bad guys. But without healthy probiotics, which our immune system has relied on for millions of years, there is no training.

Should our family's probiotics not be available for this training, we are in trouble. Cesarean sections, for example, will prevent our bodies from coming into contact with mother's probiotics from the birthing canal. Should we then be deprived of her breast milk, we will also miss out on these important probiotics that help train our immune system.

This scenario can result in a variety of situations. Our immune system may launch against the wrong things, including "good" proteins that give us nourishment. It may also launch against even the slightest difference in our air or what we might touch. This is called *sensitization*. The body's immune system becomes overly sensitized to things it should become tolerant to.

The other thing that can happen without the right probiotics is that the baby's brush barrier will not form properly, with the right mix of tight junctions and desmosomes. The intestines may then let into the body large molecules and toxins that the immune system

THE SCIENCE OF LEAKY GUT SYNDROME

knows it cannot handle. Once the immune system "sees" these invaders, it will launch an inflammatory attack in order to purge them, while alerting the body that it has been invaded (Pierce and Klinman 1977).

Illustrating this, researchers from Finland's University of Tampere Medical School (Majamaa and Isolauri 1997) found that the probiotic *Lactobacillus* GG (ATCC 53103) promotes IgA immunity, prevents increased intestinal permeability, and helps control antigen absorption. They gave *Lactobacillus* GG with whey formula or whey without probiotics to 27 children with atopic eczema and cow's milk allergy. They also gave *Lactobacillus* GG to mothers of 10 breast-fed infants with atopic eczema and cow's milk allergy.

The atopic dermatitis symptoms improved significantly during the one-month study period among infants and mothers treated with the probiotics. Probiotic-treated infants also showed decreased levels of alpha 1-antitrypsin while the non-probiotic group did not. The probiotic-treated groups also had lower levels of intestinal permeability. The researchers concluded: *"These results suggest that probiotic bacteria may promote endogenous barrier mechanisms in patients with atopic dermatitis and food allergy, and by alleviating intestinal inflammation, may act as a useful tool in the treatment of food allergy."*

This role played by probiotics to mediate and moderate potential allergens appears critical during the first few months of life, when the mucosal epithelial layer, the intestinal barrier and the immune system are all still in development. Probiotics increase plasma levels IL-10 and total IgA in children with allergic predisposition. Both of these immunoglobulins are central to intestinal immunity and preventing intestinal permeability and the hypersensitive allergic response.

University of Helsinki researchers (Salmi *et al.* 2010) studied 35 infants with atopic eczema, of which 16 had milk allergies. They gave the infants Lactobacillus rhamnosus GG or a placebo. After four weeks, they found that the intestinal organic acids of the milk allergy children began to look more like the non-allergic infants.

Researchers from Germany's Royal Veterinary and Agricultural University (Rosenfeldt *et al.* 2004) wanted to find out if probiotics could reverse intestinal inflammation and strengthen intestinal barrier function in 41 allergic children. Probiotics *Lactobacillus rhamnosus*

19070-2 and *Lactobacillus reuteri* DSM 12246 were given to the children for six weeks—who displayed symptoms of moderate and severe allergic atopic dermatitis. Intestinal permeability was quantified using the lactulose-mannitol test. Gastrointestinal symptoms were also analyzed. Before the probiotic treatment, the researchers found that lactulose-to-mannitol ratios were high, indicating increased intestinal permeability. After the probiotic treatment, the probiotic group's lactulose-to-mannitol ratios were significantly lower. The probiotic group also experienced a significant decrease in gastrointestinal symptoms and eczema symptoms. The researchers concluded: "The study suggests that probiotic supplementation may stabilize the intestinal barrier function."

Remember the research from the University of Turku (Kalliomäki and Isolauri 2002) mentioned earlier. This clinical trial showed that probiotic supplementation reduced atopic eczema risk by 50% among children. They concluded by saying: "Probiotics have also been shown to reverse increased intestinal permeability and to reduce antigen load in the gut by degrading and modifying macromolecules."

As infants wean from breast milk, they can also pick up a host of probiotic colonies from drinking raw milk or by feeding on yogurt or kefir. These will introduce still new probiotics into the intestines. The probiotics will all help increase baby's oral tolerance and further develop the intestinal barrier.

Probiotic Enemies

The parade of infective microorganisms and infectious diseases in our rather sterile society continues despite our dramatically-increased use of prescriptive and over the counter antibiotics, antifungals, antivirals, antiseptic soaps and cleaning disinfectants.

The use of antibiotics has soared over the past few decades—suspiciously over the same period that food sensitivities have also soared. Today, over 3,000,000 pounds of pure antibiotics are taken by humans annually in the United States. This is complemented by the approximately 25,000,000 pounds of antibiotics given to animals each year.

Meanwhile, many of these antibiotics either are given in vain or are ineffectual. The Centers for Disease Control states that, "Almost half of patients with upper respiratory tract infections in the U.S. still receive antibiotics from their doctor." This said, the CDC also warns that "90% of upper respiratory infections, including children's ear infections, are viral, and antibiotics don't treat viral infection. More than 40% of about 50 million prescriptions for antibiotics each year in physicians' offices were inappropriate."

Indeed, the growing use of antibiotics has also created a Pandora's box of *superbugs*. As bacteria are repeatedly hit with the same antibiotic, they learn to adapt. Just as any living organism does (yes, bacteria are alive), bacteria learn to counter and resist repeatedly utilized antibiotics. As a result, many bacteria today are resistant to a variety of antibiotics. This is because bacteria tend to adjust to their surroundings. If they are attacked enough times with a certain challenge, they are likely to figure out how to avoid it and thrive despite it.

This has been the case for a number of other new antibiotic-resistant strains of bacteria. They have simply evolved to become stronger and more able to counteract these antibiotic measures.

This phenomenon has created *multi-drug resistant organisms*. Some of the more dangerous MDROs include species of *Enterococcus, Staphylococcus, Salmonella, Campylobacter, Escherichia coli*, and others. Superbugs such as MRSA are only the tip of the bacterial iceberg.

Another growing infectious bacterium is *Clostridium difficile*. This bacterium will infect the intestines of people of any age. Among children, this is one of the world's biggest killers—causing acute, watery diarrhea. It is also a growing infection among adults. Every year *C. difficile* infects tens of thousands of people in the U.S. according to the Mayo Clinic. Worse, *C. difficile* are increasingly becoming resistant to antibiotics and infections from clostridia are growing in incidence each year.

Medical researchers from the Norwegian University of Science and Technology (Mai *et al.* 2010) found that early antibiotic use increased the likelihood of allergies at age eight. Over 3,300 children were studied for antibiotic use and respiratory conditions at the ages of two months, one year, four years and eight years old. Of all groups, 43% of the children received antibiotics. A third of the children had a respiratory infection, including pneumonia, bronchitis or otitis. The researchers found that those who used antibiotics during their first year of life had increased rates of wheeze and eczema by age eight.

Dysbiosis of the Intestines

Dysbiosis is a state where the body has an imbalance between probiotic populations and pathogenic bacteria populations. In other words, the system is being overrun by the pathogenic bacteria and there are not enough probiotics in place to control their populations. When the body is lacking probiotics, or is overgrown with pathobiotic populations, there is typically an intestinal infection of some type. The extent of the infection, of course, depends upon the type of pathogenic bacteria present, and their populations in proportion to probiotic populations.

Many disorders can be traced back to dysbiosis. Some are direct and obvious, and some are not so obvious, and often appear as other disorders. In general, most digestive disorders are either caused by or accompanied by a lack of balanced intestinal probiotic populations. There are several types of dysbiosis.

We can usually detect *putrefaction dysbiosis* from the incidence of slow bowel movement. Symptoms of putrefaction dysbiosis include depression, diarrhea, fatigue, memory loss, numbing of hands and feet, sleep disturbances, joint pain and muscle weakness. Many of these disorders and others are often due directly to the overgrowth of pathobiotics and their endotoxins. The bacteria are burdening the blood stream with endotoxin waste products and neurotoxins; infecting cells, joints, nerves, brain tissues and other regions of the body.

Another overgrowth issue is *fermentation dysbiosis*. This is often evidenced by bloating, constipation, diarrhea, fatigue, and gas; and the faulty digestion of carbohydrates, grains, proteins and fiber. This is also a result of pathobiotic overgrowth, but in this type of dysbiosis, yeasts are prevalent among the overgrowth populations. As we know from baking bread, yeast will ferment quickly in warm, humid environments.

A body with low probiotic populations will create havoc for the immune system. *Deficiency dysbiosis* is related to an absence of probiotics, leading to damaged intestinal mucosa. This can lead to irritable bowel syndrome, food sensitivities, and intestinal permeability.

The lack of probiotics allows the intestinal wall to come into contact with foreign molecules. This can open up the junctions between the intestinal cells.

This can in turn lead to the entry of these toxins along with larger more complex food particles into the bloodstream—such as larger peptides and protein molecules—as we have discussed. Because these molecules are not normally found in the blood stream, the immune system identifies them as foreigners. The body then launches an inflammatory immune response, leading to *sensitization dysbiosis*. Linked to probiotic deficiency, sensitization dysbiosis causes food and chemical sensitivities, acne, connective tissue disease and psoriasis. Intestinal permeability has also been suspected in a variety of lung and joint infections.

The obvious signs of dysbiosis include hormonal imbalances and mood swings, high cholesterol, vitamin B deficiencies, frequent gas and bloating, indigestion, irritable bowels, easy bruising of the skin, constipation, diarrhea, vaginal infections, reduced sex drive, prostate enlargement, food sensitivities, chemical sensitivities, bladder infections, allergies, rhinovirus and rotavirus infections, influenza, and various histamine-related inflammatory syndromes such as rashes, asthma and skin irritation.

Illustrating the connection between probiotics and allergic skin response, Denmark children ages one to thirteen years old who were diagnosed with atopic dermatitis were given freeze-dried *L. rhamnosus* 19070-2 and *L. reuteri* DSM 122460 probiotics for six weeks. The children were then examined for symptoms. Among the probiotic groups, 56% reported improved eczema symptoms, compared to 15% among the control groups (Rosenfeldt *et al.* 2003).

Connection Between Allergies, Probiotics and IIPS

Probiotics mechanisms have been increasingly connected to inflammatory and allergic responses. They play a critical role in maintaining the epithelial barrier function of the intestinal tract. We've shown that allergies increase with intestinal permeability. Without an adequate intestinal barrier, larger food molecules, endotoxins and microorganisms can enter the bloodstream more easily. These increase the body's total toxin burden, making the immune system more sensitive.

Finnish researchers (Ouwehand *et al.* 2009) gave 47 children with birch pollen allergies *Lactobacillus acidophilus* NCFM and *Bifidobacterium lactis* Bl-04 or a placebo for four months, beginning before the birch pollen season. The probiotic group had significantly less sinus congestion, and lower numbers of nasal membrane eosinophils.

Researchers from Finland's University of Turku (Kirjavainen *et al.* 2003) gave 35 infants with milk allergies *Lactobacillus* GG or a placebo for 5.5 months. The researchers concluded that: "Supplementation of infant formulas with viable but not heat-inactivated LGG is a potential approach for the management of atopic eczema and cow's milk allergy."

The British medical publication *Lancet* published a study (Kalliomäki *et al.* 2001) where 132 children with a high risk of atopic eczema were given either a placebo or *Lactobacillus rhamnosus* GG during their first two years of life. While 31 of 68 of the children receiving the placebo contracted atopic eczema, only 14 of 64 children receiving the probiotic developed atopic eczema by the end of the study.

University of Helsinki researchers (Viljanen *et al.* 2005) treated 230 milk-allergic infants *Lactobacillus* GG, four probiotic strains, or a placebo for four weeks. Among IgE-sensitized allergic children, the LGG provoked a reduction in symptoms while the placebo group did not.

Researchers from Sweden's Umeå University (West *et al.* 2009) fed Lactobacillus F19 or a placebo to 179 infants with allergic eczema from four months to 13 months old. The placebo group had double the incidence of eczema at 13 months than the probiotic group. The probiotic group as a whole also tested with more balanced Th1/Th2 ratios—with greater Th1 levels than the placebo group.

Allergy Hospital researchers from Helsinki University (Kuitunen *et al.* 2009) gave a probiotic blend of two lactobacilli, bifidobacteria, propionibacteria and prebiotics, or a placebo to mothers of 1,223 infants with a high risk of allergies during the last month of pregnancy term. Then they gave their infants the dose from birth until six months of age. They evaluated the children at five years of age for allergies. Of the 1,018 infants who completed the dosing, 891 were evaluated after five years. Allergies among the cesarean-birth children were nearly half in the probiotic group compared to the placebo group (24.3% versus 40.5%).

University of Milan researchers (Arslanoglu *et al.* 2008) found that a mixture of prebiotics galactooligosaccharides (GOS) and fructooligosaccharides (FOS) reduces allergy incidence. A mix of these or a placebo were given with formula for the first six months after birth to 134 infants. The incidence of dermatitis, wheezing, and allergic urticaria in the prebiotic group was half of what was found among the placebo group. The researchers concluded that: "The observed dual protection lasting beyond the intervention period suggests that an immune modulating effect through the intestinal flora modification may be the principal mechanism of action."

Researchers from Finland's National Public Health Institute (Piirainen *et al.* 2008) found that *Lactobacillus rhamnosus* GG fed to pollen-allergic persons for 5-½ months resulted in lower levels of pollen-specific IgE, higher levels of IgG and higher levels of IgA in the saliva. This is consistent with lower sensitivity, greater immunity, and a greater tolerance for pollens and foods.

Researchers from the Medical School at Finland's University of Tampere (Majamaa and Isolauri 1997) gave *Lactobacillus* GG (ATCC 53103) or placebo to 27 infants allergic to milk. The probiotic group showed significant improvement of allergic symptoms after one month of treatment. This and levels of fecal tumor necrosis factor-alpha gave cause for the researchers to conclude that: "These results suggest that probiotic bacteria may promote endogenous barrier mechanisms in patients with atopic dermatitis and food allergy, and by alleviating intestinal inflammation, may act as a useful tool in the treatment of food allergy."

Probiotics balance levels of pro and anti-inflammatory cytokines. They reduce antigens by digesting or otherwise modifying proteins and other food molecules. Probiotics can reverse increased intestinal permeability among children with food allergies. They enhance IgA responses, which are often dysfunctional in food allergy children. Probiotics also normalize the gut microenvironment (Laitinen and Isolauri 2006).

Probiotics improve the intestinal barrier function. They reduce the production of proinflammatory cytokines (Miraglia del Giudice and De Luca 2004).

Research from Sweden's Linköping University (Böttcher *et al.* 2008) gave *Lactobacillus reuteri* or a placebo to 99 pregnant women from gestational week 36 until infant delivery. The babies were followed for two years after birth, and analyzed for eczema, allergen sensitization and immunity markers. Probiotic supplementation lowered TGF-beta2 levels in mother's milk and babies' feces, and slightly increased IL-10 levels in mothers' colostrum. Lower levels of TGF-beta2 are associated with lower sensitization and lower risk of IgE-associated eczema.

German researchers (Grönlund *et al.* 2007) tested 61 infants and mother pairs for allergic status and bifidobacteria levels from 30-35 weeks of gestation and from one-month old. Every mother's breast milk contained some type of bifidobacteria, with *Bifidobacterium longum* found most frequently. However, only the infants of allergic, atopic mothers had colonization with *B. adolescentis*. Allergic mothers also had significantly less bifidobacteria in their breast-milk than non-allergic mothers.

Japanese scientists (Xiao *et al.* 2006) gave 44 patients with Japanese cedar pollen allergies *Bifidobacterium longum* BB536 for 13 weeks. The probiotic group had significantly decreased symptoms of rhinorrhea (runny nose) and nasal blockage versus the placebo group. The probiotic group also had decreased activity among plasma T-helper type 2 (Th2) cells and reduced symptoms of Japanese cedar pollen allergies. The researchers concluded that the results "suggest the efficacy of BB536 in relieving JCPsis symptoms, probably through the modulation of Th2-skewed immune response."

Researchers from the Wellington School of Medicine and Health Sciences at New Zealand's University of Otago (Wickens *et al.* 2008) studied the association between probiotics and eczema in 474 children. Pregnant women took either a placebo, *Lactobacillus rhamnosus* HN001, or *Bifidobacterium animalis* subsp *lactis* strain HN019 starting from 35 weeks gestation, and their babies received the same treatment from birth to two years old. The probiotic infants given *L. rhamnosus* had significantly lower incidence of eczema compared with infants taking the placebo. There was no significant difference between the *B. animalis* group and the placebo group, however.

Researchers from Japan's Kansai Medical University Kouri Hospital (Hattori *et al.* 2003) gave 15 children with atopic dermatitis either *Bifidobacterium breve* M-16V or a placebo. After one month, the probiotic group had a significant improvement of allergic symptoms.

Japanese scientists (Ishida *et al.* 2003) gave a drink with *Lactobacillus acidophilus* strain L-92 or a placebo to 49 patients with perennial allergic rhinitis for eight weeks. The probiotic group showed significant improvement in runny nose and watery eyes symptoms, along with decreased nasal mucosa swelling and redness compared to the placebo group. These results were also duplicated in a follow-up study (2005) of 23 allergy sufferers by some of the same researchers.

Researchers from Tokyo's Juntendo University School of Medicine (Fujii *et al.* 2006) gave 19 preterm infants placebo or *Bifidobacterium breve* supplementation for three weeks after birth. Anti-inflammatory serum TGF-beta1 levels in the probiotic group were elevated on day 14 and remained elevated through day 28. Messenger RNA expression was enhanced for the probiotic group on day 28 compared with the placebo group. The researchers concluded that: "These results demonstrated that the administration of B. breve to preterm infants can up-regulate TGF-beta1 signaling and may possibly be beneficial in attenuating inflammatory and allergic reactions in these infants."

Scientists from Britain's Institute of Food Research (Ivory *et al.* 2008) gave *Lactobacillus casei* Shirota (LcS) to 10 patients with seasonal allergic rhinitis. The researchers compared immune status with daily ingestion of a milk drink with or without live *Lactobacillus casei* over a period of five months. Blood samples were tested for plasma IgE and grass pollen-specific IgG by an enzyme immunoassay. Patients treated with the *Lactobacillus casei* milk showed significantly reduced levels of antigen-induced IL-5, IL-6 and IFN-gamma production compared with the placebo group. Levels of specific IgG also increased and IgE decreased in the probiotic group. The researchers concluded that: "These data show that probiotic supplementation modulates immune responses in allergic rhinitis and may have the potential to alleviate the severity of symptoms."

Researchers from the Skin and Allergy Hospital at the University of Helsinki (Kukkonen *et al.* 2007) studied the role of probiotics and allergies with 1,223 pregnant women carrying children with a high-risk of allergies. A placebo or lactobacilli and bifidobacteria combination with GOS was given to the pregnant women for two to four weeks before delivery, and their babies continued the treatment after birth. At two years of age, the infants in the probiotic group had 25% fewer cases of eczema and 34% few cases of atopic eczema.

The same researchers from the Skin and Allergy Hospital and Helsinki University Central Hospital (Kukkonen *et al.* 2009) studied the immune effects of feeding probiotics to pregnant mothers. In all, 925 pregnant mothers were given a placebo or a combination of *Lactobacillus rhamnosus* GG and LC705, *Bifidobacterium breve* Bb99, and *Propionibacterium freudenreichii* ssp. *shermanii* for four weeks prior to delivery. Their infants were given the same formula together with prebiotics, or a placebo for six months after birth. During the infants' six-month treatment period, antibiotics were prescribed less often among the probiotic group by 23%. In addition, respiratory infections occurred less frequently among the probiotic group through the two-year follow-up period (even after treatment had stopped) compared to the placebo group (an average of 3.7 infections versus 4.2 infections).

Finnish scientists (Kirjavainen *et al.* 2002) gave 21 infants with early onset atopic eczema a placebo or *Bifidobacterium lactis* Bb-12. Serum IgE concentration correlated directly to *Escherichia coli* and bacteroide counts, indicating the association between these bacteria with atopic sensitization. The probiotic group had a decrease in the numbers of *Escherichia coli* and bacteroides after treatment.

Sonicated *Streptococcus thermophilus* cream was applied to the forearms of 11 patients with atopic dermatitis for two weeks. This led to a significant increase of skin ceramide levels, and a significant improvement of their clinical signs and symptoms—including erythema, scaling and pruritus (Di Marzio *et al.* 2003).

Japanese researchers (Odamaki *et al.* 2007) gave yogurt with *Bifidobacterium longum* BB536 or plain yogurt to 40 patients with Japanese cedar pollinosis for 14 weeks. *Bacteroides fragilis* significantly changed with pollen dispersion. The ratio of *B. fragilis* to bifidobacteria also increased significantly during pollen season among the placebo group but not in the *B. longum* group. Peripheral blood mononuclear cells from the patients indicated that *B. fragilis* microorganisms induced significantly more Th2 cell cytokines such as interleukin-6, and fewer Th1 cell cytokines such as IL-12 and interferon. The researchers concluded that: "These results suggest a relationship between fluctuation in intestinal microbiota and pollinosis allergy. Furthermore, intake of BB536 yogurt appears to exert positive influences on the formation of anti-allergic microbiota."

Scientists from the Department of Oral Microbiology at Japan's Asahi University School of Dentistry (Ogawa *et al.* 2006) studied skin allergic symptoms and blood chemistry of healthy human volunteers during the cedar pollen season in Japan. After supplementation with *Lactobacillus casei*, pro-inflammatory activity of cedar pollen-specific IgE, chemokines, eosinophils and interferon-gamma levels all decreased among the probiotic group.

Researchers from the School of Medicine and Health Sciences in Wellington, New Zealand (Sistek *et al.* 2006) gave *Lactobacillus rhamnosus* and *Bifidobacteria lactis* or placebo to 59 children with established atopic dermatitis. They found that food-sensitized atopic children responded significantly better to probiotics than did other atopic dermatitis children.

French scientists (Passeron *et al.* 2006) found that atopic dermatitis children improved significantly after three months of *Lactobacillus rhamnosus* treatment, based on SCORAD (symptom) levels of 39.1 before and 20.7 afterward.

Scientists from Finland's National Public Health Institute (Piirainen *et al.* 2008) gave a placebo or *Lactobacillus rhamnosus* GG to 38 patients with atopic eczema for 5.5 months—starting 2.5 months before birch pollen season. Saliva and serum samples taken before and after indicated that allergen-specific IgA levels increased significantly among the probiotic group versus the placebo group (using the enzyme-linked immunosorbent assay (ELISA)). Allergen-specific IgE levels correlated positively with stimulated IgA and IgG in saliva, while they correlated negatively in the placebo group. The researchers concluded that: "L. rhamnosus GG displayed "immunostimulating effects on oral mucosa seen as increased allergen specific IgA levels in saliva."

Children with cow's milk allergy and IgE-associated dermatitis were given a placebo or *Lactobacillus rhamnosus* GG and a combination of four other probiotic bacteria (Pohjavuori *et al.* 2004). The IFN-gamma by PBMCs at the beginning of supplementation was significantly lower among cow's milk allergy infants. However, cow's milk allergy infants receiving *L. rhamnosus* GG had significantly increased levels of IFN-gamma, showing increased tolerance.

The British medical publication *Lancet* published a study (Kalliomäki *et al.* 2003) where 107 children with a high risk of atopic eczema were given either a placebo or *Lactobacillus rhamnosus* GG during their first two years of life. Fourteen of 53 children receiving the probiotic developed atopic eczema, while 25 of 54 of the children receiving the placebo contracted atopic eczema by the end of the study.

In a study from the University of Western Australia School of Pediatrics (Taylor *et al.* 2006), 178 children born of mothers with allergies were given either *Lactobacillus acidophilus* or a placebo for the first six months of life. Those given the probiotics showed reduced levels of IL-5 and TGF-beta in response to polyclonal stimulation (typical for allergic responses), and significantly lower IL-10 responses to vaccines as compared with the placebo group. These results illustrated that the probiotics had increased allergen resistance among the probiotic group of children.

Researchers from the Department of Otolaryngology and Sensory Organ Surgery at Osaka University School of Medicine in Japan (Tamura *et al.* 2007) studied allergic response in chronic rhinitis patients. For eight weeks, patients were given either a placebo or *Lactobacillus casei* strain Shirota. Those with moderate-to-severe nasal symptom scores at the beginning of the study who were given probiotics experienced significantly reduced nasal symptoms.

IIPS, Probiotics and Irritable Bowel Disorders

As discussed earlier, the risk of irritable bowel syndrome (IBS), Crohn's disease, and other intestinal conditions increases dramatically with IIPS. This relates to the fact that IIPS allows toxins and large macromolecules access to the intestinal tissue inside the intestinal barrier. As they access this region, the immune system launches an inflammatory response to kick out these intruders.

Most of these conditions are considered autoimmune diseases. However, the concept that the body's immune system is attacking itself for no reason is illogical. There are reasons the immune system might target cells from within the body. These can range from the cells being damaged by environmental toxins, endotoxins, oxidative (free) radicals, viruses, to the immune system itself being damaged.

Thus, while we can see that the inflammatory condition is launching an attack upon the body's own cells, the attack is taking place for good reason: The intruders that would have been normally blocked by the intestinal barrier are now making contact with the intestinal cells. As this contact is made, the intestinal cells become altered and/or damaged. As this takes place, the immune cells (such as T-cells) identify that the intestinal cells have been compromised. This results in an immune launch against the intestinal cells and subsequent inflammation—causing the irritation notable in irritable bowel disorders.

How can probiotics help?

The research illustrates that probiotics directly attack foreign invaders like bacteria, viruses and fungi before they can reach and damage the cells of the intestinal walls. Probiotics can also bind to oxidative radicals formed by many types of toxins. Probiotics will also line the intestinal cells, creating a barrier for toxins to enter the blood. They secrete lactic acid and other biochemicals that prevent endotoxin microorganisms from flourishing. Probiotics will also signal the immune system with the identities of pathogens, and then assist in their eradication.

These capabilities of our intestinal probiotics not only reduce the contact our intestinal cells have with these irritating molecules: They also encourage the rebuilding of the desmosomes, reducing the gaps (pores) between our intestinal cells. With less irritation, our body's intestines can begin to rebuild, in other words.

Deficiencies of probiotics in the intestines usually result in overgrowths of pathogenic microorganisms like *Clostridia* spp., *E. coli*, *H. pylori* and *Candida* spp. These damage the cells of the intestinal wall and produce endotoxins that poison intestinal cells. These can damage the brush barrier of the intestines and result in intestinal permeability and an increased risk of food sensitivities.

Here is some research supporting these conclusions:

Researchers from the Medical University of Warsaw (Gawrońska *et al.* 2007) investigated 104 children who had functional dyspepsia, irritable bowel syndrome, or functional abdominal pain. They gave the children either placebo or *Lactobacillus rhamnosus* GG. for four weeks. The probiotic group had overall treatment success (25% versus 9.6%) compared to the placebo group. The IBS probiotic group had even more treatment success compared to the placebo IBS group (33% versus 5%). The probiotic group also had significantly reduced pain frequency.

French researchers (Drouault-Holowacz *et al.* 2008) gave probiotics or a placebo to 100 patients with irritable bowel syndrome. Between the first and fourth weeks of treatment, the probiotic group had significantly less abdominal pain (42% versus 24%) than the placebo group.

Researchers from Poland's Curie Regional Hospital (Niedzielin *et al.* 2001) gave *Lactobacillus plantarum* 299V or placebo to 40 IBS patients. IBS symptoms significantly improved for 95% of the probiotic patients versus just 15% of the placebo group.

Forty IBS patients took *Lactobacillus acidophilus* SDC 2012, 2013 or a placebo for four weeks in research at the Samsung Medical Center and Korea's Sungkyunkwan University School of Medicine (Sinn *et al.* 2008). The probiotic group had a 23% reduction in pain and discomfort while the placebo group showed no improvement.

Scientists from Italy's University of Parma (Fanigliulo *et al.* 2006) gave *Bifidobacterium longum* W11 or rifaximin (an IBS medication) to 70 IBS patients for two months. The probiotic patients reported fewer symptoms and greater improvement than the rifaximin patients. The researchers commented: "The abnormalities observed in the colonic flora of IBS suggest, in fact, that a probiotic approach will ultimately be justified."

Researchers from the University of Helsinki (Kajander *et al.* 2008) treated 86 patients with IBS with either a placebo or a combination of *Lactobacillus rhamnosus* GG, *L. rhamnosus* Lc705, *Propionibacterium freudenreichii* subsp. *Shermanii* JS and *Bifidobacterium animalis* subsp. *lactis*. After five months, the probiotic group had a significant reduction of IBS symptoms, especially with respect to distension and abdominal pain. The researchers concluded that: "This multis-pecies probiotic seems to be an effective and safe option to alleviate symptoms of irritable bowel syndrome, and to stabilize the intestinal microbiota."

Scientists from the Canadian Research and Development Centre for Probiotics and The Lawson Health Research Institute in Ontario (Lorea Baroja *et al.* 2007) studied 20 IBS patients, 15 Crohn's patients, five ulcerative colitis patients, and 20 healthy volunteers. All subjects were given a yogurt supplemented with *Lactobacillus rhamnosus* GR-1 and *L. reuteri* RC-14 for 30 days. IBS inflammatory markers were tested in the bloodstream. CD4(+) CD25(+) T-cells increased significantly among the probiotic IBS group. Tumor necrosis factor (TNF)-alpha(+)/interleukin (IL)-12(+) monocytes decreased for all the groups except the IBS probiotic group. Myeloid DC decreased among most probiotic groups, but was also stimulated in IBS patients. Serum IL-12, IL-2(+) and CD69(+) T-cells also decreased in probiotic IBS patients. The researchers also concluded that: "Probiotic yogurt intake was associated with significant anti-inflammatory effects…"

Researchers from the General Hospital of Celle (Plein and Hotz 1993) gave *Saccharomyces boulardii* or placebo to 20 Crohn's disease patients with diarrhea flare-ups. After ten weeks, the probiotic group had a significant reduction in bowel movement frequency compared with the control group. The control group's bowel movement frequency rose in the tenth week and then subsided to initial frequency levels—consistent with flare-ups.

In another study from Finland (Kajander *et al.* 2005), a placebo or combination of *Lactobacillus rhamnosus* GG, *L. rhamnosus* LC705, *Bifidobacterium breve* Bb99 and *Propionibacterium freudenreichii* subsp. *shermanii* JS was given to of 103 patients with IBS. The total symptom score (abdominal pain + distension + flatulence + borborygmi) was 7.7 points lower among the probiotic group. This represented a 42% reduction in the symptoms of the probiotic group compared with a 6% reduction of symptoms among the placebo group.

In a study from Yonsei University College of Medicine in Korea (Kim *et al.* 2006), 40 irritable bowel syndrome patients were given either a placebo or a combination of *Bacillus subtilis* and *Streptococcus faecium* for four weeks. The severity and frequency of abdominal pain decreased significantly in the probiotic group.

Researchers from Sweden's Lund University Hospital (Nobaek *et al.* 2000) gave 60 patients with irritable bowel syndrome either a placebo or daily rose-hip drink with *Lactobacillus plantarum* for four weeks. Enterococci levels increased among the placebo group but were unchanged in the test group. Flatulence was significantly reduced among the probiotic group compared with the placebo group. At a 12-month follow-up, the probiotic group maintained significantly better overall GI symptoms and function than the placebo group.

New York scientists (Hun 2009) gave 44 IBS patients either a placebo or *Bacillus coagulans* GBI-30 for eight weeks. The probiotic group experienced significant improvements in abdominal pain and bloating symptoms versus the placebo group.

Scientists at Ireland's University College in Cork (O'Mahony *et al.* 2005) studied 77 irritable bowel syndrome patients with abnormal IL-10/IL-12 ratios—indicating a proinflammatory, Th1 status. The patients were given a placebo, *Lactobacillus salivarius* UCC4331 or *Bifidobacterium infantis* 35624 for eight weeks. IBS symptoms were logged daily and assessed weekly. Tests included quality of life, stool microbiology, and blood samples to test peripheral blood mononuclear cell release of inflammatory cytokines interleukin (IL)-10 and IL-12. Patients who took *B. infantis* 35624 had a significantly greater reduction in abdominal pain and discomfort, bloating and distention, and bowel movement difficulty, compared to the other groups. IL-10/IL-12 ratios—indicative of Th1 proinflammatory metabolism—were also normalized in the probiotic *B. infantis* group.

Researchers from the Umberto Hospital in Venice in Italy (Saggioro 2004) studied probiotics on seventy adults with irritable bowel syndrome. They were given 1) a placebo; 2) a combination of *Lactobacillus plantarum* and *Bifidobacterium breve*; or 3) a combination of *Lactobacillus plantarum* and *Lactobacillus acidophilus* for four weeks. After 28 days of treatment, pain scores measuring different abdominal regions decreased among the probiotic groups by 45% and

49% respectively, versus 29% for the placebo group. The IBS symptom severity scores decreased among the probiotic groups after 28 days by 56% and 55.6% respectively, versus 14% among the placebo group.

Sixty-eight patients with irritable bowel syndrome were treated at the TMC Hospital in Shizuoka, Japan (Tsuchiya *et al.* 2004) with either placebo or a combination of *Lactobacillus acidophilus*, *Lactobacillus helveticus* and *Bifidobacteria* for twelve weeks. The probiotic treatment was either "effective" or "very effective" in more than 80% of the IBS patients. In addition, less than 5% of the probiotic group reported the treatment as "not effective," while more than 40% of the placebo patients reported their placebo treatment as "not effective." The probiotic group also reported significant improvement of bowel habits.

Researchers from Britain's University of Manchester School of Medicine (Whorwell *et al.* 2007) gave a placebo or *Bifidobacterium infantis* 35624 to 362 primary care women with irritable bowel syndrome in a large-scale, multicenter study. After four weeks of treatment, *B. infantis* was significantly more effective than the placebo in reducing bloating, bowel dysfunction, incomplete evacuation, straining, and the passing of gas.

Scientists from Denmark's Hvidovre Hospital and the University Hospital of Copenhagen (Wildt *et al.* 2006) gave 29 colitis-IBS patients either *Lactobacillus acidophilus* LA-5 and *Bifidobacterium animalis* subsp. *lactis* BB-12, or a placebo for twelve weeks. The probiotic treatment group had a decrease in bowel frequency from 32 per week to 23 per week. Furthermore, the probiotic group had an average reduction in the frequency of liquid stools from six days per week to one day per week.

Scientists at Poland's Jagiellonian University Medical College (Zwolińska-Wcisło *et al.* 2006) tested 293 ulcer patients, 60 patients with ulcerative colitis, 12 patients with irritable bowel syndrome and 72 patients with other gastrointestinal issues. Compared to placebo, *Lactobacillus acidophilus* supplementation resulted in a lessening of symptoms, a reduction of fungal colonization, and increased levels of immune system cytokines TNF-alpha and IL-1 beta.

Medical researchers from Finland's University of Helsinki (Kajander *et al.* 2007) sought to understand the mechanism of probiotics' proven ability to reduce IBS symptoms. They gave either a placebo or a combination of *Lactobacillus rhamnosus* GG, *Lactobacillus rhamnosus* Lc705, *Propionibacterium freudenreichii* subsp. *shermanii* JS and *Bifidobacterium breve* Bb99 to 55 irritable bowel syndrome patients. After six months of treatment, composition of feces and intestinal microorganism content illustrated a significant drop in glucuronidase levels in the probiotic group compared to the placebo group. The researchers concluded that there was a complexity of different factors, and so far unknown mechanisms explaining, "the alleviation of irritable bowel syndrome symptoms by the multispecies probiotic."

Probiotics and Other Digestive Conditions

Chronic digestive problems, which include bloating, indigestion, and cramping are often symptoms of IBS, Crohn's disease or colitis. These diseases (IBS, etc.) are also typically accompanied by chronic pain and intestinal inflammation, however. Occasional indigestion, bloating and cramping is often associated with a developing case of dysbiosis caused by antibiotic use, poor diet, or an overgrowth of specific pathogenic microorganisms. Enzyme deficiency can be caused by probiotic deficiencies. Probiotics produce a number of enzymes, including protease and lipase—necessary for the break down of proteins and fats. Poor digestion is often the result of a lack of these and other enzymes. Gastrointestinal difficulties in general are often caused by dysbiosis. This can include an overgrowth of yeasts, pathogenic bacteria or both. Here are a few of the many studies showing that digestion can improve with probiotic use:

French researchers (Guyonnet *et al.* 2009) fed *Bifidobacterium lactis* DN-173010 with yogurt strains for two weeks to 371 adults reporting digestive discomfort. After two weeks, 82.5% of the probiotic group reported improved digestive symptoms compared to 2.9% of the control group.

Another group of French scientists (Diop *et al.* 2008) gave 64 volunteers with high levels of stress and incidental gastrointestinal symptoms either a placebo or *Lactobacillus acidophilus* Rosell-52 and *Bifidobacterium longum* for three weeks. At the end of the three weeks, the stress-related gastrointestinal symptoms of abdominal pain, nausea and vomiting decreased by 49% among the probiotic group.

Probiotics, Polyps, Diverticulosis and Diverticulitis

Polyps, diverticulosis and diverticulitis are abnormalities within the intestines or colon. They have been associated with Crohn's, IBS and ulcerative colitis, as well as increased food sensitivities. They also have been seen forming seemingly without other disease pathologies.

Diverticulosis is the bulging of sections of the intestines. When a bulging area weakens and bursts, that is called diverticulitis. A polyp, on the other hand, is a growth on the inside of the intestinal wall. These may be either benign or cancerous. All of these conditions are associated with intestinal probiotics, because healthy probiotic colonies are essential to the health of the intestinal wall. We can see the evidence from the research:

Scientists from Sweden and Ireland (Rafter *et al.* 2007) gave placebo or *Lactobacillus rhamnosus* GG and *Bifidobacterium lactis* Bb12 to 43 polyp patients (who also had surgery for their removal) for 12 weeks. The probiotics significantly reduced colorectal proliferation and improved epithelial barrier function (reducing intestinal permeability) among the polyp patients. Testing also showed decreased exposure to intestinal genotoxins among the probiotic polyp patient group.

Researchers from The Netherlands' University Hospital Maastricht (Goossens *et al.* 2006) gave *Lactobacillus plantarum* 299v or a placebo to 29 polyp patients twice a day for two weeks. Fecal sample examinations and biopsies were collected during colonoscopy. *L. plantarum* 299v significantly increased probiotic bacteria levels from fecal tests and from rectal biopsies. Ascending colon populations were not significantly greater, however.

Researchers from the Digestive Endoscopy Unit at Italy's Lorenzo Bonomo Hospital (Tursi *et al.* 2008) treated 75 patients with symptomatic diverticulosis. Mesalazine and/or *Lactobacillus casei* DG were given for 10 days each month. Of the 71 patients that completed the study, 66 (88%) were symptom-free after 24 months. The researchers concluded that mesalazine and/or *Lactobacillus casei* were effective in maintaining diverticulosis remission for an extended period, assuming continued treatment.

Probiotics and Ulcers

Ulcers often relate directly to food sensitivities because ulcer symptoms can worsen after eating certain foods. Also, some food sensitivities are a direct result of an ulcerated condition in the stomach or duodenum—allowing undigested food molecules access to upper intestinal cells. Some food intolerances are the direct result of an ulcer, as the food is rejected by the gastric cells. In allergies and other intolerances, the sensitivity may be the result of food molecules not being digested enough or not being correctly modified by probiotics, acids, bile, proteases and other biochemicals of the stomach and intestines.

Until only recently, medical scientists and physicians were certain that ulcers were caused by too much acid in the stomach and the eating of spicy foods. This assumption has been debunked over the past two decades, as researchers have confirmed that at least 80% of all ulcers are associated with *Helicobacter pylori* infections.

While acidic foods and gastrin produced by the stomach wall are also implicated by symptoms of heartburn and acid reflux, we know that a healthy stomach has a functional barrier that should prevent these normal food and gastric substances from harming the cells of the stomach wall. This barrier is called the mucosal membrane. This stomach's mucosal membrane contains a number of mucopolysaccharides and phospholipids that, together with secretions from intestinal and oral probiotics, protect the stomach cells from acids, toxins and bacteria invasions.

Helicobacter pylori damage the mucosal membrane that protects the stomach's gastric cells, and directly irritate the tissues. This damage produces the symptoms of heartburn.

As doctors and researchers work to eradicate *H. pylori*, which infects billions of people worldwide, they are finding that *H. pylori* is becoming increasingly resistant to many of the antibiotics used in prescriptive treatment. Research from Poland's Center of Gastrology (Ziemniak 2006) investigated antibiotic use on *Helicobacter pylori* infections: 641 *H. pylori* patients were given various antibiotics typically applied to *H. pylori*. The results indicated that *H. pylori* had developed a 22% resistance to clarithromycin and 47% resistance to metronidazole. Worse, a 66% secondary resistance to clarithromycin and metronidazole was found, indicating *H. pylori*'s increasing resistance to antibiotics.

H. pylori bacteria do not always cause ulcers. In fact, only a small percentage of *H. pylori* infections actually become ulcerative. Meanwhile, there is some evidence that *H. pylori*—like *E. coli* and *Candida albicans*—may be a normal resident in a healthy intestinal tract, assuming they are properly balanced and managed by strong legions of probiotics.

There is strong evidence that confirms the ability probiotics have in controlling and managing *H. pylori* overgrowths. We will also see that probiotics have the ability to arrest ulcerative colitis and even mouth ulcers:

Researchers from the Academic Hospital at Vrije University in The Netherlands (Cats *et al.* 2003) gave either a placebo or *Lactobacillus casei* Shirota to 14 *H. pylori*-infected patients for three weeks. Six additional *H. pylori*-infected subjects were used as controls. The researchers determined that *L. casei* significantly inhibits *H. pylori* growth. This effect was more pronounced for *L. casei* grown in milk solution than in the DeMan-Rogosa-Sharpe medium (a probiotic broth developed by researchers in 1960).

Mexican hospital researchers (Sahagún-Flores *et al.* 2007) gave 64 *Helicobacter pylori*-infected patients antibiotic treatment with or without *Lactobacillus casei* Shirota. *Lactobacillus casei* Shirota plus antibiotic treatment was 94% effective and antibiotic treatment alone was 76% effective.

Researchers from the Department of Internal Medicine and Gastroenterology at Italy's University of Bologna (Gionchetti *et al.* 2000) gave 40 ulcerative colitis patients either a placebo or a combination of four strains of lactobacilli, three strains of bifidobacteria, and one strain of *Streptococcus salivarius* subsp. *thermophilus* for nine months. The patients were tested monthly. Three patients (15%) in the probiotic group suffered relapses within the nine months, versus 20 (100%) in the placebo group.

Italian scientists from the University of Bologna (Venturi *et al.* 1999) also gave 20 patients with ulcerative colitis a combination of three bifidobacteria strains, four lactobacilli strains and *Streptococcus salivarius* subsp. *thermophilus* for 12 months. Fecal samples were obtained at the beginning, after 10 days, 20 days, 40 days, 60 days, 75 days, 90 days, 12 months and 15 days after the (12 months) end of the treatment period. Fifteen of the 20 treated patients achieved and maintained remission from ulcerative colitis during the study period.

British researchers from the University of Dundee and Ninewells Hospital Medical School (Furrie *et al*. 2005) gave 18 patients with active ulcerative colitis either B. *longum* or a placebo for one month. Clinical examination and rectal biopsies indicated that sigmoidoscopy scores were reduced in the probiotic group. In addition, mRNA levels for human beta defensins 2, 3, and 4 (higher in active ulcerative colitis) were significantly reduced among the probiotic group. Inflammatory cytokines tumor necrosis factor alpha and interleukin-1alpha were also significantly lower in the probiotic group. Biopsies showed reduced inflammation and the regeneration of epithelial tissue within the intestines among the probiotic group.

Scientists from Italy's Raffaele University Hospital (Guslandi *et al*. 2003) gave *Saccharomyces boulardii* or placebo to 25 patients with ulcerative colitis unsuitable for steroid therapy, for four weeks. Of the 24 patients completing the study, 17 attained clinical remission—confirmed endoscopically.

Researchers from Switzerland's University Hospital in Lausanne (Felley *et al*. 2001) gave fifty-three patients with ulcerative H. *pylori* infection milk with L. *johnsonii* or placebo for three weeks. Those given the probiotic drink had a significant H. *pylori* density decrease, reduced inflammation and less gastritis activity from H. *pylori*.

Lactobacillus reuteri ATCC 55730 or a placebo was given to 40 H. *pylori*-infected patients for four weeks by researchers from Italy's Università degli Studi di Bari (Francavilla *et al*. 2008). L. *reuteri* effectively suppressed H. *pylori* infection, decreased gastrointestinal pain, and reduced other dyspeptic symptoms.

Scientists from the Department of Internal Medicine at the Catholic University of Rome (Canducci *et al*. 2000) tested 120 patients with ulcerative H. *pylori* infections. Sixty patients received a combination of antibiotics rabeprazole, clarithromycin and amoxicillin. The other sixty patients received the same therapy together with a freeze-dried, inactivated culture of *Lactobacillus acidophilus*.

The probiotic group had an 88% eradication of *H. pylori* while the antibiotic-only group had a 72% eradication of *H. pylori*.

Scientists from the University of Chile (Gotteland *et al.* 2005) gave 182 children with *H. pylori* infections placebo, antibiotics or probiotics. *H. pylori* were completely eradicated in 12% of those who took *Saccharomyces boulardii*, and in 6.5% of those given *L. acidophilus*. The placebo group had no *H. pylori* eradication.

Researchers from Japan's Kyorin University School of Medicine (Imase *et al.* 2007) gave *Lactobacillus reuteri* strain SD2112 in tablets or a placebo to 33 *H. pylori*-infected patients. After four and eight weeks, *L. reuteri* was significantly decreased *H. pylori* among the probiotic group.

In a study of 347 patients with active *H. pylori* infections (ulcerous), half the group was given antibiotics and the other half was given antibiotics with yogurt (*Lactobacillus acidophilus* HY2177, *Lactobacillus casei* HY2743, *Bifidobacterium longum* HY8001, and *Streptococcus thermophilus* B-1). The yogurt plus antibiotics group had significantly more eradication of the *H. pylori* bacteria, and significantly fewer side effects than the antibiotics group (Kim *et al.* 2008).

Lactobacillus brevis (CD2) or placebo was given to 22 *H. pylori*-positive dyspeptic patients for three weeks before a colonoscopy by Italian medical researchers (Linsalata *et al.* 2004). A reduction in the UBT delta values and subsequent bacterial load ensued. *L. brevis* CD2 stimulated a decrease in gastric ornithine decarboxylase activity and polyamine. The researchers concluded: *"Our data support the hypothesis that L. brevis CD2 treatment decreases H. pylori colonization, thus reducing polyamine biosynthesis."*

Thirty *H. pylori*-infected patients were given either probiotics *Lactobacillus acidophilus* and *Bifidobacterium bifidum* or placebo for one and two weeks following antibiotic treatment by British researchers (Madden *et al.* 2005). Those taking the probiotics had a recovery of normal intestinal microflora, damaged during antibiotic treatment. The researchers also observed that those taking the probiotics throughout the two weeks showed more normal and stable microflora than did those groups taking the probiotics for only one out of the two weeks.

Researchers at the Nippon Medical School in Tokyo (Fujimori *et al.* 2009) gave 120 outpatients with ulcerative colitis either a placebo; *Bifidobacterium longum;* psyllium (a prebiotic); or a combination of *B. longum* and psyllium (synbiotic) for four weeks. C-reactive protein (pro-inflammatory) decreased significantly only with the synbiotic group, from 0.59 to 0.14 mg/dL. In addition, the synbiotic therapy resulted in significantly better scores on symptom and quality-of-life assessments.

Scientists from the Department of Medicine at Lausanne, Switzerland's University Hospital (Michetti *et al.* 1999) tested 20 human adults with ulcerative *H. pylori* infection with *L. acidophilus johnsonii.* The probiotic was taken with the antibiotic omeprazole in half the group and alone (with placebo) in the other group. The patients were tested at the start, after two weeks of treatment, and four weeks after treatment. Both groups showed significantly reduced *H. pylori* levels during and just following treatment. However, the probiotic-only group tested better than the antibiotic group during the fourth week after the treatment completion.

Medical scientists from the Kaohsiung Municipal United Hospital in Taiwan (Wang *et al.* 2004) studied 59 volunteer patients infected with *H. pylori*. They were given either probiotics (*Lactobacillus* and *Bifidobacterium* strains) or placebo after meals for six weeks. After the six-week period, the probiotic treatment *"effectively suppressed H. pylori,"* according to the researchers.

In the Polish study mentioned earlier (Ziemniak 2006), 641 *H. pylori* patients were given either antibiotics alone or probiotics with antibiotics. The two antibiotic-only treatment groups had 71% and 86% eradication of *H. pylori*, while the antibiotic-probiotic treatment group had 94% eradication.

Researchers from the Cerrahpasa Medical Faculty at Istanbul University (Tasli *et al.* 2006) gave 25 patients with Behçet's syndrome (chronic mouth ulcers) six *Lactobacillus brevis* CD2 lozenges per day at intervals of 2-3 hours. After one and two weeks, the number of ulcers significantly decreased.

Dysbiosis and Inflammation

As we've discussed earlier, when the immune system is prone to inflammatory response, it will respond with more hypersensitivity to macromolecules and other food elements that gain entry to the intestinal wall. In such a condition, the immune system is overreacting. Research has confirmed that these conditions are characterized by an increase in T-cell helper-2 cells (Th2); outside of their normal balance with Th1 cells. This sets up the hair-trigger immune system.

Research shows that probiotics produce a balance among the immune system. Let's see some of the evidence:

Researchers from the Department of Clinical Sciences at Spain's University of Las Palmas de Gran Canaria (Ortiz-Andrellucchi *et al.* 2008) studied the ability of *Lactobacillus casei* DN114001 to modulate immunity factors among lactating mothers and their babies. *L. casei* or a placebo was given to expecting mothers for six weeks. T helper-1 and T helper-2 (Th1/ Th2) levels were tested from breast-fed colostrum, early milk (10 days) and mature milk (45 days). Allergic episodes among the newborns were also observed throughout their first six months of life. Among the probiotic group, T-cell and B-cell levels were increased, and natural killer cells were significantly increased. Furthermore, Th1/Th2 ratios were more balanced (anti-inflammatory) among the probiotic group.. Levels of the proinflammatory cytokine TNF-alpha was decreased in maternal milk. Significantly fewer gastrointestinal issues occurred among the breast-fed children of the probiotic mother group as well.

Japanese scientists (Hirose *et al.* 2006) gave *Lactobacillus plantarum* strain L-137 or placebo to 60 healthy men and women, average age 56, for twelve weeks. Increased Con A-induced proliferation (acquired immunity), increases in IL-4 production by CD4+ T-cells, and a more balanced Th1:Th2 ratio was seen in the probiotic group. Quality of life scores were also higher among the probiotic group.

Gluten Sensitivities and Leaky Gut

Celiac disease—an inflammatory immune response to the gliadin protein in gluten—has been increasing over the past few years, and research is illustrating that celiac disease is more prevalent than previously considered.

Gluten sensitivities also appear to be increasing, with more and more people in western countries—especially in the U.S.—opting for gluten-free diets. This typically comes from a sense many have had that the gluten foods in their diet produce intestinal irritations, including bloating and indigestion. For this reason, the term "gluten-free" has become ubiquitous among health food stores and consumers.

In a study from George Washington University School of Medicine (Bakshi *et al.* 2012), researchers found that probiotics provide a viable solution for gluten digestion and intestinal health—and likely their absence provides the smoking gun for the cause of gluten sensitivities.

The reality is that grain-based foods have been part of the human diet for millions of years, and some of the healthiest diets – including the Mediterranean Diet—contain gracious quantities of wheat and other whole grains. This is not to mention of course the fiber content among whole grains and the research that has shown foods rich in fiber reduce heart disease and other metabolic disorders.

And many traditional societies—producing the diets of a majority of the world's population, many of which are known for long lifespan—have grains as the cornerstone of their diet. These cultures also come with an absence of a history of intestinal problems.

This leads to the logical question: Has humanity really been poisoning itself with wheat and other gluten-containing grains (including barley, rye and others)? In a word, no.

The fact is, humanity has been eating these grains for thousands of years, and it has genetically, biologically and probiotically adapted to eating these foods.

Significant research focus and several teams of investigators have confirmed that the inflammatory response to gliadin—initiated with an interleukin-15 mediated response—is inhibited by healthy intestinal probiotics.

In fact, intestinal probiotics break down gliadin into healthy, non-inflammatory components.

A 2012 paper by three medical school professors studied the various means by which the effects of celiac disease may be mitigated – by inhibiting the inflammatory response. The paper's authors include two professors who are gastroenterology professors at George Washington University School of Medicine, Anita Bakshi, M.D. and Sindu Stephen, M.D. Two other clinical M.D.s co-authored the research.

The researchers focused first upon the mechanisms of wheat gliadin protein upon the intestinal cells—which produce inflammation and intestinal permeability. These include the activation of a CD4+ T-cell response among the intestinal cells—which induces the secretion of a protein called zonulin. Zonulin then stimulates an increase in the spaces in the tight junctions between the intestinal cells, creating gut permeability.

This opening between intestinal cells is accompanied by an even greater inflammatory response as the immune system responds to larger proteins having potential contact with the bloodstream.

While there are a number of studies that have shown these effects, the researchers singled out a few studies that clearly and specifically illustrated how intestinal probiotics in a healthy body will inhibit this process by breaking down gluten through protease (enzyme) activity.

In one of these, Irish researchers found that two enzymes produced from probiotic bacteria—prolyl endopeptidase and endoprotease B—were able to break down gluten into non-reactive elements, completely sidestepping the possible intestinal response.

This research was confirmed in a clinical setting by scientists at the Celiac Sprue Research Foundation in Palo Alto, California. Here 20 celiac patients were given small doses of gluten with and without (double-blind, randomized, cross-over) being pretreated with one of these probiotic-produced enzymes—prolyl endopeptidase. The cross-over study utilized two 14-day treatment periods in total, in a staged format.

The pretreatment with the enzyme allowed a majority of the celiac patients to avoid malabsorption of carbohydrates and fats—a typical symptom of celiac sprue response.

The researchers concluded that:

> *"Pretreatment of gluten with prolyl endopeptidase avoided the development of fat or carbohydrate malabsorption in the majority of those patients who developed fat or carbohydrate malabsorption after a 2-week gluten challenge."*

In a series of studies from Finland's University of Tampere Medical School, researchers tested the probiotics strains *Lactobacillus fermentum* and *Bifidobacterium lactis* with gluten digestion and the inflammatory effects of gliadin.

They found these live probiotics were both able to inhibit the inflammation response among sensitive intestinal (Caco-2) cells. In both instances the probiotics prevented the inflammatory response as well as prevented the formation of "membrane ruffles."

The researchers stated:

> "B. lactis inhibited the gliadin-induced increase dose-dependently in epithelial permeability, higher concentrations completely abolishing the gliadin-induced decrease in transepithelial resistance."

This of course means the probiotics reduced the amount of intestinal damage caused by the inflammatory response related to the gluten ingestion.

And in their conclusion, the researchers stated:

> "We conclude thus that live B. lactis bacteria can counteract directly the harmful effects exerted by coeliac-toxic gliadin and would clearly warrant further studies of its potential as a novel dietary supplement in the treatment of coeliac disease."

While the inflammatory response in celiac sprue is typically described as being the result of a genetic abnormality, intestinal irritation and indigestion to gluten in non-celiac people provokes similar mechanisms of inflammation—though not as vigorous—and not linked with genetic abnormality (yet).

The UGW researchers concluded after reviewing the research that: "Inclusion of probiotics appears to be able to reduce the damage caused by eating gluten-contaminated foods and may even accelerate mucosal healing after the initiation of a gluten-free diet."

These results have been confirmed by other research. In a 2013 study from Argentina's University of Buenos Aires tested a probiotic supplement with 22 adults with celiac disease. The patients were given either capsules with the probiotic *Bifidobacterium infantis* or a placebo for 3 weeks.

Those taking the probiotic supplement had significantly lower levels of indigestion, constipation and other intestinal symptoms as gauged by the Gastrointestinal Symptom Rating Scale. Levels of IgA antibodies to gluten were also lower among the probiotic group.

The researchers stated:

> "The study suggests that B. infantis may alleviate symptoms in untreated celiac disease."

Certainly adult celiac patients are dealing with a dramatically heightened genetic response to the gluten protein, which is significantly greater than what is experienced by those even with some gluten sensitivity. And we cannot necessarily suggest that the inflammatory immune response of a celiac sprue patient can be completely eliminated by gliadin enzymes released by probiotics, which break down those gliadin proteins. This is because the gliadin genetic imprint may still be recognized by the immune system—producing the antibody-driven inflammatory response.

However, the non-genetic immune response that produces some bloating and/or indigestion for non-celiac people sensitive to gluten has many of the same mechanisms—especially when it comes to creating intestinal permeability. And the research is showing that even among celiac patients, symptoms of gluten intolerance are reduced. So it would only be logical to conclude—as have many researchers – that gluten sensitivities outside of celiac disease may be alleviated with healthy intestinal flora.

We also have only been looking through a narrow beam of research investigating only a few enzymes and probiotics. A healthy human intestine is a microcosm of thousands of strains of probiotic bacteria which produce a myriad of enzymes that assist our body with the digestion of nature's foods. So we are merely scratching the surface, yet the surface truly reveals the culprits involved.

After reviewing the research (before this last study), the GW medical professors supported this conclusion by stating:

"Supplementation with a variety of bacterial strains can help inhibit gluten/gliadin-induced damage in the small intestine."

The research clearly identifies the smoking gun for the growth of intestinal irritability and gluten insensitivity: The steady and growing destruction of healthy probiotics within our intestines through an unbridled use of antibiotics and antiseptics. This lack of probiotics exposes the intestines to large unbroken gliadin molecules the intestines are not intended to contend with. Healthy probiotic colonies would otherwise break these gliadins down into components our intestines were designed to deal with.

When we examine the evidence: The fact that gluten sensitivities have been growing as the use of antibiotics and antiseptics have become increasingly utilized together with the findings that enzymes produced by probiotics break down gluten and gliadin into non-toxic constituents, we can only arrive at the conclusion that our gut microflora has everything to do with wheat and other gluten sensitivities.

And with this conclusion, avoiding all forms of gluten in our diets can not only be an arduous and close to impossible task—but it may become unnecessary if we learn how to maintain healthy intestinal probiotics.

Grains Feed Our Probiotics

The reality is that grain foods containing gluten actually feed our probiotics and reduce the risk of dysbiosis. A number of studies have determined that gluten grains—and wheat in particular—also provide critical nourishment (prebiotics) for our intestinal probiotics. This has now been established in a number of laboratory and human clinical studies over the past couple of years.

In research led by Professor of Food Microbial Sciences at the UK's University of Reading, Dr. Glenn Gibson, 55 healthy men and women were given different doses of a wheat bran for three weeks. Those eating more wheat bran showed an increase in healthy probiotic bifidobacteria in their intestines and colons.

Another study led by Dr. Gibson tested 40 adults, and found the same conclusion: A polysaccharide named arabino-xylan-oligosaccharide—a component of wheat bran—was found to be the prebiotic. After many additional studies, it has been confirmed that arabino-xylan-oligosaccharide is critical for the health of our intestinal probiotics – and this nutrient is now considered a prebiotic.

(Bakshi *et al.* 2012; Pyle *et al.* 2005; Lindfors *et al.* 2008; Stenman *et al.* 2009; Smecuol *et al.* 2013; Maki *et al.* 2012; Walton *et al.* 2012; Grant *et al.* 2001; Farkas 2005; Ostlund 2003; Cara *et al.* 1992; Demidov *et al.* 2008).

Chapter Five

Leaky Gut Solutions

Throughout this book we have discussed a variety of issues that weaken the immune system as well as damage intestinal mucosal membranes and the intestinal barrier. Is this a coincidence?

The fact is, the intestinal barrier is *part* of the body's immune system. It is the body's most important first and/or second line of defense against invading microorganisms and toxins. This barrier also prevents larger, undigested food molecules from penetrating the body's tissues and invoking a hypersensitive response.

Now that we have thoroughly investigated the causes of the breakdown of the mucosal membrane and intestinal barrier, let's also lay out a variety of strategies to reverse increased intestinal permeability. These will range from dietary strategies to herbs, probiotics, water and exercise. While some of these may not directly heal the barrier, most will strengthen the immune system to help detoxify the body of some of the elements that weaken the mucosal membrane and brush barrier.

Stimulating the immune system and decreasing our toxin load will have a combined effect upon our intestinal health: They will stimulate healthier mucosal secretions that will better protect our intestinal cells. They will also speed up the healing process required to repair intestinal tissue damage and rebuild the tight junctions between our intestinal cells. These are the ultimate functions of the immune system: protect us from toxins and foreigners, and rebuild any damage that takes place. Let's lay out some strategies that help accomplish these objectives:

Herbal Medicine for IIPS

Here we will summarize some of the herbs that traditional doctors from different disciplines have utilized to curb intestinal irritation and intestinal disorders. Most of them work by stimulating healthy intestinal mucosal membranes, which in turn close the gaps in the intestinal walls.

This presentation of the science and traditional use of medical herbs utilizes the medical science and research of numerous researchers, scientists and physicians trained in herbal medicines. Here the traditional clinical use of herbal medicine has been derived from a number of *Materia Medica* texts from various traditions or otherwise documented clinical uses of these herbs upon large populations over thousands of years. Unless otherwise noted in the text, this information utilizes the following reference materials (see Reference section for complete citations):

Agarwal *et al.* 1999; Bensky *et al.* 1986; Chopra *et al.* 1956; Ellingwood 1983; Fecka 2009; Foster and Hobbs 2002; Frawley and Lad 1988; Gray-Davidson 2002; Griffith 2000; Gundermann and Müller 2007; Halpern and Miller 2002; Henih and Ladna 1980; Hobbs 2003; Hoffman 1990; Konrad *et al.* 2000; Lad 1984; LaValle 2001; Lininger *et al.* 1999; Mabey 1988; Mehra 1969; Melzig 2004; Miceli *et al.* 2009; Mindell and Hopkins 1998; Murray and Pizzorno 1998; Nadkarni and Nadkarni 1908/1975; Newall *et al.* 1996; Newmark and Schulick 1997; O'Connor and Bensky 1981; Potterton 1983; Schulick 1996; Schauenberg and Paris 1977; Schutz *et al.* 2006; Shi *et al.* 2008; Shishodia *et al.* 2008; Sung *et al.* 1999; Thieme 1996; Tierra 1992; Tierra 1990; Tiwari 1995; Tisserand 1979; Tonkal and Morsy 2008; Vila *et al.* 2002; Weiner 1969; Weiss 1988; Miceli *et al.* 2009; Wang and Huan 1998; Williard 1992; Williard and Jones 1990; Wood 1997.

Aloe vera

Aloe has been used traditionally for inflammation, constipation, wound healing, skin issues, ulcers and intestinal issues for at least five thousand years. Aloe's constituents include anthraquinones, barbaloins and mucopolysaccharides, which help replenish and thicken the mucosal membranes.

Bittersweet - *Solanum dulcamara*

This creeping shrub that grows along streams and bogs has been used extensively in traditional Western herbal medicine for all varieties of allergic epithelial issues and inflammatory conditions. It has been used for rheumatism and circulatory problems. The alkaloid solamine and the glucoside dulcamarin have been recognized as its active constituents, solasodine appears to be intricately involved in stimulating corticoid production, and the production of mucosal membranes.

Perhaps it is for this reason that many traditional herbalists have recommended bittersweet in cases of allergic skin conditions and mucous membrane issues. We should note that one of its constituents, solanine, can be poisonous in significant amounts. Therefore, as in all herbal products, consultation with a health professional is suggested before use.

Black Pepper - *Piper nigrum*

While *Piper nigrum* is considered Ayurvedic, it is probably one of the most common spices used in Western foods. In fact, the world probably owes its use of Black pepper in foods to Ayurveda.

Black pepper is used in a variety of Ayurvedic formulations because of its anti-inflammatory action. Ayurvedic doctors describe Black pepper as a stimulant, expectorant, carminative (expulsing gas), anti-inflammatory and analgesic. It has been used traditionally for a variety of intestinal issues, as well as rheumatism, bronchitis, coughs, asthma, sinusitis, gastritis and other histamine-related conditions. It is also thought to stimulate a healthy mucosal membrane among the stomach and intestines.

Black pepper used as a spice to increase taste is certainly not unhealthy, but it takes a significantly greater and consistent dose to produce its anti-inflammatory effects.

A traditional Ayurvedic prescription for gastroesophageal reflux or GERD, for example, is to take Black pepper in a warm glass of water on an empty stomach first thing in the morning over a period of time. This dose of Black pepper, according to Ayurveda, stimulates mucosal secretion, and purifies the mucosal membranes of the stomach and intestines.

Researchers from South Korea's Wonkwang University (Bae *et al.* 2010) found that the *Piper nigrum* extract piperine significantly inhibited inflammatory responses, including leukocytes and TNF-alpha.

Boswellia (Frankincense)

The medicinal Boswellia species include *Boswellia serratta, Boswellia thurifera,* and *Boswellia spp.* (other species). Boswellia contains a variety of active constituents, including a number of boswellic acids, diterpenes, ocimene, caryophyllene, incensole acetate, limonene and lupeolic acids.

The genus of *Boswellia* includes a group of trees known for their fragrant sap resin that grow in Africa and Asia. Frankincense was extensively used in ancient Egypt, India, Arabia and Mesopotamia thousands of years ago, as an elixir that relaxed and healed the body's aches and pains. The gum from the resin was applied as an ointment for rheumatic ailments, urinary tract disorders, and on the chest for bronchitis and general breathing problems. It is classified in Ayurveda as bitter and pungent.

Over the centuries, boswellia has been used as an internal treatment for a wide variety of ailments, including intestinal issues, ulcers, heartburn, bronchitis, asthma, arthritis, rheumatism, anemia, allergies and a variety of infections. Its properties are described as stimulant, diaphoretic, anti-rheumatic, tonic, analgesic, antiseptic, diuretic, demulcent, astringent, expectorant, and antispasmodic.

Boswellia has also shown to be beneficial for esophagitis and GERD.

In two studies, boswellic acids extracted from Boswellia were found to have significant anti-inflammatory action. The trials revealed that Boswellia inhibited the inflammation-stimulating LOX enzyme (5-lipoxygenase) and thus significantly reduced the production of inflammatory leukotrienes (Singh *et al.* 2008; Ammon 2006).

Another study (Takada *et al.* 2006) showed that boswellic acids inhibited cytokines and suppressed cell invasion through NF-kappaB inhibition.

Indian researchers found that Boswellia successfully treated ulcerative colitis in rats (Singh *et al.* 2008).

Boswellia also inhibits inflammation. In an *in vitro* study also from the University of Maryland's School of Medicine (Chevrier *et al.* 2005), boswellia extract proved to modulate the balance between Th1 and Th2 cytokines. This illustrated Boswellia's ability to strengthen the immune system and increase tolerance.

A similar-acting Ayurvedic herb is Guggul. Guggul is another gum derived from the resin of a tree—*Commiphora mukul.*

Bupleurum - *Bupleurum chinense; Bupleurum falcatum*
Bupleurum has also been called Hare's Ear, Saiko and Thorowax. Bupleurum belongs in the Umbelliferae family, and thus is related to fennel, dill, cumin, coriander and others—and exerts similar medicinal effects.

The root is typically used, and its constituents include triterpe-noid saponins called saikosides, flavonoids such as rutin, and sterols such as bupleurumol, furfurol and stigmasterol. The saikosides in Bupleurum have been known to boost liver function and reduce liver toxicity, as well as strengthen the mucosal membrane integrity.

This last effect appears to be the result of a special class of constituents called saikosaponins. Like other saponins, these have a balancing and protective effect upon the intestinal tissues.

Calendula (marigold) - *Calendula officinalis*

Marigold flowers, as beautiful as they are, provide potent anti-septic and antibacterial properties according to research and clinical application. It is also been used for ulcers and heartburn, due both to its soothing effects and antibacterial properties.

Calendula contains a variety of flavonoids, saponins, mucilage and bitter compounds. It has been used traditional herbalists for healing wounds, and ulcerative conditions. Its antimicrobial effects have been shown to inhibit Candida species as well.

Cayenne *Capiscium frutescens or Capiscium annum*

This red pepper contains the alkaloid capsacin—known to re-duce the amount of substance P in nerves, thereby reducing pain transmission. Cayenne also has the distinction of stimulating the production of mucosal membranes among the esophagus and di-gestive tract. It also stimulates the production of gastric acids at the same time—increasing digestion.

Capiscium contains capsaicinoids; various carotenoids such as zeaxanthin, beta-cryptoxanthin, and beta-carotene steroid gly-cosides, vitamins A & C and volatile oils; and at least twenty-three flavonoids including quercetin, luteolin and chysoeriol. These con-stituents work together to provide a number of anti-inflammatory benefits.

Researchers from Singapore's National University Hospital found that those who ate the most foods containing chili powder also contained the least incidence of ulcers.

Cayenne is known to increase circulation; increase detoxifica-tion; stimulate appetite; increase liver and heart function; stimulate the immune system and increase metabolic function. It is also a recognized antibacterial and antiviral agent. Some research has compared cayenne's antiseptic abilities to that of an antibiotic. Its actions have also been described as carminative, alterative, hemostatic, anthelmintic, stimulant, expectorant, antiseptic and diaphoric.

Comfrey - *Symphtum officinale*

Comfrey has been a favorite among traditional European herbalists for thousands of years. It contains mucilate (mucilage), allontoin, glycosides, saponins, triterpenoids, tannins, alkaloids and many other components.

Because of its saponin and mucilage content, comfrey is considered strengthening for mucous membranes throughout the body, including the esophagus and stomach wall. It is used as a poultice for healing skin wounds, and it is steeped into a tea infusion for digestive conditions.

Comfrey has been shown to inhibit prostaglandins and slow pain, while helping to rebuild the mucosal membranes. For this reason, Comfrey has been recommended for intestinal disorders for many centuries, and has a long history of success with no side effects.

Chamomile - *Matricaria recutita*

Chamomile has been shown to effectively relieve inflamed and irritated mucosal membranes, especially those within the esophagus, stomach and intestines. Chamomile is also anti-inflammatory and has been found to benefit digestion in general.

Chamomile contains alpha-biasabolol, matricin, apingenin, luteolin, quercetin, azulene and others.

Some of these effects seem to come from the azulene—found to relax the smooth muscles around the intestines. Azulene also relaxes the smooth muscles around the airways as well.

Chamomile has also been used to soothe anxiety with success.

Chinese Licorice and Common Licorice

Glycyrrhiza uralensis is also called Chinese Licorice. It is not the common Licorice (*Glycyrrhiza glabra*) known in Western and Ayurvedic herbalism. However, the two plants have nearly identical uses and constituents. So this discussion also serves *Glycyrrhiza glabra*.

Chinese licorice is known in Chinese medicine as giving moisture and balancing heat to mucosal membranes of the airways and digestive tract. It is also soothing to the throat and eases muscle spasms. The root is described as antispasmodic.

A Bulgarian study (Korlarski *et al.* 1987) gave deglycyrrhized licorice extract to 80 patients, and found that 75% experienced relief from GERD symptoms.

Due to adrenal effects, many natural physicians have suggested that the deglycyrrhized form of licorice extract is better suited for GERD sufferers.

Researchers from New York's Mount Sinai School of Medicine (Jayaprakasam *et al.* 2009) extensively investigated the anti-asthmatic properties of *Glycyrrhiza uralensis*. They found that *G. uralensis* had five major flavonoids: liquiritin, liquiritigenin, isoliquiritigenin, dihydroxyflavone, and isoononin. Liquiritigenin, isoliquiritigenin, and dihydroxyflavone were found to suppress airway inflammation via inhibiting eotaxin. Eotaxin stimulates the release of eosinophils to asthmatic airways during inflammation.

Licorice also contains glactomannan, triterpene saponins, glycerol, glycyrrhisoflavone, glycybenzofuran, cyclolicocoumarone, glycybenzofuran, cyclolicocoumarone, licocoumarone, glisoflavone, cycloglycyrrhisoflavone, licoflavone, apigenin, isokaempferide, glycycoumarin, isoglycycoumarin, glycyrrhizin and glycyrrhetinic acid (Li *et al.* 2010; Huang *et al.* 2010).

One of its main active constituents, isoliquiritigenin, has been shown to be a H2 histamine antagonist (Stahl 2008). Chinese Licorice has been shown to prevent the IgE binding that signals the release of histamine. This essentially disrupts the histamine inflammatory process while modulating immune system responses (Kim *et al.* 2006).

Another important constituent, glycyrrhizin, is a potent anti-inflammatory biochemical. It has also been shown to halt the breakdown of cortisol produced by the body. Let's consider this carefully. Like cortisone, cortisol inhibits the inflammatory process by interrupting interleukin cytokine transmission. If cortisol is prevented from breaking down, more remains available in the bloodstream to keep a lid on inflammation.

This combination of constituents gives Licorice aldosterone-like effects. This means that the root balances the production and maintenance of steroidal corticoids. A recent study by University of Edinburgh researchers (Al-Dujaili *et al.* 2012) found, for example, that licorice ingestion reduced cortisone levels in saliva.

Glycyrrhizin and other constituents in licorice (such as licochalcone A) have also been found to alter inflammatory cytokines such as IL-6, which in turn moderate inflammation and pain (Honda *et al.* 2012).

These effects in turn stimulate the secretion of healthy of mucosal membranes. This is confirmed by animal research that has confirmed that Licorice is anti-allergic, and decreases anaphylactic response, and balances electrolytes and inflammatory edema (Lee *et al.* 2010; Gao *et al.* 2009).

Cumin Seed - *Cuminum cyminum*

Cuminum cyminum has a long history of use among European and Asian herbalists. It is described as antispasmodic and carminative, so it tends to soothe inflammatory responses. Cumin has been used traditionally to ease abdominal cramping and gas.
Cumin seed contains mucilage, gums and resins. Traditional herbalists consider these constituents primarily responsible for Cumin's ability to help strengthen the mucosal membranes. This makes Cumin part of a strategy to rebuild the mucosal membranes of the digestive tract.

Dandelion - *Taraxum officinale, Taraxum mongolicum, Taraxum spp.*

Dandelion has hundreds of active constituents, including aesculetin, aesculin, arabinopyranosides, arnidiol, artemetin, B vitamins, benzyl glucoside, beta amyrin, beta-carboline, alkaloids, beta-sitosterol, bitter principle, boron, caffeic acid, caffeic acid ethyl, various esters, calcium, chicoric acid, chlorogenic acid, chlorophylls, choline, cichorin, coumaric acid, coumarin, deacetylmatricarin, di-glucopyranoside, dihydroconiferin, dihydrosyringin, dihydroxylbenzoic, acid, esculetin, eudesmanolides, faradiol, four steroids, furulic acid, gallic acid, gallicin, genkwanin-lutinoside, germacranolide acids, glucopyranosides, glucopyranosyl-arabinopyranoside, glucopyranosyl-glucopyranoside, glucopyranosyl-xyloypyranoside, guaianolide, hesperetin, hesperidin, indole alkaloids, inulin, ionone, iron, isodonsesquitin A, isoetin, isoetin-glucopyranosyl, lactupicrine, lu-penol acetate, lutein, luteolin, luteolin-7-O-, gluccoside, magnesium, mannans, mongolicumin A, mongolicumin B, monocaffeyltartaric, acid, monoterpenoid, myristic acid, pyridine derivative, palmitic acid, pectin, phi-taraxasteryl acetate, phosphorus, p-hydroxybenzoic acid, p-hydroxyphenylacetic, acid, polyphenoloxidase, polysaccha-rides, potassium, quercetins, rufescidride, scopoletin, sesquiterpene, sesquiterpene ketolac-, tone, sesquiterpene lactones, seventeen anti-oxidants, several caffeoylquinic , acids, several luteolins, silicon, so-dium, sonchuside A, steroid complexes, stigmasterol, syringic acid, syringin, tannins, taraxacin, taraxacoside, taraxafolide, taraxafolin-B, taraxasterol, taraxasteryl acetate, taraxerol, taraxinic acid beta-, glu-copyranosyl, taraxinic acid, derivatives, taraxol, thirteen benzenoids, trime-thyl ether, triterpenoids, violaxanthin, vit. A (7000 IU/oz), vitamin C, vitamin D, vitamin K, xyloypyranosides, and zinc.

As such, it is no surprise that dandelion has the ability to strengthen the immune system and the mucosal membranes.

It has also been used to treat stomach problems, and is thought to reduce blood pressure. In Chinese medicine, dandelion is known to clear heat, more specifically in the liver, kidney and skin. Dande-lion has been used to increase urine excretion, and reduce pain and inflammation. Yet it also contains an abundance of potassium—which balances its diuretic effect (as potassium is lost during heavy urination). It has been documented as a blood and digestive tonic, laxative, stomachic, alterative, cholagogue, diuretic, choleretic, anti-inflammatory, antioxidant, anti-carcinogenic, analgesic, anti-hyperglycemic, anti-coagulation and prebiotic.

In a 2007 study from researchers at the College of Pharmacy at the Sookmyung Women's University in Korea (Jeon *et al.* 2008), dandelion was found to reduce inflammation, leukocytes, vascular permeability, abdominal cramping, pain and COX levels among exudates and *in vivo*.

Dandelion was found to stimulate fourteen different strains of probiotic bifidobacteria—important components of the immune system that inhibit pathogenic bacteria (Trojanova *et al.* 2004).

Other studies have illustrated that dandelion inhibits both inter-leukin IL-6 and TNF-alpha—both inflammatory cytokines (Seo *et al.* 2005).

Dandelion was shown to stimulate the liver's production of glutathione (GST)—an important component of mucosal membranes (Petlevski *et al.* 2003).

Another study by University of British Columbia researchers showed that dandelion extract was capable of reducing copper radicals—showing its ability to reduce heavy metals in the body (Hu and Kitts 2003).

Dandelion increased the liver's production of superoxide dismutase and catalase, increasing the liver's ability to purify the blood of toxins (Cho *et al.* 2001).

Dandelion illustrated the ability to inhibit IL-1 and inflammation in Kim *et al.* (2000) and Takasaki *et al.* (1999).

In a study of 24 patients with chronic colitis, pains in the large intestine vanished in 96% of the patients by the 15th day after being given a blend of herbs including Dandelion (Chakŭrski *et al.* 1981).

Both the leaves and the root of Dandelion have been used to reduce heartburn among some traditional medicines.

Evening Primrose - *Oenothera spp.*

Another herb known by traditional herbalists to be beneficial for allergic or inflamed epithelial tissues. The seeds are rich in gamma-linolenic acid (GLA)—a fatty acid known to slow inflammatory responses of prostaglandins, especially those relating to epithelial hypersensitivity. The oil from Evening primrose can be taken internally in capsules or as oil. Herbalists give it credit for being helpful for epithelial permeability issues.

Fennel - *Foeniculum vulgare*

Foeniculum vulgare contains anetholes, caffeoyl quinic acids, carotenoids, vitamin C, iron, B vitamins, and rutins. Ayurvedic and traditional herbalists from many cultures have used Fennel to relieve digestive discomfort, gastritis, gas, abdominal cramping, bloating and irritable bowels; and to treat asthmatic hypersensitivities. Fennel stimulates bile production. Bile digests fats and other nutrients, increasing their bioavailability.

One of Fennel's constituents, called anethole, is known to suppress pro-inflammatory tumor necrosis factor alpha (TNF-a). This inhibition slows excessive immune response. The combination of anethole and antioxidant nutrients such as rutin and carotenoids in Fennel also strengthen immune response while increasing tolerance.

Fennel is not appropriate for pregnant moms, because it has been known to promote uterine contractions. As with any herbal supplement, Fennel should be used under the supervision of a health professional. Those with birch allergies should also be aware that they may also be sensitive to Fennel. (The same goes for Cumin, Caraway, Carrot seed and a few others).

Gentian - *Gentiana lutea*

This traditional herb is also known as bitter root, and has been referred to by traditional herbalists as a "bitter."

Typically the root is used, which contains various glycosides, including amarogentin, gentiopicrin, sweitiamarin and others, as well as alkaloids like gentianine and gentialutine, triterpenes, and several xanthones.

Root bitters have been used to increase appetite, stimulate bile secretions and stimulate mucosal secretions. It has been shown in research to be anti-inflammatory and used to stem fevers.

Ginger *Zingiber officinalis*

Ginger is one of the most powerful natural digestive aids, with thousands of years of use in Ayurveda and Chinese Medicine. In Ayurveda—the oldest medical practice still in use—ginger is the most recommended botanical medicine. As such, ginger is referred to as *vishwabhesaj*—meaning "universal medicine"—by Ayurvedic physicians. As mentioned earlier, an accumulation of studies and chemical analyses in 2000 determined that ginger has at least 477 active constituents.

As in all botanicals, each constituent will stimulate a slightly different mechanism—often moderating the mechanisms of other constituents. Many of ginger's active constituents have anti-inflammatory and/or pain-reducing effects. Research has illustrated that ginger inhibits COX and LOX enzymes in a balanced manner (Grzanna *et al.* 2005; Schulick 1996; and others). This allows for a gradual reduction of inflammation and pain without the negative GI side effects that accompany NSAIDs. Ginger also stimulates circulation, inhibits various infections, and strengthens the liver. It also stimulates the submucosal glands to produce healthy mucous membranes.

Ginger has been used as a treatment for various digestive disorders, as well as rheumatoid arthritis, respiratory ailments, fevers, nausea, colds, flu, hepatitis, liver disease, headaches and many digestive ailments to name a few. Herbalists classify ginger as analgesic, tonic, expectorant, carminative, antiemetic, stimulant, anti-inflammatory, and antimicrobial.

Whole ginger is clinically proven to reduce nausea, stomach-ache, ulcers and many other gastrointestinal problems. These effects combine with its inflammation-reduction effects.

Many remedies use ginger extract. Through extraction, many constituents are often lost. Some are sensitive to heat and light. Others are sensitive to ethanol or methanol extraction methods. Therefore, during the pulverization, dehydration and refining process used to make ginger extract, there is a great likelihood that many constituents will not remain in the extract.

In other words, it is suggested that ginger be consumed only in its raw form. Fresh ginger root can be purchased at practically any grocery or health food store. It then can be washed like any other fresh food, and then grated onto a salad or other dish. If it is put onto a cooked dish, it is recommended that it be put in after the cooking. Just grate onto the food before serving. Ginger root can also be bitten into and chewed raw, and it can also make a nice tea—not steeped too long of course.

Goldenseal - *Hydrastis canadensis*

Goldenseal is also called yellow root and Indian turmeric. Typically the root is used. Goldenseal contains a number of alkaloids, one of the most effective being berberine. It also contains hydrastine, resins and various volatile oils.

Goldenseal is well-known among North American Indians and early Americans, who used it for curing digestive cramping, fevers, infections and inflammation. It is considered to have a rejuvenative effect upon mucosal membranes and those supporting glands and tissue systems.

Berberine has been found in a number of studies to be antibiotic and anti-inflammatory. Its antibiotic effect may well be one reason for its usefulness with peptic ulcers, as it combats *H. pylori* growth.

Goldenseal is very potent, and most herbalists advise that it be used no more than five days in a row before taking a break. It can then be resumed. Berberine has also been advised not to use during pregnancy.

Herbs that have similar activity as goldenseal include **Barberry, Oregon Grape** and to some extent, **Yarrow.**

Jujube - *Ziziphus zizyphus*

The Jujube plant produces a delicious sweet date that tastes very much like a sweet apple. The fruit has many different properties in traditional medicine. It has been used to stimulate the immune system. It has been used to reduce stress, reduce inflammation, sooth indigestion, and repeal GERD.

Jujube contains a variety of constituents, including mucilage, ceanothic acid, alphitolic acid, zizyberanal acid, zizyberanalic acid, zizyberanone, epiceanothic acid, ceanothenic acid, betulinic acid, oleanolic acid, ursolic acid, zizyberenalic acid, maslinic acid, tetracosanoic acid, kaempferol, rutin, quercetin and others.

These constituents suggest the extensive support that this fruit can render for asthma sufferers with regard to rebuilding the mucosal membranes, reducing inflammation, relaxing the mind and nerves, and vitalizing damaged intestinal tissues.

Long Pepper - *Piper longum*

The related Ayurvedic herb, *Piper longum,* has similar properties and constituents as Black pepper. It is used to inhibit the inflammation and histamine activity that results in lung and sinus congestion. Like Black pepper, Long pepper is also known to strengthen digestion by stimulating the secretion of the mucosal membranes within the stomach and intestines. It is also said to stimulate enzyme activity and bile production.

One study by researchers from India's Markandeshwar University (Kumar *et al.* 2009) found that the oil of Long pepper fruit significantly reduced inflammation.

Mallow - *Malva silvestris*

Malva silvestris grows throughout Europe and has enjoyed an extensive and popular reputation among Western and Middle Eastern traditional medicines as a demulcent herb: It soothes irritated tissues. Mallow contains polysaccharides, asparagine and mucilage—which stimulates a balance and coating among the body's mucosal membranes. The leaves are typically used.

The mucilage is primarily composed by polysaccharides. These include beta-D-galactosyl, beta-D-glucose, and beta-D-galactoses.

Mallow has been clinically used for sore throats, heartburn, dry sinuses, and irritable bowels.

This herb has also been used in decoctions by European herbalists for allergic skin responses and eczema. For this reason, Swiss doctors during the World Wars would apply mallow compresses onto skin rashes with good success.

Mallow's leaves, flowers and roots are all used. It is an emollient and demulcent, rendering the ability to soften and coat, while stimulating healthy mucous among the airways.

Mallow has been documented among traditional medicines to successfully treat digestive conditions, sinusitis and asthma.

Marsh Mallow - *Althaea officinalis*

Marsh mallow—also called marshmallow—has similar properties and constituents as the *Malva verticillata* L (Mallow). It belongs in the same family, Malvaceaea, and has similar constituents.

Marsh mallow has also been reputed among traditional medicines around the world. This is because it contains mucilage, which supports and stimulates a healthy mucosal membrane.

For this reason, Marsh mallow is considered a demulcent: its leaves soothe irritated sore throats, heartburn, dry sinuses, and irritable bowels.

The leaves, flowers and roots are all used in healing. Marsh mallow is known to be emollient, which gives it properties that soften and coat practically any membrane within the body, including the sinuses, throat, stomach, intestines, urinary tract and of course, the esophagus.

The root of the Marsh mallow will contain up to 35% mucilage. It also contains a variety of long-chain polysaccharides. Extracts use cold water, so they dissolve the mucilage without the starches. For this reason, tea infusions for drinking and gargling using Marsh mallow often use cold water overnight, although it can also be steeped for 15-20 minutes using hot water.

Meadowsweet - *Spiraea ulmaria, Filipendula ulmaria, Spiraea betulifolia, Filipendula glaberrima, Filipendula vulgaris*

Also sometimes called *Queen of the Meadow,* this perennial bush grows throughout Europe and North America in damp grasslands and by streams in the forests.

Meadowsweet also contains numerous constituents, including multiple types of salicins, avicularin, coumarin, ellagitannins, volatile oils, eugenol, gallic acid, gaultherin, hydrolysable rugosin, hyperoside, meth-oxybenzaldehyde, monotropitin, mucilage, opiraein, phenolic glycodides, phenylcarboxylic acids, pireine, quercetin, rugosins, rutin, spiraein, spiraeoside, tannins and many others.

It has small, sweet-smelling white flowers that bloom in the summer. Its flowers, leaves and root extracts have been used to reduce digestive discomfort, fevers, aches, pains and inflammation for thousands of years. The Egyptians, Greeks, Romans and Northern Europeans were known to have utilized meadowsweet extracts for the treatment of rheumatism, infection of the urinary tract and abdominal discomfort. North American Indians used meadowsweet for bleeding, intestinal cramping, kidney issues, gastritis, colds and menstrual pain. Traditional herbalist Dr. Nicholas Culpeper wrote that meadowsweet "helps in the speedy recovery from cholic disorders and removes the instability and constant change in the stomach." [Cholic refers to increased bile acids.]

It is meadowsweet's soothing mucilage effects that provide much of its benefit in gastritis, esophagitis and GERD. The mucilage adds tone and thickness to our mucosal membranes, providing protection for our cells.

According to herbalist Richard Mabey, the tannin and mucilage content in meadowsweet moderate the adverse gastrointestinal side effects of isolated salicylates. For this reason, it is often used for heartburn, hyperacidity, acid reflux, gastritis and ulcers.

A purified version of salicin was isolated from meadowsweet in 1830 by Swiss Johann Pagenstecher. This led to the production of acetylsalicylic acid by the Bayer Company, now known by its common name of aspirin. The root of the word aspirin, "spirin" is derived from meadowsweet's genus name *Spiraea*.

The tannins within meadowsweet have been documented to have beneficial effects upon digestion as well. Thus, meadowsweet is often recommended for digestive disorders such as gastritis, GERD, indigestion, diarrhea and colitis. Meadowsweet is also often recommended for the removal of excess uric acid because of its diuretic and detoxifying effects. It has been used for kidney stones as well.

Herbalist David Hoffman documents its ability to reduce excess acidity in the stomach and ease nausea. Meadowsweet has been described as astringent, aromatic, antacidic, cholagogue (increasing bile flow), demulcent (soothing and providing mucilage), stomachic (tonic to digestive tract), and analgesic. The German Commission E monograph suggests the flower and herb for pain relief.

Unlike its pharmaceutical alternatives, meadowsweet flower extracts exhibit liver-protective effects against toxic hepatitis. Meadowsweet has been found to stimulate a normalization of liver enzymes, liver antioxidant effects. It also proved to normalize lipid peroxidation (cholesterol production) within the liver (Shilova *et al.* 2008).

Meadowsweet's phenolic extracts were found to have significant antioxidant and free radical scavenging potential (Sroka *et al.* 2005; Calliste *et al.* 2001).

Meadowsweet extract decreased inflammation, which included suppressing proinflammatory cytokines, decreasing IL-2 synthesis, and eliminating hypersensitivity *in vivo* (Churin *et al.* 2008).

Meadowsweet's antioxidant capacity was one of the highest levels in one test of 92 different phenolic plant extracts (Heinonen 1999).

Meadowsweet showed significant inhibition of several bacteria (Rauha *et al.* 2000). It was also shown to be antimicrobial by Radulović *et al.* (2007). This makes it applicable to *H. pylori* overgrowths.

Meadowsweet extract also exhibited the ability to reduce blood clotting. During *in vivo* and *in vitro* research (Liapina and Koval'chuk 1993), meadowsweet was determined to have anticoagulant (reducing clotting) and fibrinolytic (breaking down fibrin) properties, making it useful for speeding tissue healing.

Meadowsweet's anticoagulant and fibrinolytic properties were considered similar to heparin in another study (Kudriasho *et al.* 1990).

Contrasting with NSAIDs, meadowsweet was also found to be curative and preventative for acetylsalicylic acid-induced ulcers in rats (Barnaulov and Denisenko 1980).

Furthermore, meadowsweet has been found to inhibit the growth of *H. pylori*—the microorganism thought to cause or contribute to the majority of gastritis cases as well as GERD conditions (Cwikla *et al.* 2009).

Mullein - *Verbascum theapsiforme*

The leaves, flowers and herbs of *Verbascum theapsiforme* and *V. philomoides olanum* have been part of the traditional herbalist repertory for thousands of years. It is classified as a demulcent and expectorant, because it is known to soothe irritations among the airways and esophagus, and help clear thickened mucous.

Mullein's soothing and demulcent properties are due primarily to its mucilage content, which can be as high as 3%. Other constituents include saponins, which are believed to produce the expectorant properties of this herb.

Mullein has thus been used for centuries for hypersensitivity among the mucosal membranes, including coughing and bronchialspasm, skin irritations and throat infections. In all these cases, its effects have been considered soothing to epithelial cells.

Mucilage Seeds

A number of seeds are helpful for calming and settling the airways, including seeds such as Flax, Safflower, Rapeseed, Caraway, Anise, Fennel, Licorice seed, Black seed and others. Seeds contain basic compounds that offer mucilage, saponins and other polysaccharides that contribute to the health of the mucous membranes.

Not surprisingly, combinations or single versions of these seeds have been used in traditional medicine for centuries.

Pharmacology researchers from Cairo's Helwan University (Haggag *et al.* 2003) treated allergic asthmatic patients with an herbal blend containing of Anise, Fennel, Caraway, Licorice, Black seed and Chamomile—all known for their mucosal-rebuilding effects. They found that the extract significantly decreased cough frequency and intensity. It also increased lung function, with higher FEV1/FVC percentages among the asthmatic patients, as compared to those who consumed a placebo tea.

Panex Ginseng

Panex ginseng is a traditional remedy for allergies and hypersensitivity with thousands of years of use. Panax ginseng will come in white forms and red forms. The color depends upon the aging or drying technique used.

The Ginseng in the FAHF formula is termed *Radix* Ginseng or Ren shen but it is *Panex ginseng*. Depending upon how the Ginseng is cured, there are several types of Ren shen.

When Ginseng is cultivated and steamed, it is called 'red root' or Hong Shen. Ginseng root will turn red when it is oxidized or processed with steaming. Some feel that red root is better than white, but this really depends upon its intended use, the age of the root, and how it was processed. Soaking Ginseng in rock candy produces a white Ginseng that is called Bai shen. This soaking seems odd, but this has been known to increase some of its constituent levels such as superoxide and nitric oxide. When the root is simply dried, it is called 'dry root' or Sheng shaii shen. Korean Red Ginseng is soaked in a special herbal broth and then dried.

There are a number of species within the *Panax* genus, most of which also contain most of the same adaptogens, referred to as gensenosides. Most notable in the *Panex* genus is American Ginseng, *Panax quinquefolius*.

Ginseng contains camphor, mucilage, panaxosides, resins, saponins, gensenosides, arabinose and polysaccharides, among others.

Eleutherococcus senticosus, often called Siberian Ginseng, is actually not Ginseng. While it also contains adaptogens (eleutherosides), these are not the gensenoside adaptogens within Ginseng that have been observed for their ability to relieve hypersensitivity.

Researchers from Italy's Ambientale Medical Institute (Caruso *et al.* 2008) tested an herbal extract formula consisting of *Capparis spinosa, Olea europaea, Panax ginseng* and *Ribes nigrum* (Pantescal) on allergic patients. They found that allergic biomarkers, including basophil degranulation CD63 and sulphidoleukotriene (SLT) levels were significantly lower after 10 days. They theorized that these biomarkers explain the herbal formulation's *"protective effects."*

Ginseng's protective and adaptogenic effects also serve to stimulate intestinal mucosa vitality, as well as speed healing of damaged intestinal tissues.

Reishi - *Ganoderma lucidum*

This a popular medicinal mushroom. Reishi has been shown in numerous studies to significantly moderate inflammation, stimulate the mucosal membranes and aid digestion.

Reishi contains many constituents, including steroids, triterpenes, lipids, alkaloids, glucosides, coumarin glycoside, choline, betaine, tetracosanoic acid, stearic acid, palmitic acid, nonadecanoic acid, behenic acid, tetracosane, hentriacontane, ergosterol, sitosterol, ganoderenic acids, ganolucidic acids, lucidenic acids, lucidone and many more.

Ling Zhi strengthens immunity and modulates the body's tolerance and responses to allergens. Reishi has been shown to increase production of IL-1, IL-2 and natural killer cell activity. A number of studies have shown that Reishi can significantly lower IgE levels specific to allergens, and reduce inflammatory histamine levels. It has also been shown to improve lung function and has been used traditionally for bronchitis and asthma.

Recently, researchers from Japan's University of Toyama (Andoh *et al.* 2010) found that Reishi also relieves skin itching and rash *in vivo.*

Slippery Elm - *Ulmus fulva*

Slippery elm has long been used to soothe irritated throats and irritated digestive tracts. This is due to its high mucilage and mucopolysaccharide content, along with tannins, starches and others. It is considered a demulcent, and used by Northern American Indians and European herbalists for ulcers, heartburn and general stomach upset. The inner bark is typically used and has the highest mucilage content, as it adds lubrication to the mucosal membranes, giving credence to its namesake, "slippery." It is also mildly astringent, which helps stimulate digestion.

Triphala

Triphala means *"three fruits."* Triphala is a combination of three botanicals: *Terminalia chebula, Terminalia bellirica* and *Emblica officinalis.* They are also termed Haritaki, Bibhitaki and Amalaki, respectively. This combination has been utilized for thousands of years to rejuvenate the intestines, regulate digestion and balance the mucosal membranes of within the digestive tract.

The 'three fruits' also are said to produce a balance among the three doshas of *vata, pitta* and *kapha.* Each herb, in fact, relates to a particular *dosha:* Haritaki relates to *vata,* Amalaki relates to *pitta* and Bibhitaki relates to *kapha.* The three taken together comprise the most-prescribed herbal formulation given by Ayurvedic doctors for digestive issues.

This use has been justified by preliminary research. For example, in a study by pharmacology researchers from India's Gujarat University (Nariya *et al.* 2003), triphala was found to significantly reverse intestinal damage and intestinal permeability *in vivo.*

The traditional texts and the clinical use of triphala today in Ayurveda have confirmed these types of intestinal effects in humans.

We might want to elaborate a little further on Haritaki in particular. *Terminalia chebula* has been used by Ayurvedic practitioners specifically for conditions related to asthma, coughs, hoarseness, abdominal issues, skin eruptions, itchiness, and inflammation. It is also called He-Zi in traditional Chinese medicine.

Research has found that Haritaki contains a large number of polyphenols, including ellagic acids, which have significant antioxidant and anti-inflammatory properties (Pfundstein *et al.* 2010).

Turmeric - *Curcuma longa*

Turmeric can also either be considered a medicinal herb or a food-spice. It is a root (or rhizome) and a relative of ginger in the *Zingiberaceae* family. Just as we might expect from a botanical, turmeric has a large number of active constituents. The most well known of these are the curcuminoids. These include curcumin (diferuloylmethane), demethoxycurcumin and bisdemethoxycurcumin. Others include volatile oils such as tumerone, atlantone, and zingiberone, polysaccharides, proteins, and a number of resins.

These work together to stimulate the immune system along with mucosal secretions. For these reasons, turmeric is known for its anti-inflammation effects.

As stated in a recent review from the Cytokine Research Laboratory at the University of Texas (Anand 2008), studies have linked turmeric with "suppression of inflammation; angiogenesis; tumor genesis; diabetes; diseases of the cardiovascular, pulmonary, and neurological systems, of skin, and of liver; loss of bone and muscle; depression; chronic fatigue; and neuropathic pain."

Indeed, turmeric has been used for centuries for gastritis, heartburn, inflammation, gallbladder problems, diabetes, wound-healing, liver issues, hepatitis, menstrual pain, anemia, and gout. It is considered alterative, antibacterial, carminative and stimulant.

In a study on 45 patients with peptic ulcers (Prucksunand 2001), ulcers were completely resolved and absent in 76% of the group taking turmeric powder in capsules.

Other studies have also shown similar positive gastrointestinal effects of turmeric. We can conclude that not only is turmeric a known anti-inflammatory, but its *positive* gastrointestinal side effects greatly contrast the negative GI side effects of NSAIDs.

Turmeric can certainly be taken in a capsule as the above studies mention. However, because turmeric is readily available as a delicious spice, there is every reason to conclude that adding it (along with ginger) to our daily meal-plans in its raw or powdered form. This said, some herbalists, such as James LaValle, R.Ph, N.M.D., suggest that for best results turmeric should also be taken as a supplement.

Willow Bark - *Salix alba, Salix spp.*

The willow tree can grow to 75 feet tall, but many species are smaller trees and even shrubs. It has rough bark with narrow, glandular, pointed leaves and small yellow flowers. It grows along streams and fields—and often in neighborhood yards. There are some 450 species of the genus *Salix,* and most contain similar constituents. Willow species grow practically all over the world.

Willow contains numerous medicinal constituents, including various types of salicins, catechins, procyanidins, flavones, various tannins, helicon, isoquercitrin, isosalipurposide, leonuriside, luteolins, naringenin, naringin, picein, piceoside, populin, and salidroside, sisymbrifolin, tremulacin and many others.

Along with decreasing pain, Willow has been used to soothe irritated throats and digestive tracts for thousands of years by traditional herbalists from around the world. This comes from willow's mucilage effects.

Others Herbs to Consider

In addition to these herbs, several others have also been used in traditional medicine to help heartburn:

> Anise (*Pimpinella anisum*): Some similarities with licorice, stimulates mucosal integrity.
> Barberry (*Berberis vulgaris*): A bitter, with significant berberine content, which repels *H. pylori*.
> Borage (*Borago officinalis*): Relative of Chamomile, stimulates mucosal membrane integrity.
> Cinnamon (*Cinnamomum zeylanicum*): Inhibits *H. pylori* and Candida.
> Horehound (*Marrubium vulgare*): Stimulates gastric secretions and saliva secretions.
> Lavender (*Lavandula augustifolia*): Relaxes nerves and reduces stress. Also inhibits *H. pylori*.
> Lemon Balm (*Melissa officinalis*): Sedative and soothing to the digestive tract.
> Oregon Grape (*Berberis aquifolium*): Contains berberine, which inhibits *H. pylori*. Also has bitter principle, which stimulates digestion.
> Yellow Dock (*Rumex crispus*): Bitter principle stimulates secretion of gastric acids and enzymes, speeding stomach emptying.

Herbal Techniques

We've discussed a long list of herbs that can provide numerous bene-fits and healing properties that reduce the risk of intestinal permeability, increase mucosal strength and stimulate a healthy immune system. For this reason, a seasoned expert in herbal formulations can offer specific suggestions relating to ones constitution and precise level of intestinal issues.

That said, one of the strategies that many traditional physicians have utilized is to select those herbs that target the symptoms of the patient. While this might be compared to "treating the symptoms," as some pharmaceutical strategies are accused of, herbal medicines work on a much deeper level as we've discussed. While an herb's primary constituents might be productive with particular symptoms, the rest of the herb's constituents will likely also modulate the immune system's tolerance. This is its adaptogenic ability. These are the effects we have also seen among the research on herbal medicines. This *"from the outside in"* strategy produces a deeper correction of the systemic immunity issues often at the root of the problem.

We also see in many of these herbs, their ability to stimulate a healthy mucosal membrane and strengthen the intestinal barrier. These illustrate a strategy of treating from both directions: *outside-in* and *inside-out*.

Therefore, in the case of a food allergy where the primary reaction is respiratory—coughing, lung congestion, and so on—the traditional herbalist might select those anti-allergic herbs listed above that are known for their respiratory responses. Likewise, a person with allergic skin reactions would be given those herbs known to help atopic skin responses. Concurrently, the herbalist would select those herbs discussed above that modulate and strengthen the intestinal barrier and intestinal mucosal membranes to reduce the exposure of the allergen on the intestinal tissues and bloodstream.

Dosages and Methods

We have not detailed precise dosages in this section because there are many considerations when determining dosages. These include age, physical health, constitution, unique weaknesses, diet, lifestyle and other factors. Herbs should also be carefully matched, and some herbs and formulations have been known to interact with certain medications.

Therefore, it is suggested that herbs are chosen, formulated and dosed by an experienced herbalist. If there are any medications being used, the prescribing physician should be consulted.

This said, most of the herbs mentioned above, with the exception of essential oils, are safest when used as *infusions*. An infusion is simply the steeping of the fresh or dried root, bark, leaf, seed, stem or fruit in water.

In the case of most herb leaves and stems, the water is brought to a boil, and the herb can be steeped for 5-10 minutes using a strainer or tea-ball.

In the case of most roots, seeds and barks, the root can be steeped a little longer, for 10-20 minutes, depending on the herb. In some cases a seed, root or bark is better when it is soaked overnight in room temperature water.

Another strategy is to simply ingest a capsule or pressed tablet of a powdered version of the herb or herbal formulation. Liquid extracts are also available from many reputable herbal suppliers. In these cases, the literature accompanying these products should be closely examined for dosages and possible interactions. Be wary that extracts may not have the same effects as the raw or infused herb.

A number of the formulations (or their derivatives) mentioned in this section are available as encapsulated, pressed tablets or liquid extracts, together with dosage suggestions. Before using this strategy, care should be taken to assure that the herbal formulation has been ultimately designed by a reputable herbalist. Most of the popular commercial brands of herbal formulations employ professional herbalists to design their formulations. Many will also name the herbalist on the marketing material or label of the product. These should be considered more trustworthy formulations.

By far the best approach is to have an herbalist formulate and recommend herbs specific to ones constitution, symptom severity, medication and lifestyle. In the alternative, a commercial formula (such as ones discussed in this chapter) blended or overseen by a reputable herbalist, together with instructions on the packaging, can be used.

Remember, if taking pharmaceutical medications, the prescribing physician should be consulted to avoid possible interactions. Also, very small doses, gradually building up to the suggested dose, are usually recommended in the beginning to test tolerances.

Proteolytic Enzymes

As we discussed earlier, enzymes are critical components for breaking down macromolecule proteins that can slip through permeable intestines. For some of us, our body's production of enzymes and bile acids do not complete the job of cleaving proteins—breaking them into amino acids or smaller peptides the body can easily manage.

Proteolytic enzymes are produced by many plants, probiotics, and our own gastric, liver and bile system. For those with compromised digestive systems, these enzymes may not be as available as they should. In these cases, the supplementation of natural enzymes can be extremely productive while our intestinal wall is healing.

For example, chemical engineering researchers from Stanford University (Ehren *et al.* 2009) evaluated the breakdown of gluten-related proteins using two enzymes produced by probiotic microorganisms. Aspergillopepsin (ASP) produced from *Aspergillus niger* and dipeptidyl peptidase IV (DPP-IV) produced from the probiotic *Aspergillus oryzae* were tested. The two enzymes were tested on gluten-type peptides in a simulation of conditions that would resemble the digestion of whole gluten and whole-wheat bread. They found that ASP and DPP-IV collectively and effectively cleaved (broke down) the gluten-type proteins in the study.

A leading enzyme-producing company, Specialty Enzyme Biotechnology, Ltd., has led the way in the natural production of enzymes that break down gluten-foods, casein-foods and other food proteins in the digestive tract. This is a fifty year old company that produces its enzymes from natural plant sources or probiotic microorganism sources. The company and their branded subsidiary, *AST Enzymes*, now distribute a supplement geared towards gluten and casein sensitivities. According to company information and standardized independent laboratory assays, here is a list of the enzymes and their function within the body (the author has no affiliation with this company or its products):

Enzyme	Function
Dipeptidyl Peptidase IV SEB-Pro GR™	Blend of five proteases that help digest proteins. DPP-IV focuses on proline component of gliadin (glutens) and casein proteins.
Amylase I, II &	Breaks down carbohydrates and starches into dextrins and

Glucoamylase	sugars
Cellulase	Digests cellulose, a complex polysaccharide found in all plant material.
Hemicellulase and Xylanase (HemiSEB® cellulose)	Break down carbohydrates and plant polysaccharides such as hemicellulose, a major component of plant cell walls.
Alpha-Galactosidase	Breaks down complex carbohydrates such as raffinose and stachyose
Lactase	Breaks down lactose into simple sugars
Lipase	Helps break-down fats into essential fatty acids

This combination provides a ready supply of enzymes that can assist a food-sensitive person in breaking down those macromolecule proteins they may be sensitive to. As we saw in the hydrolyzed protein feeding research among infants, when large sensitized proteins were broken down, most of the children were able to consume the hydrolyzed formula. In the same way, supplemented enzymes can break down proteins the body may be sensitive to, such as gluten-related proteins, soy, milk and others.

As mentioned some plant-based foods supply enzymes that are considered proteolytic. These include bromelain, papain and nattokinase. These have also been shown to have anti-inflammatory properties.

Papain is derived directly from papayas. It is a rich source of proteolytic enzymes. The nattokinase enzyme is produced by *Bacillus natto*, the bacterium used to ferment soy Bromelain is another botanical enzyme with proteolytic and anti-inflammatory properties. Bromelain is derived from pineapple.

Probiotics also produce a significant number of our body's digestive enzymes. This is one reason why probiotics are so helpful for digestive issues, as we've discussed.

Mucosal Minerals

A number of minerals are critical to the health of our mucosal membranes and thus our intestinal health. As we discussed earlier, our mucosal membranes are ionic. They attach to and escort nutrients through the intestinal wall, and they also alkalize the membranes. They thus help shield foreigners from intestinal cell contact. There are a multitude of minerals to consider, some of the most important being potassium, calcium and magnesium.

Magnesium deficiency has been found to be at the root of a number of conditions, including intestinal irritability. This is because magnesium is a critical element used by the mucosal membranes and immune system. A body deficient in magnesium will likely be immunosuppressed. Animal studies have illustrated that magnesium deficiency leads to increased IgE counts, and increased levels of inflammation-specific cytokines. Magnesium deficiency is also associated with increased degranulation among mast/basophil/ neutrophil cells, which stimulates the allergic response.

Clinical studies have confirmed that magnesium salts appear to improve allergic skin reactions, illustrating its mucosal effects (Błach et al. 2007).

Other research has reported that dietary sulfur can significantly relieve allergy symptoms. In a multi-center open label study by researchers from Washington state (Barrager et al. 2002), 55 patients with allergic rhinitis were given 2,600 mg of methylsulfonylmethane (MSM—a significant source of sulfur derived from plants—for 30 days. Weekly reviews of the patients reported significant improvements in allergic respiratory symptoms, along with increased energy and digestive improvement. Other research has suggested that sulfur blocks the reception of histamine among histamine receptors.

Good sources of sulfur include avocado, asparagus, barley, beans, broccoli, cabbage, carob, carrots, Brussels sprouts, chives, coconuts, corn, garlic, leafy green vegetables, leeks, lentils, onions, parsley, peas, radishes, red peppers, soybeans, shallots, Swiss chard and watercress.

The other macro- and trace-minerals should not be ignored, however. For example, research has shown that zinc modulates T-cell activities (Hönscheid et al. 2009).

Numerous holistic doctors now prescribe full-spectrum mineral combinations for food sensitivities. Many have attested to the ability of these minerals to balance the inflammatory response and stimulate healthy mucosal membranes.

Good sources of the full spectrum of trace and macro minerals include mineral water, whole rock salt, spirulina and vegetables.

Diet Strategies for IIPS

Foods that our digestive tract, probiotics and immune system can easily manage with the least amount of toxic byproducts will help us rebuild our intestinal barrier and digestive immune systems.

On the other hand, those foods or drinks that are either over-processed, denatured, mixed with synthetic toxins or otherwise not intended for our body will damage our probiotic systems, damage our mucosal membranes, damage the brush barrier of our intestines—creating increased intestinal permeability—and stimulate the exaggerated immune response characteristic of food sensitivities.

So what should we be eating then?

As we summarize this information, the reader should remember that significant dietary changes done too quickly or otherwise incorrectly can have negative health consequences and even dangerous effects on a person with food sensitivities. Also note that some may be sensitive to some of the foods discussed here. Therefore, it is suggested that new foods and dietary changes be made gradually, and under the supervision of a health professional knowledgeable in diet.

Increasing Plant-Based Foods

As we covered in detail earlier, animal-heavy fatty diets discourage the colonization of our probiotics, and encourage the growth of pathogenic microorganisms that can damage our intestines and brush barrier. Fatty animal-heavy diets also produce byproducts such as phytanic acid and beta-glucuronidase that can damage our intestinal cells and mucosal membranes within the intestines.

Furthermore, the research clearly shows that people eating a significant amount of fruits and vegetables have a reduced risk of colon cancer, intestinal polyps and other intestinal issues. This is because plant-based foods discourage inflammatory responses. They support healthy mucosal membranes. Plant foods are also wholesome and nutritious, stimulating immunity. They feed our probiotics with complex polysaccharides called prebiotics. They are also a source of fiber (there is no fiber in animal foods)—critical for intestinal health.

Plant-based foods contain many antioxidants, anti-carcinogens and other nutrients that strengthen the immune system.

Diet research has revealed that diets with less animal fat produces less cancer (especially colon cancer), heart disease and other inflammatory conditions. And plant-based protein is a more digestible source of protein than animal-based proteins. This is because animal-based proteins are more complex and difficult to break down into amino acids. The body utilizes aminos and small peptides, not complex proteins. Plants provide aminos and smaller peptides in more digestible form.

As we've discussed, the complexities of digesting animal proteins produce increased levels of beta-glucuronidase, nitroreductase, azoreductase, steroid 7-alpha-dehydroxylase, ammonia, urease, cholylglycine hydrolase, phytanic acid and others. These enzymes and toxins deter our probiotics and produce intestinal inflammation.

While these effects are not typically noticeable by most of us, they become noticeable as researchers compare the intestinal health of various diets, as we discussed previously. Some of these studies also used crossover design, which means they had each group trade the other group's diet to see if the changes were consistent among both groups.

Certainly this is not to say everyone can immediately accept a completely meatless diet or a strict Mediterranean diet. This is to say that a diet that contains more plant-based foods than is currently the norm among Western industrialized countries will likely assist intestinal health in general.

Whole Foods and Antioxidants

Some of the botanical constituents known to be significantly antioxidant, immunity-strengthening and blood-purifying include *lecithin* and *octacosanol* from whole grains; *polyphenols* and *sterols* from vegetables; *lycopene* and other phytochemicals from tomatoes; *quercetin* and *sulfur/allicin* from garlic, onions and peppers; *pectin* and *rutin* from apples and other fruits; *phytocyanidins* and antioxidant *fla-*

vonoids such as *apigenin* and *luteolin* from various greenfoods; and *anthocyanins* from various fruits and even oats.

Some sea-based botanicals like kelp also contain antioxidants as well. Consider a special polysaccharide compound from kelp called *fucoidan*. Fucoidan has been shown in animal studies to significantly reduce inflammation (Cardoso *et al.* 2009; Kuznetsova *et al.* 2004).

Procyanidins are found in apples, currants, cinnamon, bilberry and many other foods. The extract of *vitis vinifera* seed (grapeseed) is one of the highest sources of bound antioxidant proanthrocyanidins and leucocyanidines called *procyanidolic oligomers*, or "PCOs." Pycnogenol also contains significant levels of PCOs.

Research has demonstrated that PCOs have protective and strengthening effects on tissues by increasing enzyme conjugation (Seo *et al.* 2001). PCOs also increase vascular wall strength (Robert *et al.* 2000).

Oxygenated carotenoids such as *lutein* and *astaxanthin* also have been shown to exhibit strong antioxidant activity. Astaxanthin is derived from the microalga *Haematococcus pluvialis,* and lutein is available from a number of foods, including spirulina.

Nearly every plant-food has some measure of some of these botanical constituents. They alkalize the blood and increase the detoxification capabilities of the liver. They help clear the blood of toxins. Foods that are particularly detoxifying and immunity-building include fresh pineapples, beets, cucumbers, apricots, apples, almonds, zucchini, artichokes, avocados, bananas, beans, leafy greens, berries, casaba, celery, coconuts, cranberries, watercress, dandelion greens, grapes, raw honey, corn, kale, citrus fruits, watermelon, lettuce, mangoes, mushrooms, oats, broccoli, okra, onions, papayas, parsley, peas, radishes, raisins, spinach, tomatoes, walnuts, and many others.

For example, the flavonoids *kaempferol* and *flavone* have been shown to block mast cell proliferation by over 80% (Alexandrakis *et al.* 2003). Sources of kaempferol include Brussels sprouts, broccoli, grapefruit and apples.

Diets with significant fiber levels also help clear the blood and tissues of toxins to support the immune system. Fiber in the diet should range from about 35 to 45 grams per day according to the recommendations of many diet experts. Six to ten servings of raw fruits and vegetables per day should accomplish this—which is even part of the USDA's recommendations. This means raw, fibrous foods can be at every meal.

Good fibrous plant sources also contain healthy *lignans* and *phytoestrogens* that help balance hormone levels, and help the body make its own natural corticoids. Foods that contain these include peas, garbanzo beans, soybeans, kidney beans and lentils.

Garlic, cayenne and onions can be added to any cooked dishes to add inflammation-inhibiting *quercetin* and other antioxidants. Cooked beans or grains can be spiced with turmeric, ginger, basil, rosemary and other anti-inflammatory spices such as cayenne.

Over the past few years, research has discovered that red, purple and blue fruits have tremendous antioxidant and anti-inflammatory benefits. Continued studies have concluded that oxidative species— free radicals—are at the root of much of the damage that burdens the immune system and triggers allergic inflammatory responses. Oxidative species come from poor diets and chemical toxins— exacerbated by stress.

The greatest and most efficient way to neutralize these oxidative radicals comes from fresh botanical foods. The method scientists and food technologists have used to measure the ability of a particular food has to neutralize free radicals is the *Oxygen Radical Absorbance Capacity Test* (ORAC). This technical laboratory study is performed by a number of scientific bodies, including the USDA and specialized labs such as Brunswick Laboratories in Massachusetts.

Research from the USDA's Jean Mayer Human Nutrition Research Center on Aging at Tufts University has suggested that a diet high in ORAC value may protect blood vessels and tissues from damage that can result in inflammation (Sofic *et al.* 2001; Cao *et al.* 1998). These tissues, of course, include the intestines.

This research and others have implicated that damage from free radicals also contributes to many disease mechanisms, which burden the immune system and result in hypersensitivity. Although antioxidants cannot be considered treatments for any disease, many studies have suggested that increased antioxidant intake supports immune function and detoxification, allowing the body to better respond with greater tolerance. Many researchers have agreed that consuming 3,000 to 5,000 ORAC units per day can have protective benefits.

ORAC Values of Selected (Raw) Fruits (USDA, 2007-2008)

Cranberry	9,382		Pomegranate	2,860
Plum	7,581		Orange	1,819
Blueberry	6,552		Tangerine	1,620
Blackberry	5,347		Grape (red)	1,260
Raspberry	4,882		Mango	1,002
Apple (Granny)	3,898		Kiwi	882
Strawberry	3,577		Banana	879
Cherry (sweet)	3,365		Tomato (plum)	389
Gooseberry	3,277		Pineapple	385
Pear	2,941		Watermelon	142

There is tremendous attention these days on two unique fruits from the Amazon rain forest and China called *acai* and *goji berry* (or wolfberry) respectively. A recent ORAC test documented by Schauss *et al.* (2006) gives acai a score of 102,700 and a test documented by Gross *et al.* (2006) gives goji berries a total ORAC of 30,300. However, subsequent tests done by Brunswick Laboratories, Inc. gives these two berries 53,600 (acai) and 22,000 (gogi) total-ORAC values.

In addition, we must remember that these are the dried berries being tested in the later case, and a concentrate of acai being tested in the former case. The numbers in the chart above are for fresh fruits. Dried fruits will naturally have higher ORAC values, because the water is evaporated—giving more density and more antioxidants per 100 grams. For example, in the USDA database, dried apples have a 6,681 total-ORAC value, while fresh apples range from 2,210 to 3,898 in total-ORAC value. This equates to a two-to-three times increase from fresh to dried. In another example, fresh red grapes have a 1,260 total-ORAC value, while raisins have a 3,037 total-ORAC value. This comes close to an increase of three times the ORAC value following dehydration.

One of the newest additions to the new high-ORAC superfruits is the maqui superberry. This is small purplish fruit grown in Chile. It is about the size of an elderberry (another good antioxidant fruit).

Part of the equation, naturally, is cost. Dried fruit and concentrates are often more expensive than fresh fruit. High-ORAC dried fruits or concentrates from açaí, gogi or maqui will also be substantially more expensive than most fruits grown domestically (especially for Americans and Europeans). Our conclusion is that local or in-country grown fresh fruits with high total-ORAC values produce the best value. Local fresh fruit offers great free radical scavenging ability, support for local farmers, and pollen proteins we are most likely more tolerant to.

By comparison, spinach—an incredibly wholesome vegetable with a tremendous amount of nutrition—has a fraction of the ORAC content of some of these fruits, at 1,515 total ORAC. It should be noted, however, that some (dehydrated) spices have incredibly high ORAC values. For example, USDA's database lists ground turmeric's total ORAC value at 159,277 and oregano's at 200,129. However, while we might only consume a few hundred milligrams of a spice per day, we can eat many grams—if not pounds—of fruit per day.

The Humble Apple

At some point, the apple rightfully gained that famous adage of "an apple a day keeps the doctor away." While often said in jest now, there is a considerable amount of truth and history to this expression. The fact is, the apple is one of the healthiest foods we could choose to eat. Apples were used for many decades by traditional country doctors for a variety of different complaints. It is reputed that apples were once part of treatments for skin eruptions, gout, biliousness, nervous disorders, diarrhea, constipation, and jaundice.

Fiber is critical to the health of our intestines, and apples have the perfect type and blend of fiber. We need between 30 and 45 grams of it per day for healthy digestion and elimination. Apples contain one of the highest levels of fiber, with a pound (two large apples or three medium apples with skin) delivering up to 10 grams. The apple also contains an almost perfect combination of both soluble fiber and insoluble fiber. We need both kinds.

The apple's soluble fiber comes in the form of pectin. Pectin is important for a number of reasons. Pectin helps reduce cholesterol because it absorbs and binds with bile and low density fatty acids in the intestine and colon, escorting these out through the colon prior to their entry into the blood stream.

The insoluble fiber in apples helps keep the intestines and colon clean, providing a natural scrubber to the intestinal wall, and along the spaces between the villi—those tiny digestive fingers of the intestine. The fiber in apples keeps the colon running smoother: helping to prevent colon polyps and irritable bowels. Apples have also been known to help regulate bowel movements.

Apples are a rich source of a number of vitamins. A pound of apples (1-2 medium-to-large apples) has up to 360 IU of vitamin A, 15-20 mg of vitamin C, and 24 grams of calcium. Apples also contain decent amounts of vitamin B6, vitamin K, B2 and B6, along with smaller amounts of B1, B3 and B5. Apples are also a great source of potassium and manganese, with respectable amounts of iron, magnesium, copper and manganese. Organic apples may contain more. Several studies have confirmed that organic fruits contain more nutrients than their conventionally-grown counterparts. All of these stimulate intestinal health.

Surprisingly apples contain a number of amino acids, the building blocks for protein. Apples contain a notable amount of leucine, lysine, valine, alanine, aspartic acid, glutamic acid, glycine, proline, and serine, along with smaller amounts of tryptophan, threonine, isoleucine, methionine, cystine, phenylalanine, tyrosine, arginine and histidine. That makes up 18 of a total of 20 possible amino acids, and all nine of the "essential" amino acids. Who would have thought of the apple as a good source of protein?

Apples contain several key antioxidants, which are known to reduce the effects of aging, promote healing, decrease inflammation, boost the immune system and help detoxify cells, blood and organs. Outside of its active antioxidants vitamin C and A, apples contain flavones such as quercetin that have a much more powerful effect in the body. Apples also contain lutein and zeaxanthin, both powerful antioxidants. These healthy range of antioxidants in apples have been attributed to helping reduce inflammatory issues such as arthritis and allergies, while helping to prevent infection and cancer cell growth.

Since many nutrients are disbursed under heat, cooking apples should be done in stainless steel or glassware at low heat. Apple juice should be approached with discrimination as well. Those with blood sugar issues might want to avoid apple juice on an empty stomach. The fructose and glucose content of apple juice is highly absorbable—not unlike white sugar. This is especially a concern with filtered apple juice, which has most or all of the pulp removed by filtration and heating. The heating and filtration process can also rob the juice of many nutrients. Fresh pressed whole apple juice with all the pulp is the best guarantee for preserving the nutrient content of the apple in juice. Second best would be unfiltered and pasteurized. Apple juice made from concentrate has probably the least desirable. The heat needed to evaporate the water reduces much of its nutrient content not to speak of its pulp and fibers.

Best eaten 'in the nude' and unpeeled, the apple is quite simply an incredible source of vitamins, minerals, protein, antioxidants and fiber. An apple a day is, well, as healthy as they say.

Whole Oats and Barley

Oats and barley are also particularly high in soluble fiber, consisting primarily of mixed linkage beta glucans - (1,3)(1,4)-beta-d-glucans. Beta-glucans are unique polysaccharides that have been the focus of much research in recent years. The American Diabetes Association recommends 40 grams of soluble fiber per day to prevent adult-onset diabetes.

Oats and barley also contain considerable amounts of protein. Oats' protein levels are also notable, at 17% - a very high quality protein with a balance of amino acids. And, they are totally free of gluten.

Oats and barley also have a number of important vitamins and minerals. They are also a good source of folate (22% adult DV in a serving for oats), pantothenic acid (21% DV), thiamin (79% DV), calcium (8% DV), iron (41% DV), magnesium (69% DV), potassium (19% DV), zinc (41% DV), copper (49% DV) and manganese (383% DV), along with other nutrients and trace elements.

Oats and barley are also good sources for healthy fats. A serving of oats contains 173 milligrams of omega-3 alpha-linolenic acids, and 3781 mg of omega-6 fatty acids. The fat content of oats -

higher than most other grains - is also balanced between monoun-saturated and polyunsaturated fats. Oats also contain a unique com-bination of glycolipids, diacylglycerols and estolides, and a number of single-, double-, triple- and tetra-bonded diacylglycerols. These unique fatty acids distinguish oats from other grains.

Oats and barley have low glycemic indexes. In oatmeal form, oats have a particularly low glycemic index of 58. Researchers have found that oats provide a 50% reduction in glycemic load or peak, because of the high viscosity of its fiber. The American Diabetes Association recommends 40 grams of soluble fiber per day to pre-vent adult-onset diabetes. Researchers have found that oats provide a 50% reduction in glycemic load or peak.

Oats reduce cholesterol. In 2007, the UK's University of Tees-side's School of Health and Social Care released a Cochrane review study comparing ten different trials reporting on oats' ability to reduce cholesterol. The study's results concluded that oats lowered total cholesterol and low density lipoproteins an average of 7.7 mg/dL and 7 mg/dL respectively. The mechanism seems to be the beta-glucans' ability to inhibit bile acid absorption.

Oats and barley reduce the risk of artery disease. Oats and bar-ley contain unique alkaloid polyphenols called avenanthramides. Recent research indicates that avenanthramides reduce incidence and complications of atherosclerosis - the scarring and inflamma-tion of the artery walls. Avenanthramides have also shown signifi-cant antioxidant capacity.

The best way to eat oats is to cook them lightly. Use either whole rolled or whole groats (also called Irish oats). Whole rolled will require very little cooking. Bring the water to a boil, put in a pinch of whole salt and then the oats at 50/50 water. Cook for less than five minutes, turn off the heat, and add your raisins, cinnamon, raw honey, strawberries, raspberries and other toppings.

Don't Squeeze the Lemons (and other Citrus)

Lemons have been recognized as healing, anti-microbial food fruits for thousands of years. They were cultivated well over 2,500 years ago, and used extensively to preserve foods and purify the blood in sickness. Traditional healers have used lemons for the treatment of arteriosclerosis, bleeding gums, ulcers, arthritis, gingivitis, warts, ringworm, skin irritations, varicose veins and other issues. Lemon also stimulates appetite and increases metabolism.

Lemon is highly acidic, but it is known for its alkalinity effects once within the body. This is because its acids, oils and antioxidants neutralize free radicals produced by toxins and lipid peroxides. Lemon also appears to stimulate elimination of toxins at a faster rate.

A lemon will contain about 5% vitamin C, more than oranges and grapefruits. This natural form of ascorbic acid, together with bioflavonoids, provides a superior form of vitamin C.

Lemons also contain calcium, phosphorus, vitamin A, protein and iron. In fact, a pound of lemons can contain as much as 274 milligrams of calcium and 3.3 grams of protein.

Lemons also contain the oils limonene, beta-pinene, citral, alpha-terpinene and alpha-pinene. These oils are known to stimulate the immune system and help clear toxins. Lemon oil is also highly antibacterial, and it has been shown to inhibit pneumococcus and meningococcus bacteria.

For this reason, it is important not to extract the juice from the lemon and leave behind other nutrients that are embedded into the fiber and inside peel portions.

Most people do just that. They extract the acidic juice, leaving behind those alkaline portions that balance its acidity. Those alkaline fibers and calcium are important in terms of the benefit that lemons bring.

For this reason, squeezing out the lemon juice and throwing away the peel and fiber is not advised. The best way to eat a lemon is to peel the outer rind off, leaving a good portion of the inner rind—where most of the oil resides—and then putting the entire fruit into a blender. And don't worry about the lemon seeds. Some of them will be chopped up, and a few partial whole seeds might have to be spit out or swallowed (better if swallowed). The end result will be delicious and nutritious.

A whole lemon minus the rind, together with other fruits and some kefir is simply delicious. The tartness usually reserved for lemons is surprisingly absent, simply because of the wholeness of the lemon addition.

This nutritional point applies to all citrus fruits. Oranges, mandarins, grapefruit and other citrus fruits all contain limonene in the peels, along with other healthy components. One category, polymethoxylated flavones have been found to provide healthy effects.

A new study has found that a polymethoxylated flavonoid called nobiletin reduces very low density cholesterol (LDL or VLDL) levels. The researchers, from the Robarts Research Institute of London and Ontario (Mulvihill et al. 2011), found that the secretion of LDL and VLDL by human liver cells was significantly inhibited by nobiletin.

They also found that the polymethoxylated flavonoid, with a chemical structure of 3'4'5,6,7,8-hexamethoxyflavone, reduced VLDL levels found in insulin resistance and atherosclerosis.

Remember that LDL and VLDL are implicated in cardiovascular disease, because they promote lipid peroxidation, which damages the arteries and many other tissue systems.

Agricultural Research Service (ARS) scientists (Manthey and Bendele 2008) who found that 3'4'3,5,6,7,8-heptamethoxyflavone (HMF), another citrus polymethoxylated flavone found in citrus peels, inhibited a precursory protein called apoprotein B found within low-density lipoprotein (LDL).

Citrus peels contain several polymethoxylated flavonoids (PMFs). Nobiletin is a O-methylated flavone. It renders a hydroxyl group that mediates a reaction called O-methylation. Methylation allows for the donation of methyl groups, which provide radical-neutralizing effects, as well as the inhibition of lipid peroxide-friendly LDL cholesterol apoprotein B. Other O-methylated flavones include tangeritin (first found in tangerine oil), wogonin (found in the herb baikal scullcap), and sinensetin, found in the Java tea herb *Orthosiphon stamineus*.

What this all means is that citrus peels are healthy for the intestines. Because they attach to radicals and LDL cholesterol, they reduce the damage these can have upon the intestinal walls. They also contain polysaccharides that provide nourishment for our probiotics.

About Juicing

Juicing has been advocated for many years by a number of health experts and nutritionists. Many have promoted juicing for detoxification and cleansing. And juicing can have its place. It is just not recommended for intestinal health.

Juicing is a suboptimal way to glean the benefits of fruits and vegetables. This is because many antioxidant nutrients are contained within the soluble and insoluble fibers in fruits and vegetables. Juicing strips out these beneficial nutrients along with their all-important fibers. Thus we lose their benefit to our intestines and the mucosal membranes of our digestive tract.

The moral here is that nature provides fiber with antioxidants for a combined effect. While antioxidants do attach and bind to toxins and neutralize radicals such as lipid peroxides, fiber attaches to LDL cholesterol in the intestines, which prevents them from becoming lipid peroxides in the first place. Fibers also attach to numerous other radicals and toxins within the intestines, flushing them out through the colon. *This prevents their entry into the bloodstream.*

While juicing is somewhat practical for hard fiber vegetables like carrots, the best strategy for most other fruits and vegetables is to make smoothies. This is basically putting the whole fruit or vegetable into a blender (after peeling in the case of oranges and the like, although orange peels are also a great cleansing nutrient), mixing with some water, a greenfood powder, and perhaps some kefir or yogurt, and then blending them up into a fruit/vegetable smoothie. For thinner consistency, simply add more water, and for thicker consistency, less water.

While juice can also be added to our smoothies, juices are not recommended in the living cleanse diet. This is because juices have been separated from their fibers, and this makes the juice not wholesome. Furthermore, many commercial juices are pasteurized or flash-pasteurized, rendering many of the enzymes and antioxidants useless, and often denatured. Furthermore, the sugars in pasteurized juices can turn to more simplified versions, rendering them unstable and acidic upon consumption and subject to becoming radicals within the body. They will also irritate the intestinal walls.

Quercetin

A number of studies have shown that quercetin inhibits the release of the inflammatory mediator histamine (Kimata *et al.* 2000). Foods rich in quercetin include onions, garlic, apples, capers, grapes, leafy greens, tomatoes and broccoli. In addition, many of the herbs listed earlier contain quercetin as an active constituent.

In other words, quercetin stimulates and balances the immune system and immune response. In a recent study, quercetin was given to Wistar rats after they were sensitized to peanuts. After a week, the rats were given either the quercetin or a placebo for four weeks. After the treatment period, the rats' histamine levels and allergen-specific IgE levels fell. More importantly, the quercetin completely inhibited anaphylaxis among the treated rats, while the untreated rats experienced no change (Shishehbor *et al.* 2010).

Over the past few years an increasing amount of evidence is pointing to the conclusion that foods with quercetin slow inflammatory response and autoimmune derangement. Researchers from Italy's Catholic University (Crescente *et al.* 2009) found that quercetin inhibited arachidonic acid-induced platelet aggregation. Arachidonic acid-induced platelet aggregation is seen in allergic inflammatory mechanisms.

Researchers from the University of Crete (Alexandrakis *et al.* 2003) found that quercetin can inhibit mast cell proliferation by up to 80%.

Organic foods contain higher levels of quercetin. A study from the University of California-Davis' Department of Food Science and Technology (Mitchell *et al.* 2007) tested flavonoid levels between organic and conventional tomatoes over a ten-year period. Their research concluded that quercetin levels were 79% higher for tomatoes grown organically under the same conditions as conventionally-grown tomatoes.

Fatty Acid Strategies

The types of fats we eat relate directly to IIPS and intestinal health because some fats are pro-inflammatory while others are anti-inflammatory. One reason that some fats are pro-inflammatory is that they oxidize more easily, producing unstable lipoperoxides. These can damage our cell membranes and the tight junctions between our intestinal cells. This doesn't mean that the pro-inflammatory fats are necessarily bad. Rather, we must have a *balance* of fats between the pro- and anti-inflammatory ones, with the balance teetering on the anti-inflammatory side.

The fat balance of our diet is also important because our cell membranes are made of different lipids and lipid-derivatives like phospholipids and glycolipids. An imbalanced fat diet therefore can lead to weak cell membranes, which leads to cells less protected and more prone to damage by oxidative radicals—and increased intestinal permeability.

Illustrating this, Danish researchers (Willemsen *et al.* 2008) tested the intestinal permeability/barrier integrity of incubated human intestinal epithelial cells with different dietary fats. The different fats included individual omega-6 oils linolenic acid (LA), gamma linolenic acid (GLA), DGLA, arachidonic acid (AA); a blend of omega-3 oils alpha-linolenic acid (ALA), eicosapentaenoic acid (EPA), docohexaenoic acid (DHA); and a blend of fats similar to the composition of human breast milk fat. The DGLA, AA, EPA, DHA and GLA oils reduced interleukin-4 mediated intestinal permeability. LA and ALA did not. The blend with omega-3 oils, *"effectively supported barrier function,"* according to the researchers. They also concluded that DGLA, AA, EPA and DHA—all long chain poly-unsaturated fats—were *"particularly effective in supporting barrier integrity by improving resistance and reducing IL-4 mediated permeability."*

Arachidonic acids in moderation are important for nutrition, and we all need them, especially in early feeding as infants. They are important factors in the inflammatory process—but in the right quantity. For this reason, our bodies convert linoleic acid to arachidonic as needed.

As we showed with the research earlier, a meat-heavy diet can over-supply arachidonic acid. Because arachidonic acid stimulates the production of pro-inflammatory prostaglandins and leucotrienes in the enzyme conversion process, too much leads to a tendency for our bodies to over-respond during an inflammatory event. Worse, a system overloaded with arachidonic acid makes halting the inflammatory process more difficult.

Interestingly, carnivorous animals cannot or do not readily convert linoleic acid (found in many common plants) to arachidonic acid, but herbivore animals do convert linoleic acid to arachidonic acid, as do humans. This conversion—on top of an animal-protein heavy diet—produces high arachidonic acid levels. On the other hand, a diet that is balanced between plant-based monounsaturates, polyunsaturates and some saturates will balance arachidonic acids with the other fatty acids.

Here is a quick review of the major fatty acids and the foods they come from:

Major Omega-3 Fatty Acids (EFAs)

Acronym	Fatty Acid Name	Major Dietary Sources
ALA	Alpha-linolenic acid	Walnuts, soybeans, flax, canola, pumpkin seeds, chia seeds
SDA	Stearidonic acid	hemp, spirulina, blackcurrant
DHA	Docosahexaenoic acid	Body converts from ALA; also obtained from certain algae, krill and fish oils
EPA	Eicosapentaenoic acid	Converts in the body from DHA

Major Omega-6 Fatty Acids (EFAs)

Acronym	Fatty Acid Name	Major Dietary Sources
LA	Linoleic acid	Many plants, safflower, sunflower, sesame, soy, almond especially
AA	Arachidonic acid	Meats, salmon
PA	Palmitoleic acid	Macadamia, palm kernel, coconut
GLA	Gamma-linolenic acid	Borage, primrose oil, spirulina

Major Omega-9 Fatty Acids

Acronym	Fatty Acid Name	Major Dietary Sources
EA	Eucic acid	Canola, mustard seed, wallflower
OA	Oleic acid	Sunflower, olive, safflower
PA	Palmitoleic acid	Macadamia, palm kernel, coconut

Major Saturated Fatty Acids

Acronym	Fatty Acid Name	Major Dietary Sources
Lauric	Lauric acid	Coconut, dairy, nuts
Myristic	Myristic acid	Coconut, butter
Palmitic	Palmitic acid	Macadamia, palm kernel, coconut, butter, beef, eggs
Stearic	Stearic acid	Macadamia, palm kernel, coconut, eggs

Essential fatty acids

EFA's are fats necessary for adequate health. Eaten in the right proportion, they can also lower inflammation and speed healing. EFA's are long-chain polyunsaturated fatty acids—longer than the linolenic, linoleic and oleic acids. The major EFAs are omega-3s—primarily alpha linolenic acid (ALA), docosahexaenoic acid (DHA) and eicosapentaenoic acid (EPA). EPA and DHA are found in algae, mackerel, salmon, herring, sardines, sablefish (black cod); and omega-6s—primarily linoleic acid, (LA), gamma-linoleic acid (GLA), palmitoleic acid (PA) and arachidonic acid (AA). The term *essential* was originally given with the assumption that these types of fats could not be assembled or produced by the body—they must be taken directly from our food supply.

This assumption, however, is not fully correct. While it is true that we need *some* of these from our diet, our bodies readily convert linoleic acid to arachidonic acid, and ALA to DHA and EPA. Therefore, these fats can be considered essential in some sense, but we do not necessarily have to consume each one of them.

Monounsaturated Fats

Monounsaturated oils are high in omega-9 fatty acids like oleic acid. A monounsaturated fatty acid has one double carbon-hydrogen bonding chain. Oils from seeds, nuts and other plant-based sources have the largest quantities of monounsaturates. Oils that have large proportions of monounsaturates such as olive oil are known to lower inflammation when replacing high saturated fat in diets. Monounsaturates also aid in skin cell health and reduce atopic skin responses.

Monounsaturated fatty acids like oleic acid have been shown in studies to lower heart attack risk, aid blood vessel health, and offer anti-carcinogenic potential. The best sources of omega-9s are olives, sesame seeds, avocados, almonds, peanuts, pecans, pistachio nuts, cashews, hazelnuts, macadamia nuts, several other nuts and their respective oils.

Polyunsaturated Fats

Polyunsaturated fats have at least two double carbon-hydrogen bonds. They come from a variety of plant and marine sources. Omega-3s ALA, DHA and EPA simply have longer chains with more double carbon-hydrogen bonds than the polyunsaturate Omega-6s. ALA, DHA and EPA are known to lower inflammation and increase artery-wall health. These *long-chain* omega-3 polyunsaturates are also considered critical for intestinal health.

The omega-6 fatty acids are the most available form of fat in the plant kingdom. Linoleic acid is the primary omega-6 fatty acid and it is found in most grains and seeds.

servin

Saturated Fats

Saturated fats have multiple fatty acids without double bonds (the hydrogens "saturate" the carbons). They are found among animal fats, and tropical oils such as coconut and palm. Milk products such as butter and whole milk contain saturated fats, along with a special type of healthy linoleic fatty acid called CLA or *conjugated linoleic acid.*

The saturated fats from coconuts and palm differ from animal saturates in that they have shorter chains. This actually gives them—unlike animal saturates—an antimicrobial quality.

Trans Fats

Trans fats are oils that either have been overheated or have undergone hydrogenation. Hydrogenation is produced by heating while bubbling hydrogen ions through the oil. This adds hydrogen and repositions some of the bonds. The "trans" refers to the positioning of part of the molecule in reverse—as opposed to "cis" positioning. The cis positioning is the bonding orientation the body's cell membranes work best with. Trans fats have been known to be a cause for increased radical species in the system; damaging artery walls; contributing to inflammation, heart disease, high LDL levels, liver damage, diabetes, and other metabolic dysfunction (Mozaffarian *et al.* 2009). Trans fat overconsumption slows the conversion of LA to GLA.

It should be noted that CLA is also a trans-fat, but this is a trans fat the body works well with—it is considered a healthy fat.

Arachidonic Acid

The science and research on arachidonic acid was discussed earlier. AA is an essential fatty acid, and research has shown that it is essential for infants while they are building their intestinal barriers. However, as we discussed, AA is pro-inflammatory, and too much of it as we age increases the burden on our immune systems, and tends to push our bodies towards hypersensitivity.

As we discussed in the last chapter, AA content is highest among animal meats, fish, fried foods and heavily-processed foods. Plant-based foods contain little or no AA.

The Anti-inflammatory Omega-3s

Research has illustrated that DHA obtained from fish oils and DHA from algae have significant therapeutic and anti-inflammatory effects. The research is so well-known that we hardly need to quote it here.

ALA is the primary omega-3 fatty acid the body can most easily assimilate. Once assimilated, the healthy body will convert ALA to omega-3s, primarily DHA, at a rate of about 7-15%, depending upon the health of the liver. One study of six women performed at England's University of Southampton (Burdge *et al.* 2002) showed a conversion rate of 36% from ALA to DHA and other omega-3s. A follow-up study of men at Southampton showed ALA conversion to the omega-3s occurred at an average of 16%.

DHA readily converts to EPA by the body. EPA degrades quickly if unused in the body. It is easily converted from DHA as needed. Our bodies store DHA and not EPA.

It appears that the anti-inflammatory effects of DHA in particular relates to a modulation of a gene factor called NF-kappaB. The NF-kappaB is involved in signaling among cytokine receptors. With more DHA consumption, the transcription of the NF-kappaB gene sequence is reduced. This seems to reduce inflammatory signaling (Singer *et al.* 2008).

Because much of the early research on the link between fatty acids and inflammatory disease was performed using fish oil, it was assumed that both EPA and DHA fatty acids reduced inflammation. Recent research from the University of Texas' Department of Medicine/Division of Clinical Immunology and Rheumatology (Rahman *et al.* 2008) has clarified it is DHA that is primarily implicated in reducing inflammation. DHA was shown to inhibit RANKL-induced pro-inflammatory cytokines, and a number of inflammation steps, while EPA did not.

The process of converting ALA to DHA and other omega-3s requires an enzyme produced in the liver called delta-6 desaturase. Some people—especially those who have a poor diet, are immune-suppressed, or burdened with toxicity such as cigarette smoke—may not produce this enzyme very well. As a result, they may not convert as much ALA to DHA and EPA.

For those with low levels of DHA—or for those with problems converting ALA and DHA—DHA microalgae can be supplemented. These algae produce significant amounts of DHA. They are the foundation for the DHA molecule all the way up the food chain, including fish. This is how fish get their DHA, in other words. Three algae species—*Crypthecodinium cohnii, Nitzschia laevis* and *Schizochytrium spp.*—are now in commercial production and available in oil and capsule form.

Microalgae-derived DHA is preferable to fish or fish oils. Fish and fish oils typically contain saturated fats and may also—depending upon their origin—contain toxins such as mercury and PCBs (though to their credit, many producers also carefully distill their fish oil). However, we should note that salmon contain a considerable amount of arachidonic acid as well (Chilton 2006). And finally, algae-derived DHA does not strain fish populations.

One study (Arterburn *et al.* 2007) measured pro-inflammatory arachidonic acid levels within the body before and after supplementation with algal DHA. It was found that arachidonic acid levels decreased by 20% following just one dose of 100 milligrams of algal DHA.

In a study by researchers from The Netherlands' Wageningen University Toxicology Research Center (van Beelen *et al.* 2007), all three species of commercially produced algal oil showed equivalency with fish oil in their inhibition of cancer cell growth. Another study (Lloyd-Still *et al.* 2007) of twenty cystic fibrosis patients concluded that 50 milligrams of algal DHA was readily absorbed, maintained DHA bioavailability immediately, and increased circulating DHA levels by four to five times.

In a randomized open-label study (Arterburn *et al.* 2008), researchers gave 32 healthy men and women either algal DHA oil or cooked salmon for two weeks. After the two weeks, plasma levels of circulating DHA were bioequivalent.

We should include that ALA, the plant-based omega-3 oil, also produces anti-inflammatory activity. In studies at Wake Forest University (Chilton *et al.* 2008), for example, flaxseed oil produced anti-inflammatory effects, along with borage oil and echium oil (both also containing GLA).

Gamma Linoleic Acid

As mentioned earlier, a wealth of studies have confirmed that GLA reduces or inhibits the inflammatory response. Leukotrienes produced by arachidonic acid stimulate inflammation, while leukotrienes produced by GLA block the conversion of polyunsaturated fatty acids to arachidonic acid. This means that GLA reduces the inflammatory response.

A healthy body will convert linoleic acid into GLA readily, utilizing the same delta-6 desaturase enzyme used for ALA to DHA conversion.

From GLA, the body produces *dihomo-gamma linoleic acid,* which cycles through the body as an eicosinoid. GLA aids in skin health, and down-regulates the inflammatory and hypersensitivity allergic response.

In addition to conversion from LA, GLA can be also obtained from the oils of borage seeds, evening primrose seed, hemp seed, and from spirulina. Excellent food sources of LA include chia seeds, seed, hempseed, grapeseed, pumpkin seeds, sunflower seeds, safflower seeds, soybeans, olives, pine nuts, pistachio nuts, peanuts, almonds, cashews, chestnuts, and their respective oils.

The conversion of LA to GLA (and ALA to DHA) is reduced by trans-fat consumption, smoking, pollution, stress, infections, and various chemicals that affect the liver.

The Healthy Fat Balance

In a meta-study by researchers from the University of Crete's School of Medicine (Margioris 2009), numerous studies showed that long-chain polyunsaturated omega-3s tend to be anti-inflammatory while omega-6 oils tend to be pro-inflammatory.

This, however, simplifies the equation too much. Most of the research on fats has also shown that most omega-6s are healthy oils, and GLA is also an omega-6. Balance is the key. Let's look at the research:

In a study by researchers from the University of Guelph in Ontario (Tulk and Robinson 2009), eight middle-aged men with metabolic disorder were tested for the inflammatory effects resulting from changing their fat content proportion between omega-3 and omega-6. The men were divided into two groups, one eating a high saturated fat diet with a proportion of 20:1 between omega-6 and omega-3, and the other eating a diet of 2:1 (high omega-3 diet). Both groups were tested before and after the diet change. Testing after the diet change showed that the high omega-3 diet did not change the inflammatory marker tests.

The proportion between omega-6s and omega-3s is thus recommended to be about one or two to one (1-2:1). The current Western American diet has been estimated to be about twenty to thirty to one (20-30:1) for the proportion between omega-6 and omega-3. This imbalance (of too much omega-6 and too little omega-3) has been associated with a number of inflammatory diseases, including arthritis, heart disease, ulcerative colitis, Crohn's disease, and others. When fat consumption is out of balance, the body's metabolism will trend towards inflammation. This is because omega-6 oils convert more easily to arachidonic acid than do omega-3s. AA seems to push the body toward the processes of inflammation (Simopoulos 1999).

We also know that reducing dietary saturated fats and increasing omega-6 polyunsaturated fats reduces inflammation, cardiovascular disease, high cholesterol and diabetes (Ros and Mataix 2008).

The relationships were cleared up in a study performed at Sydney's Heart Research Institute (Nicholls et al. 2008). Here fourteen adults consumed meals either rich in saturated fats or omega-6 polyunsaturated fats. They were tested following each meal for various inflammation and cholesterol markers. The results showed that the high saturated fat meal increased inflammatory activities and decreased the liver's production of HDL cholesterol; whereas HDL levels and the liver's anti-inflammatory capacity were increased after the omega-6 meals.

What this tells us is that the omega-3/omega-6 story is complicated by the saturated fat content of the diet and subsequent liver function. High saturated fat diets increase (bad) LDL content and reduce the anti-inflammatory and antioxidant capacities of the liver. Diets lower in saturated fat and higher in omega-6 and omega-3 fats encourage antioxidant and anti-inflammatory activity.

We also know that diets high in monounsaturated fats—such as the Mediterranean Diet—are also associated with significant anti-inflammatory effects. Mediterranean diets contain higher levels of monounsaturated fats like oleic acids (omega-9) as well as higher proportions of fruits and vegetables, and lower proportions of saturated fats (Basu *et al.* 2006).

High saturated fat diets are also associated with increased obesity, and a number of studies have shown that obesity is directly related to inflammatory diseases—including allergies as we've discussed. High saturated fat diets and diets high in trans fatty acids have also been clearly shown to accompany higher levels of inflammation and inflammatory factors such as IL-6 and CRP (Basu *et al.* 2006).

Noting the research showing the relationships between the different fatty acids and inflammation, and the condition of the liver (which can be burdened by too much saturated fat), scientists have logically arrived at a model for dietary fat consumption for a person who is either dealing with or wants to prevent inflammation-oriented diseases such as food sensitivities:

Omega-3	25%-30% of dietary fats
Omega-6+Omega-9	40%-50% of dietary fats
Saturated	5%-10% of dietary fats
GLA	10%-20% of dietary fats
Trans-Fats	0% of dietary fats

Fermented Foods

Probiotics will change the structure of foods as they ferment the food. In many cases they produce enzymes that digest and break down macromolecular versions of the sugars and proteins that we might be sensitive to. They will present to the digestive tract a different, often more digestible form of the nutrient along with numerous enzymes that aid in further digestion and assimilation.

Fermented foods also deliver to the digestive tract colonies of probiotics that can colonize and continue to help break down those food macromolecules that can cause IIPS. While fermented foods may only present temporary residents, they will typically endure for a couple of weeks, and during that time provide numerous benefits.

During that two weeks, we can eat another meal of the fermented food to help replenish those colonies.

Illustrating this, researchers from the Department of Food Science and Human Nutrition at the University of Illinois (Frias *et al.* 2008) studied the sensitivity response (or, as the researchers termed it, *"immunoreactivity"*) of soybeans in the cracked bean form and in the flour state before and after fermentation with probiotics. They fermented some of the cracked beans and flour with *Aspergillus oryzae, Rhizopus oryzae, Lactobacillus plantarum,* and *Bacillus subtilis.* These are fermenting bacteria are commonly used to make various probiotic cultured foods such as tempeh and sauerkraut.

The researchers used ELISA tests and the Western blot test to quantify IgE immunoglobulin response with human plasma. They found that all of the fermentation processes dramatically decreased the immunoreactivity of the soybeans and flours. Soy flour fermented with *L. plantarum* exhibited the highest reduction, with a 96-99% lower immunoreactivity levels. *R. oryzae* and *A. oryzae* reduced immunoreactivity by 66% and 68% respectively. *B. subtilis* produced from 81% to 86% reduction in immunoreactivity to the soy.

In addition, a positive side effect of the fermentation was the improvement of the protein quality of the soy products. After fermentation with *R. oryzae,* for example, levels of the amino acids alanine and threonine were increased, making the soy products more nutritious!

The bottom line is that this research illustrates what healthy colonies of probiotics can do within the intestinal tract. Probiotics process foods. During their processing, probiotics reduce the ability of undigested proteins to irritate the intestinal walls - including casein and gluten proteins, known to produce sensitivities to wheat and dairy.

Here is a sampling of some of the world's favorite probiotic foods:

Traditional Yogurt

Traditional yogurt is produced using *L. bulgaricus* and *S. thermophilus.* Commercial preparations sometimes include L. acidophilus, but the use of *L. acidophilus* in yogurt will rarely result in the final product containing *L. acidophilus.* This is because *L. bulgaricus* is a hardy organism, and it will easily overtake *L. acidophilus* within a culture. Note also that in commercial yogurt preparations that are pasteurized after culturing, there are few or no living probiotics remaining after pasteurization. Some manufacturers culture the milk after pasteurization. This will result in a healthy probiotic culture.

Traditional Kefir

Kefir is a traditional drink originally developed in the Caucasus region of what is now considered Southern Russia, Georgia, Armenia and Azerbaijan. Kefir uses fermented milk mixed with kefir grains that resemble little chunks of cauliflower. Kefir typically contains *L. bulgaricus* and *S. thermophilus*. Cow's milk is most used, but sheep's milk, goat's milk or deer milk can also be used.

Traditional Buttermilk

Buttermilk is a soured beverage that was originally curdled from cream. Traditional buttermilk utilizes the acids that probiotic bacteria produce for curdling. Today, forced curdling is done using commercially available acidic products such as lemon juice or vinegar. This however, does not result in the probiotic cultures of traditional buttermilk, unless of course, raw probiotic milk is utilized as a base.

This also goes for butter and cottage cheese. Both were probiotic foods until modern dairies decided that there was no value in the probiotics that naturally occur from grass-fed cows.

Traditional Kimchi

Kimchi is a fermented cabbage with a wonderful history from Korea. Kimchi was considered a ceremonial food served to emperors and ambassadors. It was also highly regarded as a healing and tonic food. There are a variety of different recipes of kimchi, depending upon the region and occasion. *Lactobacillus kimchii* is the typical probiotic colonizer, but others have also been used.

Traditional Miso

Miso is an ancient fermented food from Japan. A well-made miso will contain over 160 strains of aerobic probiotic bacteria. This is because the ingredients are perfect prebiotics for these probiotics. Miso is produced by fermenting beans and grains. Soybeans are often used, but other types of beans are also used. *Aspergillus oryzae* or koji is typically used as a fermenting base. When other beans other than soy are used, they will produce different varieties of miso. Shiromiso is white miso, kuromiso is black miso, and akamiso is red miso. They are each made with different beans. There are also various other miso recipies, many of which are highly guarded by their makers.

Traditional Shoyu

Shoyu is a traditional form of soy sauce made by blending a mixture of cooked soybeans and wheat, again with koji, or *Aspergillus oryzae*. The combination is fermented for an extended time. The aging process for shoyu is dependent upon the storage temperature and cooking methods used, and is also regarded as a secret by many producers.

Traditional Tempeh

Tempeh is an aged and fermented soybean food. It is extremely healthy and contains a combination of probiotics and naturally metabolized soy. Tempeh is made by first soaking dehulled soybeans for 10-12 hours. The beans are then cooked for 20 minutes and strained. The dry, cooked beans are then mixed with a tempeh starter containing *Rhyzopus oryzae*, *Rhizopus oligosporus* or both. The flattened and aged cake will be full with white mycelium (fungal roots) when it is ready. This tasty food can then be eaten raw, baked, or toasted.

Traditional Kombucha Tea

Traditional kombucha tea is an ancient beverage from the orient. Its use dates back many centuries: It was used by China and Taiwanese emperors, as well as Russian, and Eastern Europe peoples, where its reputation grew.

Recent research has revealed that kombucha was originally derived from kefir grains developed for fermentation. The kefir was exported to China, where the grains were added to tea with sugar rather than milk. The result was a combination of probiotic bacteria and yeasts that can include (depending upon the evolution of the mother culture) *Acetobacter xylinum*, *Acetobacter xylinoides*, *Glucobacter bluconicum, Acetobacter aceti, Saccharomycodes Ludwigii, Schizosaccharomyces pombe,* and *Picha fermentans*—and possibly some other species.

The fermenting of these organisms renders a beverage that is full of nutrients and enzymes as well as healthy probiotics. While the probiotic count may not be as high as yogurt or kefir, the range of probiotics will be wider.

Traditional Lassi

Lassi is a traditional beverage once enjoyed by kings and governors in ancient India. Lassi is still very popular in India. It is quite simple to make, as it is made with yogurt, fruit and spices. Quite simply, it is a blend of diluted yogurt with fruit pulp—often mango is used in the traditional lassi. A little salt, turmeric and sweetener give it a sweet-n-salty taste. Other spices are also sometimes used. Sugar is often added in today's versions, but honey and/or fruit would be preferable, health-wise.

Traditional Sauerkraut

Sauerkraut is a traditional German fermented food. It is made quite simply, by blending shredded cabbage and pickling salt with *Lactobacillus plantarum* and *L. brevis* fermentation cultures.

More information on probiotic foods, supplements and the science of probiotics may be found in the author's book: *Probiotics—Protection Against Infection.*

Raw vs. Pasteurized Milk

Remember the study by researchers at Switzerland's University of Basel (Waser *et al.* 2007). The researchers studied 14,893 children between the ages of five and 13 from five different European countries, including 2,823 children from farms and 4,606 children attending a Steiner School (known for its farm-based living and instruction). The researchers found that drinking farm milk was associated with decreased incidence of allergies and asthma. In other words, the raw milk was found to be the largest single determinant of this reduced allergy and asthma incidence among farm children. Why?

Raw milk from the cow contains a host of bacteria. In a healthy, mostly grass-fed cow, these bacteria are primarily probiotics. This is because a grass diet provides prebiotics that promote the cow's own probiotic colonies. Should the cow be fed primarily dried grass and dried grains, probiotic counts will be reduced, and replaced by pathogenic bacteria. As a result, most non-grass fed herds must be given lots of antibiotics to help keep their bacteria counts low. Probiotics, on the other hand, naturally keep bacteria counts down.

As a result, the non-grass fed cow's milk will have higher pathogenic bacteria counts than grass-fed cows. This means that the milk itself will also have high counts. When the non-grass-fed cow's milk is pasteurized, the heat kills most of these bacteria. The result is a milk containing dead pathogenic bacteria parts. These are primarily proteins and peptides, which get mixed with the milk and are eventually consumed with the milk.

In other words, pasteurization may kill the living pathogenic bacteria, but it does not get rid of the bacteria proteins. This might be compared to cooking an insect: If an insect landed in our soup we could surely cook it until it died. But the soup would still contain the insect parts.

Now the immune system of most people, and especially infants with their hypersensitive immune system, is trained to attack and discard pathogenic bacteria. And how does the body identify pathogenic bacteria? From their proteins.

In the case of pasteurized commercial milk, the immune system can still identify heat-killed microorganism body parts and proteins and launch an immune response against these proteins. This was shown in research from the University of Minnesota two decades ago (Takahashi *et al.* 1992).

It is not surprising that weak immune systems readily reject pasteurized cow's milk. In comparison, raw milk has far fewer microorganism content in general, most of which are probiotic in content. This was confirmed by tests done by a local California organic milk farm, who tested their raw milk against standardized tests from conventional milk farms.

In addition, pasteurization breaks apart or denatures many of the proteins and sugar molecules. This was illustrated by researchers from Japan's Nagasaki International University (Nodake *et al.* 2010), who found that when beta-lactoglobulin was conjugated with dextran-glycylglycine, its allergenicity decreased. This occurred by shielding epitope reception on cell membranes. A dextran is a very long chain of glucose molecules—a polysaccharide. In this case, the polysaccharide is joined with the amino acid, glycine.

This is not surprising. Natural whole cow's milk contains special polysaccharides called oligosaccharides. They are largely indigestible polysaccharides that feed our intestinal bacteria. Because of this trait, these indigestible sugars are called prebiotics.

Whole milk contains a number of these oligosaccharides, including oligogalactose, oligolactose, galacto-oligosaccharides (GOS) and transgalactooligosaccharides (TOS). These polysaccharides provide a number of benefits. Not only are they some of the more preferred food for probiotics: they also reduce the ability of pathogenic bacteria like *E. coli* to adhere to intestinal cells.

These oligosaccharides also provide bonds that reduce the incidence of beta-lactoglobulin, through the combination of being food for probiotics and the availability of the buffering effect of long-chain polysaccharides on radical molecules.

This reduction of beta-lactoglobulin has been directly observed in humans and animals after supplementation with probiotics (Taylor *et al.* 2006; Adel-Patient *et al.* 2005; Prioult *et al.* 2003).

Galacto-oligosaccharides are produced by conversion from enzymes in healthy cows and mothers.

The Benefits of Raw Whole Milk

While some children are sensitized to milk, milk should not be ignored as a healthy food for infants in most cases. Cow's milk contains many of the nutrients found in mother's milk. These include a host of vitamins, proteins, nucleotides, minerals, probiotics, immunoglobulins and healthy fatty acids. Raw milk also helps support the intestinal barrier.

Researchers from the University of Malawi College of Medicine (Brewster *et al.* 1997)—in Southeastern Africa—tested intestinal permeability and disease progression among 533 kwashiorkori-ridden children. Kwashiorkori is a protein assimilation disease often seen among children in poor countries, and is typically accompanied by increased intestinal permeability.

The researchers compared a local mix of maize-soya-egg to the standard milk diet given in kwashiorkor treatment. Intestinal permeability significantly improved among the milk diet group. Fatalities among the milk group were 14% versus 21% among the maize group. The maize group also experienced more infections and gained less weight compared to the milk group.

Raw whole milk is a substantial food for children, and pregnant or lactating mothers, assuming that:

> ➤ The milk comes from cows that have been primarily grass-fed. When cows eat grass, they nourish their natural probiotic colonies. They also have stronger immune systems with which to battle pathogenic microorganisms. This means that the milk that comes out will have more probiotics and fewer pathogens. When cows are grass-fed they also receive more sunlight, which increases the health of their own immune systems. Just as in the case of a healthy mother, when cows' immune systems are stronger, they will produce more nourishing milk, which is healthier for the milk consumer.

> ➤ The cows receive no synthetic or genetically modified growth hormones. Growth hormones injected into cows have been shown to produce higher levels of IGF-1 in the milk and human body after drinking milk from growth hormones-injected cows. The American Public Health Association stated in a 2009 Policy Release regarding the use of growth hormones in dairy cows, after a review of the evidence, that, *"elevated IGF-1 levels in human blood are associated with higher rates of colon, breast, and prostate cancers."* Indeed, researchers from the University of Cincinnati's College of Medicine (Biro *et al.* 2010) studied 1,239 girls from 6-8 years old. They found that girls in this age group are reaching puberty at double the rate they did just ten years ago.

> ➤ The cows receive little or no antibiotics. These antibiotics will travel through the milk into the body. Here they can weaken the immune system and set up a greater susceptibility of antibiotic-resistant microorganisms.

> ➢ The milk (from grass-fed cows) is not pasteurized. Pasteurization kills all the beneficial microorganisms cows provide that promote healthy probiotics in the gut.

At least within the United States, the consumer should check to be sure that the dairy is registered with the state and undergoes continuous microorganism control. This means the state tests the milk periodically. Also the dairy should test every batch of milk and should be able to supply their customers with test results. These should show coliform counts less than 10 bacteria per mL of milk (also the same as pasteurized milk).

For those readers whose states ban the sale of raw milk; organic milk, yogurt and kefir are probably the best alternatives. Organic milk from a smaller dairy will typically come from predominantly grass-fed cows. They will also not receive hormones or antibiotics (organic cows can receive antibiotics if they are sick, but must then be separated from the milking herd for a significant period of time).

Note that lactose-intolerant persons typically do fine with fresh raw milk from an organic dairy. This is not a guarantee, but the owner of one of the largest raw milk dairies in California has informed the author that many of his raw milk customers are lactose-intolerant.

How does this work? The probiotics in the cow have large colonies of lactobacilli. These species love to break down lactose and they produce lactase. They also consume a number of the polysaccharides in raw milk.

If pasteurized milk is the only option, it can be mixed with yogurt or kefir to increase its probiotic benefit and digestion. This will supply the microorganisms that can help break down the lactose and proteins in the milk to better prepare it for digestion.

Note that as for this and any other information, the reader should consult their health provider before making any significant changes to their diet. Any experimentation with raw milk or any other severely sensitized food should be done in the supervision of a health expert prepared to deal with severe allergic responses.

Why the big disclaimer again? This is because while this information is based upon science, food sensitivities can still be tricky and unique. It always pays to be cautious, moderate and careful.

Cabbage

One of the more productive whole foods applicable to mucosal health and the health of the intestines is cabbage. Cabbage contains a unique constituent, s-methylmethionine, also referred to as vitamin U. Through a pathway utilizing one of the body's natural enzymes, called Bhmt2, s-methylmethionine is converted to methionine and then to glutathione in a series of steps.

In this form, glutathione has been shown to stimulate the repair of the mucosal membrane within the stomach and intestines. This rebuilding of the mucosal membrane is critical to replenishing the intestinal barrier that is depleted in many food sensitive people. Glutathione has also been shown to increase liver health.

Raw cabbage or cabbage juice has been used as a healing agent for ulcers and intestinal issues for thousands of years among traditional medicines, including those of Egyptian, Ayurvedic and Greek systems. The Western world became aware of raw cabbage juice in the 1950s, when Garnett Cheney, M.D. conducted several studies showing that methylmethionine-rich cabbage juice concentrate was able to reduce the pain and bleeding associated with ulcers.

In one of Dr. Cheney's studies, 37 ulcer patients were treated with either cabbage juice concentrate or placebo. Of the 26-patient cabbage juice group, 24 patients were considered "successes," achieving an astounding 92% success rate.

In another study, medical researchers from Iraq's University Department of Surgery (Salim 1993) conducted a double-blind study of 172 patients who suffered from gastric bleeding caused by nonsteroidal anti-inflammatory drugs (NSAIDs). They gave the patients either cysteine, methylmethionine sulfonium chloride (MMSC) or a placebo. Those receiving either the cysteine or the MMSC stopped bleeding. Their conditions became *"stable"* as compared with many in the control group, who continued to bleed.

Research has found this effect to be due to the fact that s-methylmethionine stimulates the healing of cell membranes among the leaves and stems of plants that have been damaged. Antioxidants are produced for similar reasons. Plants produce antioxidants to help to protect them from damage from the sun, insects and diseases. It just so happens that what protects plants also helps heal humans.

Probiotic Supplementation Strategies

The supplementation of probiotics to stimulate intestinal cell health should follow the research. This is vital, because not all probiotic species and strains are alike. Rather, research has shown that specific species and strains, used in specific doses alongside prebiotic-rich diets are most beneficial for the intestines.

After reviewing hundreds of clinical studies, some quoted in this book and many more discussed in the author's *Probiotics–Protection Against Infection* (2009), we summarize here the probiotics that have been shown useful for decreasing intestinal permeability. Under each species, the specific effects found in the research to contribute to its being beneficial for intestinal health are listed: (refer to the author's probiotics text mentioned above for reference specifics):

Lactobacillus acidophilus

Lactobacillus acidophilus is by far the most familiar probiotic to most of us, and is also by far the most-studied probiotic species to date. They are one of the main residents of the human gut, although supplemented strains may still be transient. In addition to helping digest lactose, probably the most important benefit of *L. acidophilus* is their ability to inhibit the growth of pathogenic intestinal microorganisms such as *Candida albicans*, *Escherichia coli*, *Helicobacter pylori*, *Salmonella*, *Shigella* and *Staphylococcus* species.

The research has shown that under certain conditions *L. acidophilus:*

➤ Help digest milk
➤ Reduce stress-induced GI problems
➤ Inhibit *E. coli*
➤ Reduce infection from rotavirus
➤ Reduce necrotizing enterocolitis
➤ Reduce intestinal permeability
➤ Control *H. pylori*
➤ Modulate PGE2 and IgA
➤ Reduce dyspepsia
➤ Modulate IgG
➤ Relieve and inhibit IBS and colitis
➤ Inhibit and control *Clostridium* spp.
➤ Inhibit *Bacteroides* spp.
➤ Inhibit *Candida* spp. Overgrowths
➤ Reduce allergic response

➢ Decrease allergic symptoms
➢ Inhibit upper respiratory infections

Lactobacillus helveticus

L. helveticus was made popular by cheese-makers from Switzerland. The Latin word *Helvetia* refers to Switzerland. *L. helveticus* is used to make Swiss cheese and other varietals, as it produces lactic acid but not other probiotic metabolites that can often make cheese taste bitter or sour.

The research has shown that under certain conditions *L. helveticus*:

➢ Normalize gut colonization similar to breast-fed infants among formula-fed infants

Lactobacillus salivarius

L. salivarius are residents of most humans. They are found in the mouth, small intestines, colon, and vagina. They are hardy bacteria that can live in both oxygen and oxygen-free environments. *L. salivarius* is one of the few bacteria species that can also thrive in salty environments. *L. salivarius* produce prolific amounts of lactic acid, which makes them hardy defenders of the teeth and gums. They also produce a number of antibiotics, and are speedy colonizers.

The research has shown that under certain conditions *L. salivarius*:

➢ Inhibit mutans streptococci in the mouth
➢ Reduce dental carries
➢ Reduce gingivitis and periodontal disease
➢ Reduce mastitis
➢ Reduce risk of strep throat caused by *S. pyogenes*
➢ Reduce ulcerative colitis and IBS
➢ Inhibit *E. coli*
➢ Inhibit *Salmonella* spp.
➢ Inhibit *Candida albicans*

Lactobacillus casei

L. casei are transient bacteria within the human body, but are residents of cow intestines. Thus they are readily found in naturally raw milk and colostrum. *L. casei* have been reported to reduce allergy symptoms and increase immune response. This is accomplished by their regulating the immune system's CHS, CD8 and T-cell responsiveness—an effect seen among immunosuppressed patients. *L. casei* are also competitive bacteria that will overtake other probiotics in a combined supplement. So it is best to supplement *L. casei* individually.

The research has shown that under certain conditions *L. casei*:

➢ Inhibit pathogenic microbial infections
➢ Reduce occurrence, risk and symptoms of IBS
➢ Inhibit severe systemic inflammatory response syndrome
➢ Inhibit respiratory tract infections
➢ Inhibit bronchitis
➢ Maintain remission of diverticular disease
➢ Inhibit *H. pylori* (and ulcers)
➢ Reduce allergy symptoms
➢ Inhibit *Pseudomonas aeruginosa*
➢ Decrease milk intolerance
➢ Increase CD3+ and CD4+
➢ Increase phagocytic activity
➢ Support liver function
➢ Decrease proinflammatory cytokine TNF-alpha
➢ Strengthen the immune system
➢ Inhibit and reduce diarrhea episodes
➢ Stimulate cytokine interleukin-1beta (IL-1b)
➢ Stimulate interferon-gamma
➢ Inhibit *Clostridium difficile*
➢ Reduce asthma symptoms
➢ Reduce constipation
➢ Decrease beta-glucuronidase
➢ Stimulate natural killer cell activity (NK-cells)
➢ Increase IgA levels
➢ Increase lymphocytes
➢ Decrease IL-6 (pro-inflammatory)
➢ Increase IL-12 (stimulates NK-cells)
➢ Reduce lower respiratory infections
➢ Inhibit *Candida* overgrowth
➢ Inhibit vaginosis
➢ Prevent colorectal tumor growth
➢ Restore NK-cell activity in smokers
➢ Stimulate the immune system among the elderly
➢ Increase CD56 lymphocytes
➢ Decrease rotavirus infections
➢ Decrease colds and influenza
➢ Reduce risk of bladder cancer
➢ Increase (good) HDL-cholesterol

➢ Decrease triglycerides
➢ Decrease blood pressure
➢ Inhibit viral infections
➢ Inhibit malignant pleural effusions secondary to lung cancer
➢ Reduce cervix tumors when used in combination radiation therapy
➢ Inhibit tumor growth of carcinomatous peritonitis/stomach cancer
➢ Break down nutrients for bioavailability

Lactobacillus rhamnosus

Much of the research on this species has been done on a particular strain, *L. rhamnosus* GG. *L. rhamnosus* GG have been shown in numerous studies to significantly stimulate the immune system and inhibit allergic inflammatory response as noted earlier. This is not to say, however, that non-GG strains will not perform similarly. In fact, studies with *L. rhamnosus* GR-1, *L. rhamnosus* 573/L, and *L. rhamnosus* LC705 strains have also showed positive results. The GG strain is trademarked by the Valio Ltd. Company in Finland and patented in 1985 by two scientists, Dr. Sherwood Gorbach and Dr. Barry Goldin, who also led most of the exhaustive research on this strain.

The research has shown that under certain conditions *L. rhamnosus:*_

➢ Inhibit a number of pathogenic microbial infections
➢ Improve glucose control
➢ Reduce risk of respiratory infections
➢ Decrease beta-glucosidase
➢ Reduce eczema
➢ Reduce colds and flu
➢ Strengthen the immune system
➢ Increase IgA levels in mucosal membrane
➢ Increase IgA levels in mothers breast milk
➢ Inhibit *Pseudomonas aeruginosa* infections in respiratory tract
➢ Inhibit *Clostridium difficile*
➢ Inhibit enterobacteria
➢ Reduce IBS symptoms
➢ Decrease IL-12, IL-2+ and CD69+ T-cells in IBS
➢ Reduce constipation
➢ Reduce the risk of colon cancer
➢ Modulate skin IgE sensitization
➢ Inhibit *H. pylori* (ulcer-causing)
➢ Reduce atopic dermatitis in children
➢ Increase Hib IgG levels in allergy-prone infants
➢ Reduce colic

➢ Stimulate IgM, IgA and IgG levels (modulates IgE)
➢ Stabilize intestinal barrier function (decreased permeability)
➢ Increase INF-gamma
➢ Modulate IL-4
➢ Help prevent atopic eczema
➢ Reduce *Streptococcus mutans*
➢ Stimulate tumor killing activity among NK-cells
➢ Stimulate IL-10 (anti-inflammatory)
➢ Reduce inflammation

Lactobacillus reuteri

L. reuteri is a species found residing permanently in humans. As a result, most supplemented strains attach fairly well, though temporarily, and stimulate colony growth for resident *L. reuteri* strains. *L. reuteri* will colonize in the stomach, duodenum and ileum regions. *L. reuteri* will also significantly modulate the immune response of the gastrointestinal mucosal membranes. This means that *L. reuteri* are useful for many of the same digestive ailments that *L. acidophilus* are also effective for. *L. reuteri* also have several other effects, including the restoration of our oral cavity bacteria. They also produce a significant amount of antibiotics.

The research has shown that under certain conditions *L. reuteri*:

➢ Reduce pro-inflammatory cytokines
➢ Stimulate growth and feeding among preterm infants
➢ Inhibit and suppress *H. pylori*
➢ Decrease dyspepsia
➢ Reduce nausea
➢ Reduce flatulence
➢ Reduce diarrhea (rotavirus and non-rotavirus)
➢ Reduce TGF-beta2 in breast-feeding mothers (reducing eczema)
➢ Reduce salivary *mutans streptococcus*
➢ Strengthen the immune system
➢ Reduce plaque on teeth
➢ Decrease symptoms of IBS
➢ Increase (inflammatory) CD4+ and CD25 T-cells (in IBS)
➢ Decrease (inflammatory) TNF-alpha and IL-12 (in IBS)
➢ Reduce eczema-specific IgEs in infants
➢ Reduce infant colic
➢ Reduce colds and influenza
➢ Stabilize intestinal barrier function (intestinal permeability)
➢ Decrease atopic dermatitis

Lactobacillus plantarum

L. plantarum has been part of the human diet for thousands of years. They are used in numerous fermented foods, including sauerkraut, gherkins, olive brines, sourdough bread, Nigerian ogi and fufu, kocha from Ethiopia, sour mifen noodles from China, Korean kim chi and other traditional foods. *L. plantarum* are also found in dairy and cow dung.

L. plantarum is a hardy strain. The bacteria have been shown to survive all the way through the intestinal tract. Temperature for optimal growth is 86-95 degrees F. *L. plantarum* are not permanent residents, however. When supplemented, they vigorously attack pathogenic bacteria, and create an environment hospitable for incubated resident strains to expand before departing. *L. plantarum* also produce lysine, and a number of antibiotics including lactolin. They also strengthen the mucosal membrane and reduce intestinal permeability.

**The research has shown that under certain conditions, *L. plantarum:*

➢ Strengthen the immune system
➢ Help restore healthy liver enzymes (alcohol-induced liver injury)
➢ Reduce frequency and severity of respiratory diseases
➢ Reduce intestinal permeability
➢ Inhibit various intestinal pathobiotics (incl. *Clostridium difficile*)
➢ Reduce Th2 (inflammatory) levels and increase Th1/Th2 ratio
➢ Reduce inflammatory responses
➢ Reduce symptoms of multiple traumas among injured patients
➢ Reduce fungal infections
➢ Reduce IBS symptoms
➢ Reduce pancreatic sepsis (infection)
➢ Reduce (inflammatory) interleukin-6 (IL-6) levels
➢ Decrease flatulence

Lactobacillus bulgaricus

We owe the *bulgaricus* name to Ilya Mechnikov, who named it after the Bulgarians—who used the bacteria to make the fermented milks that produced the original kefirs apparently related to their extreme longevity. In the 1960s and 1970s Russian researchers, notably Dr. Ivan Bogdanov and others, began focused research on *L. bulgaricus*. Early studies indicated antitumor effects. As the research progressed into Russian clinical research and commercialization, it became obvious that even heat-killed *L. bulgaricus* cell fragments have immune system stimulating benefits.

L. bulgaricus bacteria are transients that assist in *bifidobacteria* colony growth. They significantly stimulate the immune system and have antitumor effects. They also produce antibiotic and antiviral substances such as bulgarican and others. *L. bulgaricus* bacteria have also been reported to have anti-herpes properties. *L. bulgaricus* require more heat to colonize than many probiotics—at 104-109 degrees F.

The research has shown that under certain conditions *L. bulgaricus:*

➤ Reduce intestinal permeability
➤ Decrease IBS symptoms
➤ Help manage HIV symptoms
➤ Stimulate TNF-alpha
➤ Stimulate IL-1beta
➤ Decrease diarrhea (rotavirus and non-rotavirus)
➤ Decrease nausea
➤ Increase phagocytic activity
➤ Increase leukocyte levels
➤ Increase immune response
➤ Increase CD8+ levels
➤ Lower CD4+/CD8+ ratio (reducing inflammation)
➤ Increase IFN-gamma
➤ Lower total cholesterol
➤ Lower LDL levels
➤ Lower triglycerides
➤ Inhibit viruses
➤ Reduce salivary mutans in the mouth
➤ Increase absorption of dairy (lactose)
➤ Increase white blood cell counts after chemotherapy
➤ Increase IgA (immunity) to rotavirus
➤ Reduce intestinal bacteria

Bifidobacterium bifidum

These are normal residents in the human intestines, and by far the largest residents in terms of colonies. Their greatest populations occur in the colon, but also inhabit the lower small intestines. Breast milk typically contains large populations of *B. bifidum* along with other bifidobacteria. *B. bifidum* are highly competitive with yeasts such as *Candida albicans*. As a result, their populations may be decimated by large yeast overgrowths. This will also result in a number of endotoxins, including ammonia, being leached out of the colon into the bloodstream. As a result, B. *bifidum* populations are extremely important to the health of the liver, as has been illustrated in the research. They produce an array of antibiotics such as bifidin and various antimicrobial biochemicals such as formic acid. B. *bifidus* populations can also be severely damaged by the use of pharmaceutical antibiotics.

The research has shown that under certain conditions B. *bifidum*:

➢ Increase cell regeneration in alcohol-induced liver injury
➢ Stimulate immunity in very low birth weight infants
➢ Increase TGF-beta (anti-inflammatory) levels
➢ Reduce allergies
➢ Reduce H. *pylori* colonization
➢ Increase CD8+ T-cells as needed
➢ Establish infant microflora
➢ Inhibit E. *coli*
➢ Reduce intestinal bacteria infections
➢ Reduce acute diarrhea (rotavirus and non-rotavirus)

Bifidobacterium infantis

B. *infantis* are also normal residents of the human intestines—primarily among children. As implicated in the name, infants colonize a significant number of B. *infantis* in their early years. They will also colonize in the vagina, leading to the newborn's first exposure to protective probiotic bacteria. For this reason, it is important that pregnant mothers consider probiotic supplementation with B. *infantis*. B. *infantis* are largely anaerobic, and thrive within the darkest regions, where they can produce profuse quantities of acetic acid, lactic acid and formic acid to acidify the intestinal tract.

The research has shown that under certain conditions, B. *infantis*:

➢ Reduce acute diarrhea (rotavirus and non-rotavirus)
➢ Reduce or eliminate symptoms of IBS
➢ Reduce death among very low birth weight infants
➢ Increase immunity among very low birth weight infants
➢ Establish infant microflora
➢ Normalize Th1/Th2 ratio
➢ Reduce inflammatory allergic responses
➢ Normalize IL-10/IL-12 ratio

Bifidobacterium longum

B. longum are also normal inhabitants of the human digestive tract. They predominate the colon but also live in the small intestines. They are one of our top four bifidobacteria inhabitants. Like *B. infantis*, they produce acetic, lactic and formic acid. Like other bifidobacteria, they resist the growth of pathogenic bacteria, and thus reduce the production of harmful nitrites and ammonia. *B. longum* also produce B vitamins. Healthy breast milk contains significant *B. longum*.

The research has shown that under certain conditions *B. longum*:

➢ Reduce death among very low birth weight infants
➢ Reduce sickness among very low birth weight infants
➢ Reduce acute diarrhea (rotavirus and non-rotavirus)
➢ Reduce vomiting
➢ Reduce nausea
➢ Reduce ulcerative colitis
➢ Reduce or alleviate symptoms of IBS
➢ Stabilize intestinal barrier function (decreased permeability)
➢ Inhibit *H. pylori*
➢ Increase TGF-beta1 (anti-inflammatory) levels
➢ Decrease (inflammatory) TNF-alpha
➢ Decrease (inflammatory) IL-10 cytokines
➢ Reduce lactose-intolerance symptoms
➢ Reduce diarrhea
➢ Increase helper T-cells type2 (Th2)
➢ Increase (anti-inflammatory) IL-6
➢ Reduce (inflammatory) Th1
➢ Reduce pro-inflammatory IL-12 and interferon
➢ Stimulate healing of liver in cirrhosis
➢ Reduce constipation
➢ Reduce hypersensitivity
➢ Reduce IBS symptoms
➢ Inhibit intestinal pathogenic bacteria
➢ Decrease prostate cancer risk
➢ Decrease itching, nasal blockage and rhinitis in allergies
➢ Reduce (inflammatory) NF-kappaB
➢ Reduce (inflammatory) IL-8 levels
➢ Reduce progression of chronic liver disease
➢ Increase absorption of dairy nutrients

Bifidobacterium animalis/B. lactis

B. animalis was previously thought to be distinct from *B. lactis*, but today they are considered the same species with *B. lactis* being a subspecies of *B. animalis*. *B. lactis* has also been described as *Streptococcus lactis*. They are transient bacteria typically present in raw milk. They are also used as starters for traditional cheeses, cottage cheeses and buttermilks. They are also found among certain plants.

The research has shown that under certain conditions *B. animalis*:

➤ Reduce constipation
➤ Improve digestive comfort
➤ Decrease total cholesterol
➤ Increase blood glucose control
➤ Reduce respiratory diseases (severity and frequency)
➤ Strengthen the immune system
➤ Reduce salivary mutans in mouth
➤ Increase body weight among preterm infants
➤ Reduce (inflammatory) CRP levels
➤ Reduce (inflammatory) TNF-alpha levels
➤ Reduce acute diarrhea (rotavirus and non-rotavirus)
➤ Reduce (inflammatory) IL-10 levels
➤ Reduce (inflammatory) TGF-beta1 levels
➤ Reduce inflammatory responses
➤ Reduce (inflammatory) CDE4+CD54(+) cytokines
➤ Stimulate improvement in atopic dermatitis patients
➤ Reduce IBS symptoms
➤ Reduce diarrhea
➤ Normalize bowel movements
➤ Decrease intestinal permeability
➤ Reduce blood levels of interferon-gamma
➤ Stimulate IgA among milk-allergy infants
➤ Improve atopic dermatitis symptoms and sensitivity
➤ Inhibit *H. pylori*
➤ Reduce allergic inflammation
➤ Increase T-cell activity as needed
➤ Increase immunity among the elderly
➤ Increase absorption of dairy

Bifidobacterium breve

B. breve are also normal inhabitants of the human digestive tract—living mostly within the colon. They produce prolific acids, and also B vitamins. Like the other bifidobacteria, they also reduce ammonia-producing bacteria in the colon, aiding the health of the liver. Latin *brevis* means short.

The research has shown that under certain conditions ***B. breve:***

➤ Reduce severe systemic inflammatory response syndrome
➤ Increase resistance to respiratory infection
➤ Reduce (inflammatory) TNF-alpha
➤ Reduce (inflammatory) IL-10
➤ Reduce (inflammatory) TGF-beta1
➤ Reduce IBS symptoms
➤ Decrease (pro-colon cancer) beta-glucoronidase
➤ Inhibit *H. pylori*
➤ Increase antipoliovirus vaccination effectiveness
➤ Reduce acute diarrhea (rotavirus and non-rotavirus)
➤ Reduce allergy symptoms
➤ Increase growth weights among very low birth weight infants

Streptococcus thermophilus

Streptococcus thermophilus are common participants in yogurt making. They are also used in cheese making, and are even sometimes found in pasteurized milk. They will colonize at higher temperatures, from 104-113 degrees F. This is significant because this bacterium readily produces lactase, which breaks down lactose. (This is the only streptococci known to do this.) Like many other supplemented probiotics, *S. thermophilus* are temporary microorganisms in the human body. Their colonies will typically inhabit the system for a week or two before exiting (unless consistently consumed). During that time, however, they will help set up a healthy environment to support resident colony growth. Like other probiotics, *S. thermophilus* also produce a number of different antibiotic substances, including acids that deter the growth of pathogenic bacteria.

The research has shown that under certain conditions ***S. thermophilus:***

➤ Reduce acute diarrhea (rotavirus and non-rotavirus)
➤ Reduce intestinal permeability
➤ Inhibit *H. pylori*
➤ Help manage AIDS symptoms
➤ Increase lymphocytes among low-WBC patients
➤ Increase (anti-inflammatory) IL-1beta
➤ Decrease (inflammatory) IL-10
➤ Increase tumor necrosis factor-alpha (TNF-a)
➤ Increase absorption of dairy
➤ Decrease symptoms of IBS

➢ Inhibit *Clostridium difficile*
➢ Increase immune function among the elderly
➢ Restore infant microflora similar to breast-fed infants
➢ Increase (anti-inflammatory) CD8+
➢ Increase (anti-inflammatory) IFN-gamma
➢ Reduce acute gastroenteritis (diarrhea)
➢ Reduce baby colic
➢ Reduce symptoms of atopic dermatitis
➢ Reduce nasal cavity infections
➢ Increase HDL-cholesterol
➢ Increase growth in preterm infants
➢ Reduce intestinal bacteria
➢ Reduce upper respiratory tract infections from *Staphylococcus aureus*, *Streptococcus pneumoniae*, beta-hemolytic streptococci, and *Haemophilus influenzae*
➢ Reduce salivary mutans streptococci in the mouth
➢ Reduce flare-ups of chronic pouchitis
➢ Reduce LDL-cholesterol in overweight subjects
➢ Reduce ulcerative colitis

Saccharomyces boulardii

    S. boulardii are yeasts (fungi). They render a variety of preventative and therapeutic benefits to the body. Yet should this or another yeast colony grow too large, they can quickly become a burden to the body due to their dietary needs (primarily refined sugars) and waste products. *S. boulardii* are known to enhance IgA—which, as we've discussed, will typically reduce IgE atopic sensitivities. This is likely why this probiotic helps clear skin disorders. *S. boulardii* also help control diarrhea, and have been shown to be helpful in Crohn's disease and irritable bowel issues. *S. boulardii* have also been shown to be useful in combating cholera bacteria (*Vibrio cholerae*).

The research has shown that under certain conditions *S. boulardii*:

➢ Decrease infectious *Entameba histolytica* (intestinal)
➢ Inhibit *H. pylori*
➢ Decrease intestinal permeability
➢ Decrease diarrhea infections
➢ Stimulate T-cells as needed
➢ Decrease C-reactive protein
➢ Decrease beta-glucoronidase enzyme (associated with colon cancer)
➢ Inhibit *E. coli*
➢ Reduce ulcerative colitis
➢ Reduce symptoms of Crohn's disease
➢ Reduce *Clostridium difficile*

Probiotic Supplement Considerations

The main consideration in probiotic supplementation is consuming live organisms. These are typically labeled as "CFU" which stands for *colony forming units*. In other words, live probiotics will produce new colonies once inside the intestines. Dead ones will not. So the key is keeping the probiotics alive while in the capsule and supplement bottle, until we are ready to consume them. Here are a few considerations about probiotic supplements:

Capsules

Vegetable capsules contain less moisture than gelatin or enteric-coated capsules. Even a little moisture in the capsule can increase the possibility of waking up the probiotics while in the bottle. Once woken up, they will starve and die. Enteric coating can minimally protect the probiotics within the stomach, assuming they have survived in the bottle. Some manufactures use oils to help protect the probiotics in the stomach. In all cases, encapsulated freeze-dried probiotics should be refrigerated (no matter what the label says) at all times during shipping, at the store, and at home. Dark containers also better protect the probiotics from light exposure, which can kill them.

Powders

Powders of freeze-dried probiotics are subject to deterioration due to increased exposure to oxygen and light. Powders should be refrigerated in dark containers and sealed tightly to be kept viable. They should also be consumed with liquids or food, preferably dairy or fermented dairy. If used as to insert into the vagina, a douche mixture with water and a little yogurt is preferable.

Caplets/Tablets

Some tablet/caplets have special coatings that provide viability through to the intestines without refrigeration. If not, those tablets would likely be in the same category as encapsulated products, in terms of requiring refrigeration.

Shells or Beads

These can provide longer shelf viability without refrigeration and better survive the stomach. However, because of the size of the shell, these typically come with less CFU quantity, increasing the cost of a therapeutic dose. Another drawback may be that the intestines must dissolve this thick shell. An easy test is to examine the stool to be sure that the beads or shells aren't coming out the other end whole.

Lozenges

These are new and exciting ways to supplement with probiotics. A correctly formulated chewable or lozenge can inoculate the mouth, nose and throat with beneficial bacteria to compete with and fight off pathogenic bacteria as they enter or reside in our nose, throat, mouth and even lungs. However, the probiotics in a lozenge will not likely survive the stomach acids and penetrate the intestines.

Still, lozenges are an excellent way to protect against new infections and prevent sore throats when we are traveling or working in enclosed spaces. The bacteria in a lozenge or chewable ease out as we are sucking or chewing, leaving probiotics dispersed throughout our gums and throat, rendering increased immunity. This type of supplement should still be kept sealed, airtight and cool. Refer to the author's book *Oral Probiotics* (2010) for detailed information regarding species and strategies for oral probiotic lozenges.

Liquid Supplements

There are several probiotic supplements in small liquid form. One brand has a long tradition and a hardy, well-researched strain. A liquid probiotic should be in a light-sealed, refrigerated container. It should also contain some dairy or other probiotic-friendly culture, giving the probiotics some food while they are waiting for delivery.

Probiotic Dosage

A good dosage for intestinal probiotics for prevention and maintenance can be ten to fifteen billion CFU (*colony forming units*) per day. Total intake during an illness or therapeutic period, however, will often double or triple that dosage. Much of the research shown in this text utilized 20 billion to 40 billion CFU per day, about a third of that dose for children and a quarter of that dose for infants. (*B. infantis* is often the supplement of choice for babies.)

Supplemental oral probiotic dosages can be far less (100 million to two billion), especially when the formula contains the hardy *L. reuteri*.

People who must take antibiotics for life-threatening reasons can alternate doses of probiotics between their antibiotic dosing. The probiotic dose can be at least two hours before or after the antibiotic dose. (Always consult with the prescribing doctor first.)

Remember that these dosages depend upon delivery to the intestines. Therefore, a product that passes into the stomach with little protection would likely not deliver well to the intestines. Such a supplement would likely require higher dosage to achieve the desired effects.

Hydration

The intestinal mucosal membranes are primarily water. In a dehydrated state, this mucosal membrane thins. It is for this reason that research on water drinking has found that many ulcerated conditions can be cured simply by drinking adequate water (Batmanghelidj 1997).

The immune system is also irrevocably aligned with the body's water availability. The immune system utilizes water to produce lymph fluid. Lymph fluid circulates immune cells throughout the body so that they can target specific intruders. The lymph is also used to escort toxins out of the body.

Water in general is needed to speed the removal of toxins, from every organ and tissue system.

Water also increases the availability of oxygen to cells. Water balances the level of free radicals. Water flushes and replenishes the digestive tract. Thus, water is necessary for the proper digestion of food. The gastric cells and intestinal wall cells require water for proper functioning.

Water is also intimately involved in the release of histamine. Research has revealed that increased levels of histamine are released during periods of dehydration, in order to help provide water balance within the bloodstream, tissues, kidneys and other organs (Batmanghelidj 1987 and 1990).

A rule of thumb accepted by many experts, and consistent with government studies, would be to drink one-half ounce of water per pound of body weight per day.

Drinking just any water is not advised. Care must be taken to drink water that is pure yet naturally mineralized. Research has confirmed that distilled water and soft water are not advisable. Please refer to the author's book, *Pure Water* (2010) for the specific research that concludes which types of water and filtration methods are the healthiest.

Intestinal Fortitude

This expression is often used for someone who can handle a significant amount of stress. This is often communicated with the expression of 'having guts'—given to a person who shows bravery in the face of risk.

The bottom line is that the health of our intestines are specific to our body's health, our moods and our immunity.

As we proved in the first chapter, IIPS is not only a real disorder: It is a disorder that is associated with a number of health conditions, from liver disorders to bacterial infections to cardiovascular disease, asthma and allergies. While natural physicians have discussed this condition for many decades, western medicine has tried to discredit the condition. But this did not prevent the international medical research community from precisely defining the condition, and showing its relationship to many different diseases.

We can compare the situation to the linesman of a football team. These linesman are the blockers that keep the other team's players from getting to and sacking the quarterback. If they can keep the other teams' players out, the quarterback will be able to pass the ball or hand it off safely.

Now if the linesmen are not strong enough to keep out the other team's players, the quarterback is in trouble. The linebackers of the other team will storm in and tackle the quarterback.

This is the situation with intestinal permeability. The mucosal brush barrier in the intestines is set up to keep the bad guys out of the bloodstream and tissues of the body. These bad guys range from toxins to food macromolecules to free radicals and bacteria endotoxins. Should they flood into the body, they will damage the cells and tissues of the body, causing a variety of possible disease conditions.

As we've shown, the most obvious sign of this condition is systemic inflammation. Systemic inflammation is the damage of the body's cells and tissues by toxins, radicals and infective agents. Systemic inflammation is common amongst practically every serious disease.

This text has also focused on strategies to improve our gut's mucosal membranes and intestinal health in general. These strategies are not simply the author's or anyone else's theories: They are strategies that have been proven by scientific research and clinical experience. Some of this research is from modern research, and some is from centuries of safe clinical use among literally billions of persons who have experienced intestinal issues around the world.

Whether we decide to embrace IIPS or not, it is real. And regardless of whether we apply those strategies to improve or at least maintain the intestinal brush barrier, the health of our intestines will determine our overall health and our ability to fight or avoid disease.

References and Bibliography

Abbott M, Hayward S, Ross W, Godefroy SB, Ulberth F, Van Hengel AJ, Roberts J, Akiyama H, Popping B, Yeung JM, Wehling P, Taylor SL, Poms RE, Delahaut P. Validation procedures for quantitative food allergen ELISA methods: community guidance and best practices. *J AOAC Int.* 2010 Mar-Apr;93(2):442-50.

Adel-Patient K, Ah-Leung S, Creminon C, Nouaille S, Chatel JM, Langella P, Wal JM. Oral administration of recombinant Lactococcus lactis expressing bovine beta-lactoglobulin partially prevents mice from sensitization. *Clin Exp Allergy.* 2005 Apr;35(4):539-46.

Aggarwal BB, Harikumar KB. Potential therapeutic effects of curcumin, the anti-inflammatory agent, against neurodegenerative, cardiovascular, pulmonary, metabolic, autoimmune and neoplastic diseases. *Int J Biochem Cell Biol.* 2009 Jan;41(1):40-59.

Aggarwal BB, Sung B. Pharmacological basis for the role of curcumin in chronic diseases: an age-old spice with modern targets. *Trends Pharmacol Sci.* 2009 Feb;30(2):85-94.

Agne PS, Bidat E, Agne PS, Rance F, Paty E. Sesame seed allergy in children. *Eur Ann Allergy Clin Immunol.* 2004 Oct;36(8):300-5.

Agostoni C, Fiocchi A, Riva E, Terracciano L, Sarratud T, Martelli A, Lodi F, D'Auria E, Zuccotti G, Giovannini M. Growth of infants with IgE-mediated cow's milk allergy fed different formulas in the complementary feeding period. *Pediatr Allergy Immunol.* 2007 Nov;18(7):599-606.

Ahmed T, Fuchs GJ. Gastrointestinal allergy to food: a review. *J Diarrhoeal Dis Res.* 1997 Dec;15(4):211-23.

Aho K, Koskenvuo M, Tuominen J, Kaprio J. Occurrence of rheumatoid arthritis in a nationwide series of twins. *J Rheumatol.* 1986 Oct;13(5):899-902.

Airola P. *How to Get Well.* Phoenix, AZ: Health Plus, 1974.

Akkol EK, Güvenç A, Yesilada E. A comparative study on the antinociceptive and anti-inflammatory activities of five Juniperus taxa. *J Ethnopharmacol.* 2009 Jun 6.

Alemán A, Sastre J, Quirce S, de las Heras M, Carnés J, Fernández-Caldas E, Pastor C, Blázquez AB, Vivanco F, Cuesta-Herranz J. Allergy to kiwi: a double-blind, placebo-controlled food challenge study in patients from a birch-free area. *J Allergy Clin Immunol.* 2004 Mar;113(3):543-50.

Alexander DD, Cabana MD. Partially hydrolyzed 100% whey protein infant formula and reduced risk of atopic dermatitis: a meta-analysis. *J Pediatr Gastroenterol Nutr.* 2010 Apr;50(4):422-30.

Alexandrakis M, Letourneau R, Kempuraj D, Kandere-Grzybowska K, Huang M, Christodoulou S, Boucher W, Seretakis D, Theoharides TC. Flavones inhibit Proliferation and increase mediator content in human leukemic mast cells (HMC-1). *Eur J Haematol.* 2003 Dec;71(6):448-54.

Al-Harrasi A, Al-Saidi S. Phytochemical analysis of the essential oil from botanically certified oleogum resin of Boswellia sacra (Omani Luban). *Molecules.* 2008 Sep 16;13(9):2181-9.

Almqvist C, Garden F, Xuan W, Mihrshahi S, Leeder SR, Oddy W, Webb K, Marks GB; CAPS team. Omega-3 and omega-6 fatty acid exposure from early life does not affect atopy and asthma at age 5 years. *J Allergy Clin Immunol.* 2007 Jun;119(6):1438-44.

Al-Mustafa AH, Al-Thunibat OY. Antioxidant activity of some Jordanian medicinal plants used traditionally for treatment of diabetes. *Pak J Biol Sci.* 2008 Feb 1;11(3):351-8.

Altman RD, Marcussen KC. Effects of a ginger extract on knee pain in patients with osteoarthritis. *Arthritis Rheum.* 2001 Nov;44(11):2531-8.

Amato R, Pinelli M, Monticelli A, Miele G, Cocozza S. Schizophrenia and Vitamin D Related Genes Could Have Been Subject to Latitude-driven Adaptation. *BMC Evol Biol.* 2010 Nov 11;10(1):351.

American Conference of Governmental Industrial Hygienists. *Threshold limit values for chemical substances and physical agents in the work environment.* Cincinnati, OH: ACGIH, 1986.

American Dietetic Association; Dietitians of Canada. Position of the American Dietetic Association and Dietitians of Canada: vegetarian diets. *Can J Diet Pract Res.* 2003 Summer;64(2):62-81.

Ammon HP. Boswellic acids in chronic inflammatory diseases. *Planta Med.* 2006 Oct;72(12):1100-16.

Anand P, Thomas SG, Kunnumakkara AB, Sundaram C, Harikumar KB, Sung B, Tharakan ST, Misra K, Priyadarsini IK, Rajasekharan KN, Aggarwal BB. Biological activities of curcumin and its analogues (Congeners) made by man and Mother Nature. *Biochem Pharmacol.* 2008 Dec 1;76(11):1590-611.

Anderson JL, May HT, Horne BD, Bair TL, Hall NL, Carlquist JF, Lappé DL, Muhlestein JB; Intermountain Heart Collaborative (IHC) Study Group. Relation of vitamin D deficiency to cardiovascular risk factors, disease status, and incident events in a general healthcare population. *Am J Cardiol.* 2010 Oct 1;106(7):963-8.

Anderson RC, Anderson JH. Acute toxic effects of fragrance products. *Arch Environ Health.* 1998 Mar-Apr;53(2):138-46.

Andoh T, Zhang Q, Yamamoto T, Tayama M, Hattori M, Tanaka K, Kuraishi Y. Inhibitory Effects of the Methanol Extract of Ganoderma lucidum on Mosquito Allergy-Induced Itch-Associated Responses in Mice. *J Pharmacol Sci.* 2010 Oct 8.

Andre C, Andre F, Colin L, Cavagna S. Measurement of intestinal permeability to mannitol and lactulose as a means of diagnosing food allergy and evaluating therapeutic effectiveness of disodium cromoglycate. Ann Allergy. 1987 Nov;59(5 Pt 2):127-30.

André C, André F, Colin L. Effect of allergen ingestion challenge with and without cromoglycate cover on intestinal permeability in atopic dermatitis, urticaria and other symptoms of food allergy. *Allergy*. 1989;44 Suppl 9:47-51.

André C. Food allergy. Objective diagnosis and test of therapeutic efficacy by measuring intestinal permeability. *Presse Med*. 1986 Jan 25;15(3):105-8.

Andre F, Andre C, Feknous M, Colin L, Cavagna S. Digestive permeability to different-sized molecules and to sodium cromoglycate in food allergy. *Allergy Proc*. 1991 Sep-Oct;12(5):293-8.

Angioni A, Barra A, Russo MT, Coroneo V, Dessi S, Cabras P. Chemical composition of the essential oils of Juniperus from ripe and unripe berries and leaves and their antimicrobial activity. *J Agric Food Chem*. 2003 May 7;51(10):3073-8.

Anim-Nyame N, Sooranna SR, Johnson MR, Gamble J, Steer PJ. Garlic supplementation increases peripheral blood flow: a role for interleukin-6? *J Nutr Biochem*. 2004 Jan;15(1):30-6.

Annweiler C, Schott AM, Berrut G, Chauviré V, Le Gall D, Inzitari M, Beauchet O. Vitamin D and ageing: neurological issues. *Neuropsychobiology*. 2010 Aug;62(3):139-50.

Aoki T, Usuda Y, Miyakoshi H, Tamura K, Herberman RB. Low natural killer syndrome: clinical and immunologic features. *Nat Immun Cell Growth Regul*. 1987;6(3):116-28.

Apáti P, Houghton PJ, Kite G, Steventon GB, Kéry A. In-vitro effect of flavonoids from Solidago canadensis extract on glutathione S-transferase. *J Pharm Pharmacol*. 2006 Feb;58(2):251-6.

APHA (American Public Health Association). Opposition to the Use of Hormone Growth Promoters in Beef and Dairy Cattle Production. Policy Statement: 11/10/2009. Policy Number: 20098. http://www.apha.org/advocacy/policy/id=1379. Accessed Nov. 24, 2010.

Araki K, Shinozaki T, Irie Y, Miyazawa Y. Trial of oral administration of Bifidobacterium breve for the prevention of rotavirus infections. *Kansenshogaku Zasshi*. 1999 Apr;73(4):305-10.

Argento A, Tiraferri E, Marzaloni M. Oral anticoagulants and medicinal plants. An emerging interaction. *Ann Ital Med Int*. 2000 Apr-Jun;15(2):139-43.

Arshad SH, Bateman B, Sadeghnejad A, Gant C, Matthews SM. Prevention of allergic disease during childhood by allergen avoidance: the Isle of Wight prevention study. *J Allergy Clin Immunol*. 2007 Feb;119(2):307-13.

Arslan G, Kahrs GE, Lind R, Froyland L, Florvaag E, Berstad A. Patients with subjective food hypersensitivity: the value of analyzing intestinal permeability and inflammation markers in gut lavage fluid. *Digestion*. 2004;70(1):26-35.

Arslanoglu S, Moro GE, Schmitt J, Tandoi L, Rizzardi S, Boehm G. Early dietary intervention with a mixture of prebiotic oligosaccharides reduces the incidence of allergic manifestations and infections during the first two years of life. *J Nutr*. 2008 Jun;138(6):1091-5.

Arterburn LM, Oken HA, Bailey Hall E, Hamersley J, Kuratko CN, Hoffman JP. Algal-oil capsules and cooked salmon: nutritionally equivalent sources of docosahexaenoic acid. *J Am Diet Assoc*. 2008 Jul;108(7):1204-9.

Arterburn LM, Oken HA, Hoffman JP, Bailey-Hall E, Chung G, Rom D, Hamersley J, McCarthy D. Bioequivalence of Docosahexaenoic acid from different algal oils in capsules and in a DHA-fortified food. *Lipids*. 2007 Nov;42(11):1011-24.

Asero R, Antonicelli L, Arena A, Bommarito L, Caruso B, Colombo G, Crivellaro M, De Carli M, Della Torre E, Della Torre F, Heffler E, Lodi Rizzini F, Longo R, Manzotti G, Marcotulli M, Melchiorre A, Minale P, Morandi P, Moreni B, Moschella A, Murzilli F, Nebiolo F, Poppa M, Randazzo S, Rossi G, Senna GE. Causes of food-induced anaphylaxis in Italian adults: a multi-centre study. *Int Arch Allergy Immunol*. 2009;150(3):271-7.

Asero R, Antonicelli L, Arena A, Bommarito L, Caruso B, Crivellaro M, De Carli M, Della Torre E, Della Torre F, Heffler E, Lodi Rizzini F, Longo R, Manzotti G, Marcotulli M, Melchiorre A, Minale P, Morandi P, Moreni B, Moschella A, Murzilli F, Nebiolo F, Poppa M, Randazzo S, Rossi G, Senna GE. EpidemAAITO: features of food allergy in Italian adults attending allergy clinics: a multi-centre study. *Clin Exp Allergy*. 2009 Apr;39(4):547-55.

Asero R, Mistrello G, Roncarolo D, Amato S, Caldironi G, Barocci F, van Ree R. Immunological cross-reactivity between lipid transfer proteins from botanically unrelated plant-derived foods: a clinical study. *Allergy*. 2002 Oct;57(10):900-6.

Ashrafi K, Chang FY, Watts JL, Fraser AG, Kamath RS, Ahringer J, Ruvkun G. Genome-wide RNAi analysis of Caenorhabditis elegans fat regulatory genes. *Nature*. 2003 Jan 16;421(6920):268-72.

Atkinson W, Sheldon TA, Shaath N, Whorwell PJ. Food elimination based on IgG antibodies in irritable bowel syndrome: a randomised controlled trial. *Gut*. 2004 Oct;53(10):1459-64.

Atsumi T, Tonosaki K. Smelling lavender and rosemary increases free radical scavenging activity and decreases cortisol level in saliva. *Psychiatry Res.* 2007 Feb 28;150(1):89-96.

Bachas-Daunert S, Deo SK. Should genetically modified foods be abandoned on the basis of allergenicity? *Anal Bioanal Chem.* 2008 Oct;392(3):341-6.

Badar VA, Thawani VR, Wakode PT, Shrivastava MP, Gharpure KJ, Hingorani LL, Khiyani RM. Efficacy of Tinospora cordifolia in allergic rhinitis. *J Ethnopharmacol.* 2005 Jan 15;96(3):445-9.

Baker DH. Comparative nutrition and metabolism: explication of open questions with emphasis on protein and amino acids. *Proc Natl Acad Sci U S A.* 2005 Dec 13;102(50):17897-902.

Baker SM. *Detoxification and Healing.* Chicago: Contemporary Books, 2004.

Bakshi A, Stephen S, Borum ML, Doman DB. Emerging therapeutic options for celiac disease: potential alternatives to a gluten-free diet. Gastroenterol Hepatol (N Y). 2012 Sep;8(9):582-8.

Balch P, Balch J. *Prescription for Nutritional Healing.* New York: Avery, 2000.

Ballentine R. *Diet & Nutrition: A holistic approach.* Honesdale, PA: Himalayan Int., 1978.

Ballentine R. *Radical Healing.* New York: Harmony Books, 1999.

Ballmer-Weber BK, Hoffmann A, Wüthrich B, Lüttkopf D, Pompei C, Wangorsch A, Kästner M, Vieths S. Influence of food processing on the allergenicity of celery: DBPCFC with celery spice and cooked celery in patients with celery allergy. *Allergy.* 2002 Mar;57(3):228-35.

Ballmer-Weber BK, Holzhauser T, Scibilia J, Mittag D, Zisa G, Ortolani C, Oesterballe M, Poulsen LK, Vieths S, Bindslev-Jensen C. Clinical characteristics of soybean allergy in Europe: a double-blind, placebo-controlled food challenge study. *J Allergy Clin Immunol.* 2007 Jun;119(6):1489-96.

Ballmer-Weber BK, Vieths S, Lüttkopf D, Heuschmann P, Wüthrich B. Celery allergy confirmed by double-blind, placebo-controlled food challenge: a clinical study in 32 subjects with a history of adverse reactions to celery root. *J Allergy Clin Immunol.* 2000 Aug;106(2):373-8.

Banno N, Akihisa T, Yasukawa K, Tokuda H, Tabata K, Nakamura Y, Nishimura R, Kimura Y, Suzuki T. Anti-inflammatory activities of the triterpene acids from the resin of Boswellia carteri. *J Ethnopharmacol.* 2006 Sep 19;107(2):249-53.

Bant A, Kruszewski J. Increased sensitization prevalence to common inhalant and food allergens in young adult Polish males. *Ann Agric Environ Med.* 2008 Jun;15(1):21-7.

Barau E, Dupont C. Modifications of intestinal permeability during food provocation procedures in pediatric irritable bowel syndrome. *J Pediatr Gastroenterol Nutr.* 1990 Jul;11(1):72-7.

Barnes M, Cullinan P, Athanasaki P, MacNeill S, Hole AM, Harris J, Kalogeraki S, Chatzinikolaou M, Drakonakis N, Bibaki-Liakou V, Newman Taylor AJ, Bibakis I. Crete: does farming explain urban and rural differences in atopy? *Clin Exp Allergy.* 2001 Dec;31(12):1822-8.

Barnetson RS, Drummond H, Ferguson A. Precipitins to dietary proteins in atopic eczema. *Br J Dermatol.* 1983 Dec;109(6):653-5.

Barrager E, Veltmann JR Jr, Schauss AG, Schiller RN. A multicentered, open-label trial on the safety and efficacy of methylsulfonylmethane in the treatment of seasonal allergic rhinitis. *J Altern Complement Med.* 2002 Apr;8(2):167-73.

Basu A, Devaraj S, Jialal I. Dietary factors that promote or retard inflammation. *Arterioscler Thromb Vasc Biol.* 2006 May;26(5):995-1001.

Bateman B, Warner JO, Hutchinson E, Dean T, Rowlandson P, Gant C, Grundy J, Fitzgerald C, Stevenson J. The effects of a double blind, placebo controlled, artificial food colourings and benzoate preservative challenge on hyperactivity in a general population sample of preschool children. *Arch Dis Child.* 2004 Jun;89(6):506-11.

Batista R, Martins I, Jeno P, Ricardo CP, Oliveira MM. A proteomic study to identify soya allergens—the human response to transgenic versus non-transgenic soya samples. Int *Arch Allergy Immunol.* 2007;144(1):29-38.

Batmanghelidj F. Neurotransmitter histamine: an alternative view point, *Science in Medicine Simplified.* Falls Church, VA: Foundation for the Simple in Medicine, 1990.

Batmanghelidj F. Pain: a need for paradigm change. *Anticancer Res.* 1987 Sep-Oct;7(5B):971-89.

Batmanghelidj F. *Your Body's Many Cries for Water.* 2nd Ed. Vienna, VA: Global Health, 1997.

Beasley R, Clayton T, Crane J, von Mutius E, Lai CK, Montefort S, Stewart A; ISAAC Phase Three Study Group. Association between paracetamol use in infancy and childhood, and risk of asthma, rhinoconjunctivitis, and eczema in children aged 6-7 years: analysis from Phase Three of the ISAAC programme. *Lancet.* 2008 Sep. 20;372(9643):1039-48.

Becker KG, Simon RM, Bailey-Wilson JE, Freidlin B, Biddison WE, McFarland HF, Trent JM. Clustering of non-major histocompatibility complex susceptibility candidate loci in human autoimmune diseases. *Proc Natl Acad Sci U S A.* 1998 Aug 18;95(17):9979-84.

Beddoe AF. *Biologic Ionization as Applied to Human Nutrition.* Warsaw: Wendell Whitman, 2002.

189

Beecher GR. Phytonutrients' role in metabolism: effects on resistance to degenerative processes. *Nutr Rev.* 1999 Sep;57(9 Pt 2):S3-6.

Belcaro G, Cesarone MR, Errichi S, Zulli C, Errichi BM, Vinciguerra G, Ledda A, Di Renzo A, Stuard S, Dugall M, Pellegrini I., Gizzi G, Ippolito E, Ricci A, Cacchio M, Cipollone G, Ruffini I, Fano F, Hosoi M, Rohdewald P. Variations in C-reactive protein, plasma free radicals and fibrinogen values in patients with osteoarthritis treated with Pycnogenol. *Redox Rep.* 2008;13(6):271-6.

Bell IR, Baldwin CM, Schwartz GE, Illness from low levels of environmental chemicals: relevance to chronic fatigue syndrome and fibromyalgia. *Am J Med.* 1998;105 (suppl 3A).:74-82. S.

Bell SJ, Potter PC. Milk whey-specific immune complexes in allergic and non-allergic subjects. *Allergy.* 1988 Oct;43(7):497-503.

Bellanti JA, Zeligs BJ, Malka-Rais J, Sabra A. Abnormalities of Th1 function in non-IgE food allergy, celiac disease, and ileal lymphonodular hyperplasia: a new relationship? Ann *Allergy Asthma Immunol.* 2003 Jun;90(6 Suppl 3):84-9.

Ben, X.M., Zhou, X.Y., Zhao, W.H., Yu, W.L., Pan, W., Zhang, W.L., Wu, S.M., Van Beusekom, C.M., Schaafsma, A. (2004) Supplementation of milk formula with galactooligosaccharides improves intestinal micro-flora and fermentation in term infants. *Chin Med J.* 117(6):927-931, 2004.

Benard A, Desreumeaux P, Huglo D, Hoorelbeke A, Tonnel AB, Wallaert B. Increased intestinal permeability in bronchial asthma. *J Allergy Clin Immunol.* 1996 Jun;97(6):1173-8.

Bengmark S. Curcumin, an atoxic antioxidant and natural NFkappaB, cyclooxygenase-2, lipooxygenase, and inducible nitric oxide synthase inhibitor: a shield against acute and chronic diseases. *JPEN J Parenter Enteral Nutr.* 2006 Jan-Feb;30(1):45-51.

Bengmark S. Immunonutrition: role of biosurfactants, fiber, and probiotic bacteria. Nutrition. 1998 Jul-Aug;14(7-8):585-94.

Benlounes N, Dupont C, Candalh C, Blaton MA, Darmon N, Desjeux JF, Heyman M. The threshold for immune cell reactivity to milk antigens decreases in cow's milk allergy with intestinal symptoms. *J Allergy Clin Immunol.* 1996 Oct;98(4):781-9.

Ben-Shoshan M, Harrington DW, Soller L, Fragapane J, Joseph L, St Pierre Y, Godefroy SB, Elliot SJ, Clarke AE. A population-based study on peanut, tree nut, fish, shellfish, and sesame allergy prevalence in Canada. *J Allergy Clin Immunol.* 2010 Jun;125(6):1327-35.

Ben-Shoshan M, Kagan R, Primeau MN, Alizadehfar R, Turnbull E, Harada L, Dufresne C, Allen M, Joseph L, St Pierre Y, Clarke A. Establishing the diagnosis of peanut allergy in children never exposed to peanut or with an uncertain history: a cross-Canada study. *Pediatr Allergy Immunol.* 2010 Sep;21(6):920-6.

Bensky D, Gable A, Kaptchuk T (transl.). *Chinese Herbal Medicine Materia Medica.* Seattle: Eastland Press, 1986.

Bentz S, Hausmann M, Piberger H, Kellermeier S, Paul S, Held L, Falk W, Obermeier F, Fried M, Schölmerich J, Rogler G. Clinical relevance of IgG antibodies against food antigens in Crohn's disease: a double-blind cross-over diet intervention study. *Digestion.* 2010;81(4):252-64.

Bergner P. *The Healing Power of Garlic.* Prima Publishing, Rocklin CA 1996.

Berin MC, Yang PC, Ciok L, Waserman S, Perdue MH. Role for IL-4 in macromolecular transport across human intestinal epithelium. Am J Physiol. 1999 May;276(5 Pt 1):C1046-52.

Berkow R., (Ed.) *The Merck Manual of Diagnosis and Therapy.* 16th Edition. Rahway, N.J.: Merck Research Labs, 1992.

Berseth CL, Mitmesser SH, Ziegler EE, Marunycz JD, Vanderhoof J. Tolerance of a standard intact protein formula versus a partially hydrolyzed formula in healthy, term infants. Nutr J. 2009 Jun 19;8:27.

Berteau O and Mulloy B. 2003. Sulfated fucans, fresh perspectives: structures, functions, and biological properties of sulfated fucans and an overview of enzymes active toward this class of polysaccharide. *Glycobiology.* Jun;13(6):29R-40R.

Besselink MG, van Santvoort HC, Renooij W, de Smet MB, Boermeester MA, Fischer K, Timmerman HM, Ahmed Ali U, Cirkel GA, Bollen TL, van Ramshorst B, Schaapherder AF, Witteman BJ, Ploeg RJ, van Goor H, van Laarhoven CJ, Tan AC, Brink MA, van der Harst E, Wahab PJ, van Eijck CH, Dejong CH, van Erpecum KJ, Akkermans LM, Gooszen HG; Dutch Acute Pancreatitis Study Group. Intestinal barrier dysfunction in a randomized trial of a specific probiotic composition in acute pancreatitis. *Ann Surg.* 2009 Nov;250(5):712-9.

Beyer K, Morrow E, Li XM, Bardina L, Bannon GA, Burks AW, Sampson HA. Effects of cooking methods on peanut allergenicity. *J Allergy Clin Immunol.* 2001;107:1077-81.

Bhandari U, Sharma JN, Zafar R. The protective action of ethanolic ginger (Zingiber officinale) extract in cholesterol fed rabbits. *J Ethnopharmacol.* 1998 Jun;61(2):167-71.

Bielory BP, Perez VL, Bielory L. Treatment of seasonal allergic conjunctivitis with ophthalmic corticosteroids: in search of the perfect ocular corticosteroids in the treatment of allergic conjunctivitis. *Curr Opin Allergy Clin Immunol.* 2010 Oct;10(5):469-77.

Bielory L, Lupoli K. Herbal interventions in asthma and allergy. *J Asthma.* 1999;36:1–65.

Bielory L, Russin J, Zuckerman GB. Clinical efficacy, mechanisms of action, and adverse effects of complementary and alternative medicine therapies for asthma. *Allergy Asthma Proc.* 2004;25:283–91.

Biesiekierski JR, Newnham ED, Irving PM, Barrett JS, Haines M, Doecke JD, Shepherd SJ, Muir JG, Gibson PR. Gluten causes gastrointestinal symptoms in subjects without celiac disease: a double-blind randomized placebo-controlled trial. *Am J Gastroenterol.* 2011 Mar;106(3):508-14.

Binder HJ, O'Brien WM, Spiro HM, Hollingsworth JW. Gluten and the small intestine in rheumatoid arthritis. *JAMA.* 1966 Mar 7;195(10):857-8.

Bindslev-Jensen C, Skov PS, Roggen EL, Hvass P, Brinch DS. Investigation on possible allergenicity of 19 different commercial enzymes used in the food industry. *Food Chem Toxicol.* 2006 Nov;44(11):1909-15.

Biro FM, Galvez MP, Greenspan LC, Succop PA, Vangeepuram N, Pinney SM, Teitelbaum S, Windham GC, Kushi LH, Wolff MS. Pubertal assessment method and baseline characteristics in a mixed longitudinal study of girls. *Pediatrics.* 2010 Sep;126(3):e583-90.

Bischoff SC. Food allergy and eosinophilic gastroenteritis and colitis. *Curr Opin Allergy Clin Immunol.* 2010 Jun;10(3):238-45.

Bjarnason I, MacPherson A, Hollander D. Intestinal permeability: an overview. *Gastroenterology.* 1995 May;108(5):1566-81.

Bjarnason I, Smethurst P, Clark P, Menzies I, Levi J, Peters T. Effect of prostaglandin on indomethacin-induced increased intestinal permeability in man. *Scand J Gastroenterol Suppl.* 1989;164:97-102.

Bjornsson E, Janson C, Plaschke P, Norrman E, Sjoberg O (1996) Prevalence of sensitization to food allergies in adult Swedes. *Ann Allergy Asthma Immunol.* 77: 327–332.

Blázquez AB, Mayer L, Berin MC. Thymic Stromal Lymphopoietin Is Required for Gastrointestinal Allergy but Not Oral Tolerance. *Gastroenterology.* 2010 Jun 23.

Boccafogli A, Vicentini L, Camerani A, Cogliati P, D'Ambrosi A, Scolozzi R. Adverse food reactions in patients with grass pollen allergic respiratory disease. *Ann Allergy.* 1994 Oct;73(4):301-8.

Bode C, Bode JC. Effect of alcohol consumption on the gut. *Best Pract Res Clin Gastroenterol.* 2003 Aug;17(4):575-92.

Bodinier M, Legoux MA, Pineau F, Triballeau S, Segain JP, Brossard C, Denery-Papini S. Intestinal translocation capabilities of wheat allergens using the Caco-2 cell line. *J Agric Food Chem.* 2007 May 30;55(11):4576-83.

Boehm, G., Lidestri, M., Casetta, P., Jelinek, J., Negretti, F., Stahl, B., Martini, A. (2002) Supplementation of a bovine milk formula with an oligosaccharide mixture increases counts of faecal bifidobacteria in preterm infants. *Arch Dis Child Fetal Neonatal Ed.* 86: F178-F181

Bolhaar ST, Tiemessen MM, Zuidmeer L, van Leeuwen A, Hoffmann-Sommergruber K, Bruijnzeel-Koomen CA, Taams LS, Knol EF, van Hoffen E, van Ree R, Knulst AC. Efficacy of birch-pollen immunotherapy on cross-reactive food allergy confirmed by skin tests and double-blind food challenges. *Clin Exp Allergy.* 2004 May;34(5):761-9.

Bolleddula J, Goldfarb J, Wang R, Sampson H, Li XM. Synergistic Modulation Of Eotaxin And Il-4 Secretion By Constituents Of An Anti-asthma Herbal Formula (ASHMI) In Vitro. *J Allergy Clin Immunol.* 2007;119:S172.

Bongaerts GP, Severijnen RS. Preventive and curative effects of probiotics in atopic patients. *Med Hypotheses.* 2005;64(6):1089-92.

Bongartz D, Hesse A. Selective extraction of quercetrin in vegetable drugs and urine by off-line coupling of boronic acid affinity chromatography and high-performance liquid chromatography. *J Chromatogr B Biomed Appl.* 1995 Nov 17;673(2):223-30.

Borchers AT, Hackman RM, Keen CL, Stern JS, Gershwin ME. Complementary medicine: a review of immunomodulatory effects of Chinese herbal medicines. *Am J Clin Nutr.* 1997 Dec;66(6):1303-12.

Borchert VE, Czyborra P, Fetscher C, Goepel M, Michel MC. Extracts from Rhois aromatica and Solidaginis virgaurea inhibit rat and human bladder contraction. *Naunyn Schmiedebergs Arch Pharmacol.* 2004 Mar;369(3):281-6.

Böttcher MF, Jenmalm MC, Voor T, Julge K, Holt PG, Björkstén B. Cytokine responses to allergens during the first 2 years of life in Estonian and Swedish children. *Clin Exp Allergy.* 2006 May;36(5):619-28.

Bouchez-Mahiout I, Pecquet C, Kerre S, Snégaroff J, Raison-Peyron N, Laurière M. High molecular weight entities in industrial wheat protein hydrolysates are immunoreactive with IgE from allergic patients. *J Agric Food Chem.* 2010 Apr 14;58(7):4207-15.

Boverhof DR, Gollapudi BB, Hotchkiss JA, Osterloh-Quiroz M, Woolhiser MR. A draining lymph node assay (DLNA) for assessing the sensitizing potential of proteins. *Toxicol Lett.* 2010 Mar 15;193(2):144-51.

Boyce JA, Assa'ad A, Burks AW, Jones SM, Sampson HA, Wood RA, Plaut M, Cooper SF, Fenton MJ. Guidelines for the Diagnosis and Management of Food Allergy in the United State. *Natl Instit of Health.* 2010 Dec. NIH Publ No. 11-7700.

Bradette-Hébert ME, Legault J, Lavoie S, Pichette A. A new labdane diterpene from the flowers of Solidago canadensis. *Chem Pharm Bull.* 2008 Jan;56(1):82-4.

Brandtzaeg P. Food allergy: separating the science from the mythology. *Nat Rev Gastroenterol Hepatol.* 2010 Jul;7(7):380-400.

Breuer K, Heratizadeh A, Wulf A, Baumann U, Constien A, Tetau D, Kapp A, Werfel T. Late eczematous reactions to food in children with atopic dermatitis. *Clin Exp Allergy.* 2004 May;34(5):817-24.

Brewster DR, Manary MJ, Menzies IS, Henry RL, O'Loughlin EV. Comparison of milk and maize based diets in kwashiorkor. *Arch Dis Child.* 1997 Mar;76(3):242-8.

Brighenti F, Valtueña S, Pellegrini N, Ardigò D, Del Rio D, Salvatore S, Piatti P, Serafini M, Zavaroni I. Total antioxidant capacity of the diet is inversely and independently related to plasma concentration of high-sensitivity C-reactive protein in adult Italian subjects. *Br J Nutr.* 2005 May;93(5):619-25.

Brody J. *Jane Brody's Nutrition Book.* New York: WW Norton, 1981.

Brostoff J, Gamlin L, Brostoff J. *Food Allergies and Food Intolerance: The Complete Guide to Their Identification and Treatment.* Rochester, VT: Healing Arts, 2000.

Brownstein D. *Salt: Your Way to Health.* West Bloomfield, MI: Medical Alternatives, 2006.

Brown-Whitehorn TF, Spergel JM. The link between allergies and eosinophilic esophagitis: implications for management strategies. *Expert Rev Clin Immunol.* 2010 Jan;6(1):101-9.

Bublin M, Pfister M, Radauer C, Oberhuber C, Bulley S, Dewitt AM, Lidholm J, Reese G, Vieths S, Breiteneder H, Hoffmann-Sommergruber K, Ballmer-Weber BK. Component-resolved diagnosis of kiwifruit allergy with purified natural and recombinant kiwifruit allergens. *J Allergy Clin Immunol.* 2010 Mar;125(3):687-94, 694.e1.

Buchanan AD, Green TD, Jones SM, Scurlock AM, Christie L, Althage KA, Steele PH, Pons L, Helm RM, Lee LA, Burks AW. Egg oral immunotherapy in nonanaphylactic children with egg allergy. *J Allergy Clin Immunol.* 2007 Jan;119(1):199-205.

Bucher X, Pichler WJ, Dahinden CA, Helbling A. Effect of tree pollen specific, subcutaneous immunotherapy on the oral allergy syndrome to apple and hazelnut. *Allergy.* 2004 Dec;59(12):1272-6.

Budzianowski J. Coumarins, caffeoyltartaric acids and their artifactual methyl esters from Taraxacum officinale leaves. *Planta Med.* 1997 Jun;63(3):288.

Bueno L. Protease activated receptor 2: a new target for IBS treatment. *Eur Rev Med Pharmacol Sci.* 2008 Aug;12 Suppl 1:95-102.

Bundy R, Walker AF, Middleton RW, Booth J. Turmeric extract may improve irritable bowel syndrome symptomology in otherwise healthy adults: a pilot study. *J Altern Complement Med.* 2004 Dec;10(6):1015-8.

Burdge GC, Jones AE, Wootton SA. Eicosapentaenoic and docosapentaenoic acids are the principal products of alpha-linolenic acid metabolism in young men. *B J Nutr.* 2002 Oct;88(4):355-63.

Buret AG. How stress induces intestinal hypersensitivity. *Am J Pathol.* 2006 Jan;168(1):3-5.

Burits M, Asres K, Bucar F. The antioxidant activity of the essential oils of Artemisia afra, Artemisia abyssinica and Juniperus procera. *Phytother Res.* 2001 Mar;15(2):103-8.

Burks AW, James JM, Hiegel A, Wilson G, Wheeler JG, Jones SM, Zuerlein N. Atopic dermatitis and food hypersensitivity reactions. *J Pediatr.* 1998;132(1):132-6.

Burks W, Jones SM, Berseth CL, Harris C, Sampson HA, Scalabrin DM. Hypoallergenicity and effects on growth and tolerance of a new amino acid-based formula with docosahexaenoic acid and arachidonic acid. *J Pediatr.* 2008 Aug;153(2):266-71.

Burney PG, Luczynska C, Chinn S, Jarvis D (1994) The European Community Respiratory Health Survey. *Eur Respir J.* 7: 954–960.

Busse PJ, Wen MC, Huang CK, Srivastava K, Zhang TF, Schofield B, Sampson HA, Li XM. Therapeutic effects of the Chinese herbal formula, MSSM-03d, on persistent airway hyperreactivity and airway remodeling. *J Allergy Clin Immunol.* 2004;113:S220.

Butani L, Afshinnik A, Johnson J, Javaheri D, Peck S, German JB, Perez RV. Amelioration of tacrolimus-induced nephrotoxicity in rats using juniper oil. *Transplantation.* 2003 Jul 27;76(2):306-11.

Butkus SN, Mahan LK. Food allergies: immunological reactions to food. *J Am Diet Assoc.* 1986 May;86(5):601-8.

Byrne AM, Malka-Rais J, Burks AW, Fleischer DM. How do we know when peanut and tree nut allergy have resolved, and how do we keep it resolved? *Clin Exp Allergy.* 2010 Sep;40(9):1303-11.

Cabanillas B, Pedrosa MM, Rodríguez J, González A, Muzquiz M, Cuadrado C, Crespo JF, Burbano C. Effects of enzymatic hydrolysis on lentil allergenicity. *Mol Nutr Food Res.* 2010 Mar 19.

Caffarelli C, Coscia A, Baldi F, Borghi A, Capra L, Cazzato S, Migliozzi L, Pecorari L, Valenti A, Cavagni G. Characterization of irritable bowel syndrome and constipation in children with allergic diseases. *Eur J Pediatr.* 2007 Dec;166(12):1245-52.

Caffarelli C, Petroccione T. False-negative food challenges in children with suspected food allergy. *Lancet.* 2001 Dec 1;358(9296):1871-2.

Cahn J, Borzeix MG. Administration of procyanidolic oligomers in rats. Observed effects on changes in the permeability of the blood-brain barrier. *Sem Hop.* 1983 Jul 7;59(27-28):2031-4.

Calder PC. Dietary modification of inflammation with lipids. *Proc Nutr Soc.* 2002 Aug;61(3):345-58.

Calvani M, Giorgio V, Miceli Sopo S. Specific oral tolerance induction for food. A systematic review. *Eur Ann Allergy Clin Immunol.* 2010 Feb;42(1):11-9.

Caminiti L, Passalacqua G, Barberi S, Vita D, Barberio G, De Luca R, Pajno GB. A new protocol for specific oral tolerance induction in children with IgE-mediated cow's milk allergy. *Allergy Asthma Proc.* 2009 Jul-Aug;30(4):443-8.

Campbell TC, Campbell TM. *The China Study.* Dallas, TX: Benbella Books, 2006.

Canani RB, Ruotolo S, Auricchio L, Caldore M, Porcaro F, Manguso F, Terrin G, Troncone R. Diagnostic accuracy of the atopy patch test in children with food allergy-related gastrointestinal symptoms. *Allergy.* 2007 Jul;62(7):738-43.

Canonica GW, Passalacqua G. Noninjection routes for immunotherapy. *J Allergy Clin Immunol.* 2003 Mar;111(3):437-48; quiz 449.

Cantani A, Micera M. Natural history of cow's milk allergy. An eight-year follow-up study in 115 atopic children. *Eur Rev Med Pharmacol Sci.* 2004 Jul-Aug;8(4):153-64.

Cantani A, Micera M. The prick by prick test is safe and reliable in 58 children with atopic dermatitis and food allergy. *Eur Rev Med Pharmacol Sci.* 2006 May-Jun;10(3):115-20.

Cao G, Alessio HM, Cutler RG. Oxygen-radical absorbance capacity assay for antioxidants. *Free Radic Biol Med.* 1993 Mar;14(3):303-11.

Cao G, Shukitt-Hale B, Bickford PC, Joseph JA, McEwen J, Prior RL. Hyperoxia-induced changes in antioxidant capacity and the effect of dietary antioxidants. *J Appl Physiol.* 1999 Jun;86(6):1817-22.

Cara L, Dubois C, Borel P, Armand M, Senft M, Portugal H, Pauli AM, Bernard PM, Lairon D. Effects of oat bran, rice bran, wheat fiber, and wheat germ on postprandial lipemia in healthy adults. *Am J Clin Nutr.* 1992 Jan;55(1):81-8.

Caramia G. The essential fatty acids omega-6 and omega-3: from their discovery to their use in therapy. *Minerva Pediatr.* 2008 Apr;60(2):219-33.

Carroccio A, Cavataio F, Montalto G, D'Amico D, Alabrese L, Iacono G. Intolerance to hydrolysed cow's milk proteins in infants: clinical characteristics and dietary treatment. *Clin Exp Allergy.* 2000 Nov;30(11):1597-603.

Carroll D. *The Complete Book of Natural Medicines.* New York: Summit, 1980.

Caruso M, Frasca G, Di Giuseppe PL, Pennisi A, Tringali G, Bonina FP. Effects of a new nutraceutical ingredient on allergen-induced sulphidoleukotrienes production and CD63 expression in allergic subjects. *Int Immunopharmacol.* 2008 Dec 20;8(13-14):1781-6.

Cataldo F, Accomando S, Fragapane ML, Montaperto D; SIGENP and GLNBI Working Groups on Food Intolerances. Are food intolerances and allergies increasing in immigrant children coming from developing countries? *Pediatr Allergy Immunol.* 2006 Aug;17(5):364-9.

Cats A, Kuipers EJ, Bosschaert MA, Pot RG, Vandenbroucke-Grauls CM, Kusters JG. Effect of frequent consumption of a Lactobacillus casei-containing milk drink in Helicobacter pylori-colonized subjects. *Aliment Pharmacol Ther.* 2003 Feb;17(3):429-35.

Cavaleiro C, Pinto E, Gonçalves MJ, Salgueiro L. Antifungal activity of Juniperus essential oils against dermatophyte, Aspergillus and Candida strains. *J Appl Microbiol.* 2006 Jun;100(6):1333-8.

Celakovská J, Vaněčková J, Ettlerová K, Ettler K, Bukac J. The role of atopy patch test in diagnosis of food allergy in atopic eczema/dermatitis syndrom in patients over 14 years of age. *Acta Medica (Hradec Kralove).* 2010;53(2):101-8.

Celikel S, Karakaya G, Yurtsever N, Sorkun K, Kalyoncu AF. Bee and bee products allergy in Turkish beekeepers: determination of risk factors for systemic reactions. *Allergol Immunopathol (Madr).* 2006 Sep-Oct;34(5):180-4.

Cereijido M, Contreras RG, Flores-Benítez D, Flores-Maldonado C, Larre I, Ruiz A, Shoshani L. New diseases derived or associated with the tight junction. *Arch Med Res.* 2007 Jul;38(5):465-78.

Chafen JJ, Newberry SJ, Riedl MA, Bravata DM, Maglione M, Suttorp MJ, Sundaram V, Paige NM, Towfigh A, Hulley BJ, Shekelle PG. Diagnosing and managing common food allergies: a systematic review. *JAMA.* 2010 May 12;303(18):1848-56.

Chahine BG, Bahna SL. The role of the gut mucosal immunity in the development of tolerance versus development of allergy to food. *Curr Opin Allergy Clin Immunol.* 2010 Aug;10(4):394-9.

Chaitow L, Trenev N. *ProBiotics.* New York: Thorsons, 1990.

Chaitow L. *Conquer Pain the Natural Way.* San Francisco: Chronicle Books, 2002.

Chakŭrski I, Matev M, Koĭchev A, Angelova I, Stefanov G. Treatment of chronic colitis with an herbal combination of Taraxacum officinale, Hipericum perforatum, Melissa officinaliss, Calendula officinalis and Foeniculum vulgare. *Vutr Boles.* 1981;20(6):51-4.

Chan CK, Kuo ML, Shen JJ, See LC, Chang HH, Huang JL. Ding Chuan Tang, a Chinese herb decoction, could improve airway hyper-responsiveness in stabilized asthmatic children: a randomized, double-blind clinical trial. *Pediatr Allergy Immunol.* 2006;17:316–22.

Chandra RK. Prospective studies of the effect of breast feeding on incidence of infection and allergy. *Acta Paediatr Scand.* 1979 Sep;68(5):691-4.

Chaney M, Ross M. *Nutrition.* New York: Houghton Mifflin, 1971.

Chang CI, Chen WC, Shao YY, Yeh GR, Yang NS, Chiang W, Kuo YH. A new labdane-type diterpene from the bark of Juniperus chinensis Linn. *Nat Prod Res.* 2008;22(13):1158-62.

Chang TT, Huang CC, Hsu CH. Clinical evaluation of the Chinese herbal medicine formula STA-1 in the treatment of allergic asthma. *Phytother Res.* 2006;20:342–7.

Chang TT, Huang CC, Hsu CH. Inhibition of mite-induced immunoglobulin E synthesis, airway inflammation, and hyperreactivity by herbal medicine STA-1. *Immunopharmacol Immunotoxicol.* 2006;28:683–95.

Chao A, Thun MJ, Connell CJ, McCullough ML, Jacobs EJ, Flanders WD, Rodriguez C, Sinha R, Calle EE. Meat consumption and risk of colorectal cancer. *JAMA.* 2005 Jan 12;293(2):172-82.

Chapat L, Chemin K, Dubois B, Bourdet-Sicard R, Kaiserlian D. Lactobacillus casei reduces CD8+ T cell-mediated skin inflammation. *Eur J Immunol.* 2004 Sep;34(9):2520-8.

Characterization and quantitation of Antioxidant Constituents of Sweet Pepper (Capsicum annuum - Cayenne). *J Agric Food Chem.* 2004 Jun 16;52(12):3861-9.

Charles K. Food allergies are becoming more common. *N.Y. Daily News.* 2008. May 20.

Chatzi L, Apostolaki G, Bibakis I, Skypala I, Bibaki-Liakou V, Tzanakis N, Kogevinas M, Cullinan P. Protective effect of fruits, vegetables and the Mediterranean diet on asthma and allergies among children in Crete. *Thorax.* 2007 Aug;62(8):677-83.

Chatzi L, Torrent M, Romieu I, Garcia-Esteban R, Ferrer C, Vioque J, Kogevinas M, Sunyer J. Mediterranean diet in pregnancy is protective for wheeze and atopy in childhood. *Thorax.* 2008 Jun;63(6):507-13.

Chavali SR, Weeks CE, Zhong WW, Forse RA. Increased production of TNF-alpha and decreased levels of dienoic eicosanoids, IL-6 and IL-10 in mice fed menhaden oil and juniper oil diets in response to an intraperitoneal lethal dose of LPS. *Prostaglandins Leukot Essent Fatty Acids.* 1998 Aug;59(2):89-93.

Chehade M, Aceves SS. Food allergy and eosinophilic esophagitis. *Curr Opin Allergy Clin Immunol.* 2010 Jun;10(3):231-7.

Chen HJ, Shih CK, Hsu HY, Chiang W. Mast cell-dependent allergic responses are inhibited by ethanolic extract of adlay (Coix lachryma-jobi L. var. ma-yuen Stapf) testa. *J Agric Food Chem.* 2010 Feb 24;58(4):2596-601.

Cheney G, Waxler SH, Miller IJ. Vitamin U therapy of peptic ulcer; experience at San Quentin Prison. *Calif Med.* 1956 Jan;84(1):39-42.

Chevrier MR, Ryan AE, Lee DY, Zhongze M, Wu-Yan Z, Via CS. Boswellia carterii extract inhibits TH1 cytokines and promotes TH2 cytokines in vitro. *Clin Diagn Lab Immunol.* 2005 May;12(5):575-80.

Chilton FH, Rudel LL, Parks JS, Arm JP, Seeds MC. Mechanisms by which botanical lipids affect inflammatory disorders. *Am J Clin Nutr.* 2008 Feb;87(2):498S-503S.

Chilton FH, Tucker L. *Win the War Within.* New York: Rodale, 2006.

Chin A Paw MJ, de Jong N, Pallast EG, Kloek GC, Schouten EG, Kok FJ. Immunity in frail elderly: a randomized controlled trial of exercise and enriched foods. *Med Sci Sports Exerc.* 2000 Dec;32(12):2005-11.

Choi SY, Sohn JH, Lee YW, Lee EK, Hong CS, Park JW. Characterization of buckwheat 19-kD allergen and its application for diagnosing clinical reactivity. *Int Arch Allergy Immunol.* 2007;144(4):267-74.

Choi SZ, Choi SU, Lee KR. Phytochemical constituents of the aerial parts from Solidago virga-aurea var. gigantea. *Arch Pharm Res.* 2004 Feb;27(2):164-8.

Chopra RN, Nayar SL, Chopra IC, eds. *Glossary of Indian Medicinal plants.* New Delhi: CSIR, 1956.

Christopher J. *School of Natural Healing.* Springville UT: Christopher Publ, 1976.

Chrubasik S, Pollak S. Pain management with herbal antirheumatic drugs. *Wien Med Wochenschr.* 2002;152(7-8):198-203.

Chu YF, Liu RH. Cranberries inhibit LDL oxidation and induce LDL receptor expression in hepatocytes. *Life Sci.* 2005;77(15):1892-1901. 27.

Chung SY, Butts CL, Maleki SJ, Champagne ET (2003) Linking peanut allergenicity to the processes of maturation, curing, and roasting. *J Agric Food Chem.* 51: 4273–4277.

Cingi C, Demirbas D, Songu M. Allergic rhinitis caused by food allergies. *Eur Arch Otorhinolaryngol.* 2010 Sep;267(9):1327-35.

REFERENCES AND BIBLIOGRAPHY

Clark AT, Islam S, King Y, Deighton J, Anagnostou K, Ewan PW. Successful oral tolerance induction in severe peanut allergy. *Allergy.* 2009 Aug;64(8):1218-20.

Clark AT, Mangat JS, Tay SS, King Y, Monk CJ, White PA, Ewan PW. Facial thermography is a sensitive and specific method for assessing food challenge outcome. *Allergy.* 2007 Jul;62(7):744-9.

Cobo Sanz JM, Mateos JA, Muñoz Conejo A. Effect of Lactobacillus casei on the incidence of infectious conditions in children. *Nutr Hosp.* 2006 Jul-Aug;21(4):547-51.

Codispoti CD, Levin L, LeMasters GK, Ryan P, Reponen T, Villareal M, Burkle J, Stanforth S, Lockey JE, Khurana Hershey GK, Bernstein DI. Breast-feeding, aeroallergen sensitization, and environmental exposures during infancy are determinants of childhood allergic rhinitis. *J Allergy Clin Immunol.* 2010 May;125(5):1054-1060.e1.

Cohen A, Goldberg M, Levy B, Leshno M, Katz Y. Sesame food allergy and sensitization in children: the natural history and long-term follow-up. *Pediatr Allergy Immunol.* 2007 May;18(3):217-23.

Conquer JA, Holub BJ. Dietary docosahexaenoic acid as a source of eicosapentaenoic acid in vegetarians and omnivores. *Lipids.* 1997 Mar;32(3):341-5.

Coombs RR, McLaughlan P. Allergenicity of food proteins and its possible modification. Ann Allergy. 1984 Dec;53(6 Pt 2):592-6.

Cooper GS, Miller FW, Germolec DR: Occupational exposures and autoimmune diseases. *Int Immunopharm* 2002, 2:303-313.

Cooper K. *The Aerobics Program for Total Well-Being.* New York: Evans, 1980.

Corbe C, Boissin JP, Siou A. Light vision and chorioretinal circulation. Study of the effect of procyanidolic oligomers (Endotelon). *J Fr Ophtalmol.* 1988;11(5):453-60.

Couzy F, Kastenmayer P, Vigo M, Clough J, Munoz-Box R, Barclay DV. Calcium bioavailability from a calcium- and sulfate-rich mineral water, compared with milk, in young adult women. *Am J Clin Nutr.* 1995 Dec;62(6):1239-44.

Crescente M, Jessen G, Momi S, Höltje HD, Gresele P, Cerletti C, de Gaetano G. Interactions of gallic acid, resveratrol, quercetin and aspirin at the platelet cyclooxygenase-1 level. Functional and modelling studies. *Thromb Haemost.* 2009 Aug;102(2):336-46.

Cuesta-Herranz J, Barber D, Blanco C, Cistero-Bahíma A, Crespo JF, Fernández-Rivas M, Fernández-Sánchez J, Florido JF, Ibáñez MD, Rodríguez R, Salcedo G, Garcia BE, Lombardero M, Quiralte J, Rodriguez J, Sánchez-Monge R, Vereda A, Villalba M, Alonso Díaz de Durana MD, Basagaña M, Carrillo T, Fernández-Nieto M, Tabar AI. Differences among Pollen-Allergic Patients with and without Plant Food Allergy. *Int Arch Allergy Immunol.* 2010 Apr 23;153(2):182-192.

Cummings M. *Human Heredity: Principles and Issues.* St. Paul, MN: West, 1988.

D'Auria E, Sala M, Lodi F, Radaelli G, Riva E, Giovannini M. Nutritional value of a rice-hydrolysate formula in infants with cows' milk protein allergy: a randomized pilot study. *J Int Med Res.* 2003 May-Jun;31(3):215-22.

Davies G. *Timetables of Medicine.* New York: Black Dog & Leventhal, 2000.

Davies GR, Wilkie ME, Rampton DS. Effects of metronidazole and misoprostol on indomethacin-induced changes in intestinal permeability. *Dig Dis Sci.* 1993 Mar;38(3):417-25.

Davin JC, Forget P, Mahieu PR. Increased intestinal permeability to (51 Cr) EDTA is correlated with IgA immune complex-plasma levels in children with IgA-associated nephropathies. *Acta Paediatr Scand.* 1988 Jan;77(1):118-24.

de Boissieu D, Dupont C, Badoual J. Allergy to nondairy proteins in mother's milk as assessed by intestinal permeability tests. *Allergy.* 1994 Dec;49(10):882-4.

de Boissieu D, Matarazzo P, Rocchiccioli F, Dupont C. Multiple food allergy: a possible diagnosis in breast-fed infants. *Acta Paediatr.* 1997 Oct;86(10):1042-6.

De Knop KJ, Hagendorens MM, Bridts CH, Stevens WJ, Ebo DG. Macadamia nut allergy: 2 case reports and a review of the literature. *Acta Clin Belg.* 2010 Mar-Apr;65(2):129-32.

De Lucca AJ, Bland JM, Vigo CB, Cushion M, Selitrennikoff CP, Peter J, Walsh TJ. CAY-I, a fungicidal saponin from Capsicum sp. fruit. *Med Mycol.* 2002 Apr;40(2):131-7.

de Martino M, Novembre E, Galli L, de Marco A, Botarelli P, Marano E, Vierucci A. Allergy to different fish species in cod-allergic children: in vivo and in vitro studies. *J Allergy Clin Immunol.* 1990;86:909-914.

De Smet PA. Herbal remedies. *N Engl J Med.* 2002;347:2046–2056.

Dean C. *Death by Modern Medicine.* Belleville, ON: Matrix Verite-Media, 2005.

del Giudice MM, Leonardi S, Maiello N, Brunese FP. Food allergy and probiotics in childhood. *J Clin Gastroenterol.* 2010 Sep;44 Suppl 1:S22-5.

DeMeo MT, Mutlu EA, Keshavarzian A, Tobin MC. Intestinal permeation and gastrointestinal disease. *J Clin Gastroenterol.* 2002 Apr;34(4):385-96.

Demidov LV, Manziuk LV, Kharkevitch GY, Pirogova NA, Artamonova EV. Adjuvant fermented wheat germ extract (Avemar) nutraceutical improves survival of high-risk skin melanoma patients: a randomized, pilot, phase II clinical study with a 7-year follow-up. Cancer Biother Radiopharm. 2008 Aug;23(4):477-82. doi:10.1089/cbr.2008.0486. Erratum in: Cancer Biother Radiopharm. 2008 Oct;23(5):669.

Den Hond E, Hiele M, Peeters M, Ghoos Y, Rutgeerts P. Effect of long-term oral glutamine supplements on small intestinal permeability in patients with Crohn's disease. JPEN J Parenter Enteral Nutr. 1999 Jan-Feb;23(1):7-11.

Dengate S, Ruben A. Controlled trial of cumulative behavioural effects of a common bread preservative. J Paediatr Child Health. 2002 Aug;38(4):373-6.

Derebery MJ, Berliner KI. Allergy and its relation to Meniere's disease. Otolaryngol Clin North Am. 2010 Oct;43(5):1047-58.

Desjeux JF, Heyman M. Milk proteins, cytokines and intestinal epithelial functions in children. Acta Paediatr Jpn. 1994 Oct;36(5):592-6.

DesRoches A, Infante-Rivard C, Paradis L, Paradis J, Haddad E. Peanut allergy: is maternal transmission of antigens during pregnancy and breastfeeding a risk factor? J Investig Allergol Clin Immunol. 2010;20(4):289-94.

Deutsche Gesellschaft für Ernährung. Drink distilled water? Med. Mo. Pharm. 1993;16:146.

Devaraj TL. Speaking of Ayurvedic Remedies for Common Diseases. New Delhi: Sterling, 1985.

Diesner SC, Untersmayr E, Pietschmann P, Jensen-Jarolim E. Food Allergy: Only a Pediatric Disease? Gerontology. 2010 Jan 29.

Diğrak M, Ilçim A, Hakki Alma M. Antimicrobial activities of several parts of Pinus brutia, Juniperus oxy-cedrus, Abies cilicia, Cedrus libani and Pinus nigra. Phytother Res. 1999 Nov;13(7):584-7.

Din FV, Theodoratou E, Farrington SM, Tenesa A, Barnetson RA, Cetnarskyj R, Stark L, Porteous ME, Campbell H, Dunlop MG. Effect of aspirin and NSAIDs on risk and survival from colorectal cancer. Gut. 2010 Dec;59(12):1670-9.

Diop L, Guillou S, Durand H. Probiotic food supplement reduces stress-induced gastrointestinal symptoms in volunteers: a double-blind, placebo-controlled, randomized trial. Nutr Res. 2008 Jan;28(1):1-5.

Dona A, Arvanitoyannis IS. Health risks of genetically modified foods. Crit Rev Food Sci Nutr. 2009 Feb;49(2):164-75.

Donato F, Monarca S, Premi S., and Gelatti, U. Drinking water hardness and chronic degenerative diseases. Part III. Tumors, urolithiasis, fetal malformations, deterioration of the cognitive function in the aged and atopic eczema. Ann. Ig. 2003;15:57-70.

Dooley, M.A. and Hogan S.L. Environmental epidemiology and risk factors for autoimmune disease. Curr Opin Rheum. 2003;15(2):99-103.

D'Orazio N, Ficoneri C, Riccioni G, Conti P, Theoharides TC, Bollea MR. Conjugated linoleic acid: a functional food? Int J Immunopathol Pharmacol. 2003 Sep-Dec;16(3):215-20.

Dotolo Institute. The Study of Colon Hydrotherapy. Pinellas Park, FL: Dotolo, 2003.

Drouault-Holowacz S, Bieuvelet S, Burckel A, Cazaubiel M, Dray X, Marteau P. A double blind randomized controlled trial of a probiotic combination in 100 patients with irritable bowel syndrome. Gastroenterol Clin Biol. 2008 Feb;32(2):147-52.

Ducrotté P. Irritable bowel syndrome: from the gut to the brain-gut. Gastroenterol Clin Biol. 2009 Aug-Sep;33(8-9):703-12.

Duke J. The Green Pharmacy. New York: St. Martins, 1997.

Dunstan JA, Hale J, Breckler L, Lehmann H, Weston S, Richmond P, Prescott SL. Atopic dermatitis in young children is associated with impaired interleukin-10 and interferon-gamma responses to allergens, vaccines and colonizing skin and gut bacteria. Clin Exp Allergy. 2005 Oct;35(10):1309-17.

Dunstan JA, Roper J, Mitoulas L, Hartmann PE, Simmer K, Prescott SL. The effect of supplementation with fish oil during pregnancy on breast milk immunoglobulin A, soluble CD14, cytokine levels and fatty acid composition. Clin Exp Allergy. 2004 Aug;34(8):1237-42.

Dupont C, Barau E, Molkhou P, Raynaud F, Barbet JP, Dehennin L. Food-induced alterations of intestinal permeability in children with cow's milk-sensitive enteropathy and atopic dermatitis. J Pediatr Gastroen-terol Nutr. 1989 May;8(4):459-65.

Dupont C, Barau E, Molkhou P. Intestinal permeability disorders in children. Allerg Immunol (Paris). 1991 Mar;23(3):95-103.

Dupont C, Barau E. Diagnosis of food allergy in children. Ann Pediatr (Paris). 1992 Jan;39(1):5-12.

Dupont C, Soulaines P, Lapillonne A, Donne N, Kalach N, Benhamou P. Atopy patch test for early diagno-sis of cow's milk allergy in preterm infants. J Pediatr Gastroenterol Nutr. 2010 Apr;50(4):463-4.

Dupuy P, Cassé M, André F, Dhivert-Donnadieu H, Pinton J, Hernandez-Pion C. Low-salt water reduces intestinal permeability in atopic patients. Dermatology. 1999;198(2):153-5.

Duran-Tauleria E, Vignati G, Guedan MJ, Petersson CJ. The utility of specific immunoglobulin E measure-ments in primary care. Allergy. 2004 Aug;59 Suppl 78:35-41.

D'Urbano LE, Pellegrino K, Artesani MC, Donnanno S, Luciano R, Riccardi C, Tozzi AE, Ravà L, De Benedetti F, Cavagni G. Performance of a component-based allergen-microarray in the diagnosis of cow's milk and hen's egg allergy. *Clin Exp Allergy.* 2010 Jul 13.

Duwiejua M, Zeitlin IJ, Waterman PG, Chapman J, Mhango GJ, Provan GJ. Anti-inflammatory activity of resins from some species of the plant family Burseraceae. *Planta Med.* 1993 Feb;59(1):12-6.

Dykewicz MS, Lemmon JK, Keaney DL. Comparison of the Multi-Test II and Skintestor Omni allergy skin test devices. *Ann Allergy Asthma Immunol.* 2007 Jun;98(6):559-62.

Eastham EJ, Walker WA. Effect of cow's milk on the gastrointestinal tract: a persistent dilemma for the pediatrician. *Pediatrics.* 1977 Oct;60(4):477-81.

Eaton KK, Howard M, Howard JM. Gut permeability measured by polyethylene glycol absorption in abnormal gut fermentation as compared with food intolerance. *J R Soc Med.* 1995 Feb;88(2):63-6.

Ebers GC, Kukay K, Bulman DE, Sadovnick AD, Rice G, Anderson C, Armstrong H, Cousin K, Bell RB, Hader W, Paty DW, Hashimoto S, Oger J, Duquette P, Warren S, Gray T, O'Connor P, Nath A, Auty A, Metz L, Francis G, Paulseth JE, Murray TJ, Pryse-Phillips W, Nelson R, Freedman M, Brunet D, Bouchard JP, Hinds D, Risch N. A full genome search in multiple sclerosis. *Nat Genet.* 1996 Aug;13(4):472-6.

ECRHS (2002) The European Community Respiratory Health Survey II. *Eur Respir J.* 20: 1071–1079.

Ege MJ, Herzum I, Büchele G, Krauss-Etschmann S, Lauener RP, Roponen M, Hyvärinen A, Vuitton DA, Riedler J, Brunekreef B, Dalphin JC, Braun-Fahrländer C, Pekkanen J, Renz H, von Mutius E; Protection Against Allergy Study in Rural Environments (PASTURE) Study group. Prenatal exposure to a farm environment modifies atopic sensitization at birth. *J Allergy Clin Immunol.* 2008 Aug;122(2):407-12, 412.e1-4.

Eggermont E. Cow's milk protein allergy. *Tijdschr Kindergeneeskd.* 1981 Feb;49(1):16-20.

Ehling S, Hengel M, and Shibamoto T. Formation of acrylamide from lipids. *Adv Exp Med Biol* 2005, 561:223-233.

Ehren J, Morón B, Martin E, Bethune MT, Gray GM, Khosla C. A food-grade enzyme preparation with modest gluten detoxification properties. *PLoS One.* 2009 Jul 21;4(7):e6313.

el-Ghazaly M, Khayyal MT, Okpanyi SN, Arens-Corell M. Study of the anti-inflammatory activity of Populus tremula, Solidago virgaurea and Fraxinus excelsior. *Arzneimittelforschung.* 1992 Mar;42(3):333-6.

El-Ghorab A, Shaaban HA, El-Massry KF, Shibamoto T. Chemical composition of volatile extract and biological activities of volatile and less-volatile extracts of juniper berry (Juniperus drupacea L.) fruit. *J Agric Food Chem.* 2008 Jul 9;56(13):5021-5.

El-Khouly F, Lewis SA, Pons L, Burks AW, Hourihane JO. IgG and IgE avidity characteristics of peanut allergic individuals. *Pediatr Allergy Immunol.* 2007 Nov;18(7):607-13.

Ellingwood F. *American Materia Medica, Therapeutics and Pharmacognosy.* Portland: Eclectic Medical Publ., 1983.

Elliott RB, Harris DP, Hill JP, Bibby NJ, Wasmuth HE. Type I (insulin-dependent) diabetes mellitus and cow milk: casein variant consumption. *Diabetologia.* 1999 Mar;42(3):292-6. Erratum in: Diabetologia 1999 Aug;42(8):1032.

Elwood PC. Epidemiology and trace elements. *Clin Endocrinol Metab.* 1985 Aug;14(3):617-28.

Engel, M.F., Dimethyl sulfoxide in the treatment of scleroderma. *South Med J.* 1972;65:71.

Engler RJ. Alternative and complementary medicine: a source of improved therapies for asthma? A challenge for redefining the specialty? J Allergy Clin Immunol. 2000;106:627–9.

Environmental Working Group. *Human Toxome Project.* 2007. http://www.ewg.org/sites/humantoxome/. Accessed: 2007 Sep.

EPA. *A Brief Guide to Mold, Moisture and Your Home.* Environmental Protection Agency, Office of Air and Radiation/Indoor Environments Division. EPA 2002;402-K-02-003.

Erckenbrecht J, Kienle U, Zöllner L, Wienbeck M. Effects of high dose antacids on bowel motility. *Digestion.* 1982;25(4):244-7.

Ernst E. Frankincense: systematic review. *BMJ.* 2008 Dec 17;337:a2813.

Erwin EA, James HR, Gutekunst HM, Russo JM, Kelleher KJ, Platts-Mills TA. Serum IgE measurement and detection of food allergy in pediatric patients with eosinophilic esophagitis. *Ann Allergy Asthma Immunol.* 2010 Jun;104(6):496-502.

EuroPrevall. *WP 1.1 Birth Cohort Update.* 1st Quarter 2006. Berlin, Germany: Charité University Medical Centre.

Eutamene H, Lamine F, Chabo C, Theodorou V, Rochat F, Bergonzelli GE, Corthésy-Theulaz I, Fioramonti J, Bueno L. Synergy between Lactobacillus paracasei and its bacterial products to counteract stress-induced gut permeability and sensitivity increase in rats. *J Nutr.* 2007 Aug;137(8):1901-7.

Evans P, Forte D, Jacobs C, Fredhoi C, Aitchison E, Hucklebridge F, Clow A. Cortisol secretory activity in older people in relation to positive and negative well-being. *Psychoneuroendocrinology.* 2007 Aug 7

Everhart JE. *Digestive Diseases in the United States.* Darby, PA: Diane Pub, 1994.

Exl BM, Deland U, Secretin MC, Preysch U, Wall M, Shmerling DH. Improved general health status in an unselected infant population following an allergen reduced dietary intervention programme. The ZUFF-study-programme. Part I: Study design and 6-month nutritional behaviour. *Eur J Nutr.* 2000 Jun;39(3):89-102.

FAAN. *Public Comment on 2005 Food Safety Survey: Docket No. 2004N-0516 (2005 FSS).* Fairfax, VA: Food Allergy & Anaphylaxis Network.

Faeste CK, Christians U, Egaas E, Jonscher KR. Characterization of potential allergens in fenugreek (Trigonella foenum-graecum) using patient sera and MS-based proteomic analysis. *J Proteomics.* 2010 May 7;73(7):1321-33.

Faeste CK, Jonscher KR, Sit L, Klawitter J, Lovberg KE, Moen LH. Differentiating cross-reacting allergens in the immunological analysis of celery (Apium graveolens) by mass spectrometry. *J AOAC Int.* 2010 Mar-Apr;93(2):451-61.

Fajac I, Frossard N. Neuropeptides of the nasal innervation and allergic rhinitis. *Rev Mal Respir.* 1994;11(4):357-67.

Fälth-Magnusson K, Kjellman NI, Magnusson KE, Sundqvist T. Intestinal permeability in healthy and allergic children before and after sodium-cromoglycate treatment assessed with different-sized poly-ethyleneglycols (PEG 400 and PEG 1000). *Clin Allergy.* 1984 May;14(3):277-86.

Fälth-Magnusson K, Kjellman NI, Odelram H, Sundqvist T, Magnusson KE. Gastrointestinal permeability in children with cow's milk allergy: effect of milk challenge and sodium cromoglycate as assessed with polyethyleneglycols (PEG 400 and PEG 1000). *Clin Allergy.* 1986 Nov;16(6):543-51.

Fan AY, Lao L, Zhang RX, Zhou AN, Wang LB, Moudgil KD, Lee DY, Ma ZZ, Zhang WY, Berman BM. Effects of an acetone extract of Boswellia carterii Birdw. (Burseraceae) gum resin on adjuvant-induced arthritis in lewis rats. *J Ethnopharmacol.* 2005 Oct 3;101(1-3):104-9.

Fanaro S, Marten B, Bagna R, Vigi V, Fabris C, Peña-Quintana, Argüelles F, Scholz-Ahrens KE, Sawatzki G, Zelenka R, Schrezenmeir J, de Vrese M and Bertino E. Galacto-oligosaccharides are bifidogenic and safe at weaning: A double-blind Randomized Multicenter study. *J Pediatr Gastroent Nutr.* 2009 48; 82-88

Fang SP, Tanaka T, Tago F, Okamoto T, Kojima S. Immunomodulatory effects of gyokuheifusan on INF-gamma/IL-4 (Th1/Th2) balance in ovalbumin (OVA)-induced asthma model mice. *Biol Pharm Bull.* 2005;28:829–33.

Fanigliulo L, Comparato G, Aragona G, Cavallaro L, Iori V, Maino M, Cavestro GM, Soliani P, Sianesi M, Franzè A, Di Mario F. Role of gut microflora and probiotic effects in the irritable bowel syndrome. *Acta Biomed.* 2006 Aug;77(2):85-9.

FAO/WHO Expert Committee. *Fats and Oils in Human Nutrition.* Food and Nutrition Paper. 1994;(57).

Farkas E. [Fermented wheat germ extract in the supportive therapy of colorectal cancer]. Orv Hetil. 2005 Sep 11;146(37):1925-31.

Fasano A, Berti I, Gerarduzzi T, Not T, Colletti RB, Drago S, Elitsur Y, Green PH, Guandalini S, Hill ID, Pietzak M, Ventura A, Thorpe M, Kryszak D, Fornaroli F, Wasserman SS, Murray JA, Horvath K. Prevalence of celiac disease in at-risk and not-at-risk groups in the United States: a large multicenter study. *Arch Intern Med.* 2003 Feb 10;163(3):286-92.

Fawell J, Nieuwenhuijsen MJ. Contaminants in drinking water. *Br Med Bull.* 2003;68:199-208.

Felley CP, Corthésy-Theulaz I, Rivero JL, Sipponen P, Kaufmann M, Bauerfeind P, Wiesel PH, Brassart D, Pfeifer A, Blum AL, Michetti P. Favourable effect of an acidified milk (LC-1) on Helicobacter pylori gastritis in man. *Eur J Gastroenterol Hepatol.* 2001 Jan;13(1):25-9.

Fernández-Rivas M, Garrido Fernández S, Nadal JA, Díaz de Durana MD, García BE, González-Mancebo E, Martín S, Barber D, Rico P, Tabar AI. Randomized double-blind, placebo-controlled trial of sublingual immunotherapy with a Pru p 3 quantified peach extract. *Allergy.* 2009 Jun;64(6):876-83.

Fernández-Rivas M, González-Mancebo E, Rodríguez-Pérez R, Benito C, Sánchez-Monge R, Salcedo G, Alonso MD, Rosado A, Tejedor MA, Vila C, Casas ML. Clinically relevant peach allergy is related to peach lipid transfer protein, Pru p 3, in the Spanish population. *J Allergy Clin Immunol.* 2003 Oct;112(4):789-95.

Ferrier L, Berard F, Debrauwer L, Chabo C, Langella P, Bueno L, Fioramonti J. Impairment of the intestinal barrier by ethanol involves enteric microflora and mast cell activation in rodents. *Am J Pathol.* 2006 Apr;168(4):1148-54.

Filipowicz N, Kamiński M, Kurlenda J, Asztemborska M, Ochocka JR. Antibacterial and antifungal activity of juniper berry oil and its selected components. *Phytother Res.* 2003 Mar;17(3):227-31.

Filteau SM, Rollins NC, Coutsoudis A, Sullivan KR, Willumsen JF, Tomkins AM. The effect of antenatal vitamin A and beta-carotene supplementation on gut integrity of infants of HIV-infected South African women. *J Pediatr Gastroenterol Nutr.* 2001 Apr;32(4):464-70.

Finkelman FD, Boyce JA, Vercelli D, Rothenberg ME. Key advances in mechanisms of asthma, allergy, and immunology in 2009. *J Allergy Clin Immunol.* 2010 Feb;125(2):312-8.

REFERENCES AND BIBLIOGRAPHY

Fiocchi A, Restani P, Bernardo L, Martelli A, Ballabio C, D'Auria E, Riva E. Tolerance of heat-treated kiwi by children with kiwifruit allergy. *Pediatr Allergy Immunol.* 2004 Oct;15(5):454-8.

Fiocchi A, Travaini M, D'Auria E, Banderali G, Bernardo L, Riva E. Tolerance to a rice hydrolysate formula in children allergic to cow's milk and soy. *Clin Exp Allergy.* 2003 Nov;33(11):1576-80.

Fiocchi, A; Restani, P; Riva, E; Qualizza, R; Bruni, P; Restelli, AR; Galli, CL. Meat allergy: I. Specific IgE to BSA and OSA in atopic, beef sensitive children. *J Am Coll Nutr.* 1995 14: 239-244.

Flammarion S, Santos C, Guimber D, Jouannic L, Thumerelle C, Gottrand F, Deschildre A. Diet and nutritional status of children with food allergies. *Pediatr Allergy Immunol.* 2010 Jun 14.

Flandrin, J, Montanari M. (eds.). *Food: A Culinary History from Antiquity to the Present.* New York: Penguin Books, 1999.

Fleischer DM, Conover-Walker MK, Christie L, Burks AW, Wood RA. Peanut allergy: recurrence and its management. *J Allergy Clin Immunol.* 2004 Nov;114(5):1195-201.

Flinterman AE, Pasmans SG, den Hartog Jager CF, Hoekstra MO, Bruijnzeel-Koomen CA, Knol EF, van Hoffen E. T cell responses to major peanut allergens in children with and without peanut allergy. *Clin Exp Allergy.* 2010 Apr;40(4):590-7.

Flinterman AE, van Hoffen E, den Hartog Jager CF, Koppelman S, Pasmans SG, Hoekstra MO, Bruijnzeel-Koomen CA, Knulst AC, Knol EF. Children with peanut allergy recognize predominantly Ara h2 and Ara h6, which remains stable over time. *Clin Exp Allergy.* 2007 Aug;37(8):1221-8.

Food allergy continues to increase. *Child Health Alert.* 2010 Jan;28:2.

Forbes EE, Groschwitz K, Abonia JP, Brandt EB, Cohen E, Blanchard C, Ahrens R, Seidu L, McKenzie A, Strait R, Finkelman FD, Foster PS, Matthaei KI, Rothenberg ME, Hogan SP. IL-9- and mast cell-mediated intestinal permeability predisposes to oral antigen hypersensitivity. *J Exp Med.* 2008 Apr 14;205(4):897-913.

Forestier C, Guelon D, Cluytens V, Gillart T, Sirot J, De Champs C. Oral probiotic and prevention of Pseudomonas aeruginosa infections: a randomized, double-blind, placebo-controlled pilot study in intensive care unit patients. *Crit Care.* 2008;12(3):R69.

Forget P, Sodoyez-Goffaux F, Zappitelli A. Permeability of the small intestine to 51Cr EDTA in children with acute gastroenteritis or eczema. *J Pediatr Gastroenterol Nutr.* 1985 Jun;4(3):393-6.

Forget-Dubois N, Boivin M, Dionne G, Pierce T, Tremblay RE, Pérusse D. A longitudinal twin study of the genetic and environmental etiology of maternal hostile-reactive behavior during infancy and toddlerhood. *Infant Behav Dev.* 2007

Foster S, Hobbs C. *Medicinal Plants and Herbs.* Boston: Houghton Mifflin, 2002.

Fox RD, *Algoculture.* Doctorate Disseration, 1983 Jul.

Francavilla R, Lionetti E, Castellaneta SP, Magistà AM, Maurogiovanni G, Bucci N, De Canio A, Indrio F, Cavallo L, Ierardi E, Miniello VL. Inhibition of Helicobacter pylori infection in humans by Lactobacillus reuteri ATCC 55730 and effect on eradication therapy: a pilot study. *Helicobacter.* 2008 Apr;13(2):127-34.

Frawley D, Lad V. *The Yoga of Herbs.* Sante Fe: Lotus Press, 1986.

Fremont S, Moneret-Vautrin DA, Franck P, Morisset M, Croizier A, Codreanu F, Kanny G. Prospective study of sensitization and food allergy to flaxseed in 1317 subjects. *Eur Ann Allergy Clin Immunol.* 2010 Jun;42(3):103-11.

Frias J, Song YS, Martínez-Villaluenga C, González de Mejia E, Vidal-Valverde C. Immunoreactivity and amino acid content of fermented soybean products. *J Agric Food Chem.* 2008 Jan 9;56(1):99-105.

Fu G, Zhong Y, Li C, Li Y, Lin X, Liao B, Tsang EW, Wu K, Huang S. Epigenetic regulation of peanut allergen gene Ara h 3 in developing embryos. *Planta.* 2010 Apr;231(5):1049-60.

Fujimori S, Gudis K, Mitsui K, Seo T, Yonezawa M, Tanaka S, Tatsuguchi A, Sakamoto C. A randomized controlled trial on the efficacy of synbiotic versus probiotic or prebiotic treatment to improve the quality of life in patients with ulcerative colitis. *Nutrition.* 2009 May;25(5):520-5.

Furrie E, Macfarlane S, Kennedy A, Cummings JH, Walsh SV, O'neil DA, Macfarlane GT. Synbiotic therapy (Bifidobacterium longum/Synergy 1) initiates resolution of inflammation in patients with active ulcerative colitis: a randomised controlled pilot trial. *Gut.* 2005 Feb;54(2):242-9.

Furuhjelm C, Warstedt K, Larsson J, Fredriksson M, Böttcher MF, Fälth-Magnusson K, Duchén K. Fish oil supplementation in pregnancy and lactation may decrease the risk of infant allergy. *Acta Paediatr.* 2009 Sep;98(9):1461-7.

Gagnier JJ, DeMelo J, Boon H, Rochon P, Bombardier C. Quality of reporting of randomized controlled trials of herbal medicine interventions. *Am J Med.* 2006;119:1–11.

Galli E, Ciucci A, Cersosimo S, Pagnini C, Avitabile S, Mancino G, Delle Fave G, Corleto VD. Eczema and food allergy in an Italian pediatric cohort: no association with TLR-2 and TLR-4 polymorphisms. *Int J Immunopathol Pharmacol.* 2010 Apr-Jun;23(2):671-5.

Gamboa PM, Cáceres O, Antepara I, Sánchez-Monge R, Ahrazem O, Salcedo G, Barber D, Lombardero M, Sanz ML. Two different profiles of peach allergy in the north of Spain. *Allergy.* 2007 Apr;62(4):408-14.

Gao X, Wang W, Wei S, Li W. Review of pharmacological effects of Glycyrrhiza radix and its bioactive compounds. *Zhongguo Zhong Yao Za Zhi.* 2009 Nov;34(21):2695-700.

Garcia Gomez LJ, Sanchez-Muniz FJ. Review: cardiovascular effect of garlic (Allium sativum). *Arch Latinoam Nutr.* 2000 Sep;50(3):219-29.

Gardner ML. Gastrointestinal absorption of intact proteins. Annu Rev Nutr. 1988;8:329-50.

Gareau MG, Jury J, Yang PC, MacQueen G, Perdue MH. Neonatal maternal separation causes colonic dysfunction in rat pups including impaired host resistance. *Pediatr Res.* 2006 Jan;59(1):83-8.

Garzi A, Messina M, Frati F, Carfagna L, Zagordo L, Belcastro M, Parmiani S, Sensi L, Marcucci F. An extensively hydrolysed cow's milk formula improves clinical symptoms of gastroesophageal reflux and reduces the gastric emptying time in infants. *Allergol Immunopathol (Madr).* 2002 Jan-Feb;30(1):36-41.

Gastrointestinal permeability in food-allergic children. *Nutr Rev.* 1985 Aug;43(8):233-5.

Gawande S, Kale A, Kotwal S. Effect of nutrient mixture and black grapes on the pharmacokinetics of orally administered (-)epigallocatechin-3-gallate from green tea extract: a human study. *Phytother Res.* 2008 Jun;22(6):802-8.

Gawrońska A, Dziechciarz P, Horvath A, Szajewska H. A randomized double-blind placebo-controlled trial of Lactobacillus GG for abdominal pain disorders in children. *Aliment Pharmacol Ther.* 2007 Jan 15;25(2):177-84.

Geha RS, Beiser A, Ren C, Patterson R, Greenberger PA, Grammer LC, Ditto AM, Harris KE, Shaughnessy MA, Yarnold PR, Corren J, Saxon A. Multicenter, double-blind, placebo-controlled, multiple-challenge evaluation of reported reactions to monosodium glutamate. *J Allergy Clin Immunol.* 2000 Nov;106(5):973-80.

Gerez IF, Shek LP, Chng HH, Lee BW. Diagnostic tests for food allergy. Singapore Med J. 2010 Jan;51(1):4-9.

Ghadioungui P. (transl.) *The Ebers Papyrus.* Academy of Scientific Research. Cairo, 1987.

Ghayur MN, Gilani AH. Ginger lowers blood pressure through blockade of voltage-dependent calcium Channels acting as a cardiotonic pump activator in mice, rabbit and dogs. *J Cardiovasc Pharmacol.* 2005 Jan;45(1):74-80.

Giampietro PG, Kjellman NI, Oldaeus G, Wouters-Wesseling W, Businco L. Hypoallergenicity of an extensively hydrolyzed whey formula. *Pediatr Allergy Immunol.* 2001 Apr;12(2):83-6.

Gibbons E. *Stalking the Healthful Herbs.* New York: David McKay, 1966.

Gibson RA. Docosa-hexaenoic acid (DHA) accumulation is regulated by the polyunsaturated fat content of the diet: Is it synthesis or is it incorporation? *Asia Pac J Clin Nutr.* 2004;13(Suppl):S78.

Gibson, G.R., McCartney, A.L., Rastall, R.A. (2005) Prebiotics and resistance to gastrointestinal infections. *Br J of Nutr.* 93, Suppl. 1, pp31-34.

Gill HS, Rutherfurd KJ, Cross ML, Gopal PK. Enhancement of immunity in the elderly by dietary supplementation with the probiotic Bifidobacterium lactis HN019. *Am J Clin Nutr.* 2001 Dec;74(6):833-9.

Gillman A, Douglass JA. What do asthmatics have to fear from food and additive allergy? *Clin Exp Allergy.* 2010 Sep;40(9):1295-302.

Gionchetti P, Rizzello F, Venturi A, Brigidi P, Matteuzzi D, Bazzocchi G, Poggioli G, Miglioli M, Campieri M. Oral bacteriotherapy as maintenance treatment in patients with chronic pouchitis: a double-blind, placebo-controlled trial. *Gastroenterology.* 2000 Aug;119(2):305-9.

Glück U, Gebbers J. Ingested probiotics reduce nasal colonization with pathogenic bacteria (Staphylococcus aureus, Streptococcus pneumoniae, and b-hemolytic streptococci. *Am J. Clin. Nutr.* 2003;77:517-520.

Gohil K, Packer L. Bioflavonoid-Rich Botanical Extracts Show Antioxidant and Gene Regulatory Activity. *Ann N Y Acad Sci.* 2002:957:70-7.

Goldin BR, Adlercreutz H, Dwyer JT, Swenson L, Warram JH, Gorbach SL. Effect of diet on excretion of estrogens in pre- and postmenopausal women. *Cancer Res.* 1981 Sep;41(9 Pt 2):3771-3.

Goldin BR, Adlercreutz H, Gorbach SL, Warram JH, Dwyer JT, Swenson L, Woods MN. Estrogen excretion patterns and plasma levels in vegetarian and omnivorous women. *N Engl J Med.* 1982 Dec 16;307(25):1542-7.

Goldin BR, Swenson L, Dwyer J, Sexton M, Gorbach SL. Effect of diet and Lactobacillus acidophilus supplements on human fecal bacterial enzymes. *J Natl Cancer Inst.* 1980 Feb;64(2):255-61.

Goldstein JL, Aisenberg J, Zakko SF, Berger MF, Dodge WE. Endoscopic ulcer rates in healthy subjects associated with use of aspirin (81 mg q.d.) alone or coadministered with celecoxib or naproxen: a randomized, 1-week trial. *Dig Dis Sci.* 2008 Mar;53(3):647-56.

Golub E. *The Limits of Medicine.* New York: Times Books, 1994.

Gonipeta B, Parvataneni S, Paruchuri P, Gangur V. Long-term characteristics of hazelnut allergy in an adjuvant-free mouse model. *Int Arch Allergy Immunol.* 2010;152(3):219-25.

Gonlachanvit S. Are rice and spicy diet good for functional gastrointestinal disorders? *J Neurogastroenterol Motil.* 2010 Apr;16(2):131-8.

González Alvarez R, Arruzazabala ML. Current views of the mechanism of action of prophylactic antiallergic drugs. *Allergol Immunopathol (Madr).* 1981 Nov-Dec;9(6):501-8.

González-Pérez A, Aponte Z, Vidaurre CF, Rodríguez LA. Anaphylaxis epidemiology in patients with and patients without asthma: a United Kingdom database review. *J Allergy Clin Immunol.* 2010 May;125(5):1098-1104.e1.

Goossens DA, Jonkers DM, Russel MG, Stobberingh EE, Stockbrügger RW. The effect of a probiotic drink with Lactobacillus plantarum 299v on the bacterial composition in faeces and mucosal biopsies of rectum and ascending colon. *Aliment Pharmacol Ther.* 2006 Jan 15;23(2):255-63.

Gordon BR. Patch testing for allergies. *Curr Opin Otolaryngol Head Neck Surg.* 2010 Jun;18(3):191-4.

Gotteland M, Araya M, Pizarro F, Olivares M. Effect of acute copper exposure on gastrointestinal permeability in healthy volunteers. *Dig Dis Sci.* 2001 Sep;46(9):1909-14.

Gotteland M, Cruchet S, Verbeke S. Effect of Lactobacillus ingestion on the gastrointestinal mucosal barrier alterations induced by indometacin in humans. *Aliment Pharmacol Ther.* 2001 Jan;15(1):11-7.

Gotteland M, Poliak L, Cruchet S, Brunser O. Effect of regular ingestion of Saccharomyces boulardii plus inulin or Lactobacillus acidophilus LB in children colonized by Helicobacter pylori. *Acta Paediatr.* 2005 Dec;94(12):1747-51.

Govers MJ, Termont DS, Lapré JA, Kleibeuker JH, Vonk RJ, Van der Meer R. Calcium in milk products precipitates intestinal fatty acids and secondary bile acids and thus inhibits colonic cytotoxicity in humans. *Cancer Res.* 1996 Jul 15;56(14):3270-5.

Grant J, Mahanty S, Khadir A, MacLean JD, Kokoskin E, Yeager B, Joseph L, Diaz J, Gotuzzo E, Mainville N, Ward BJ. Wheat germ supplement reduces cyst and trophozoite passage in people with giardiasis. *Am J Trop Med Hyg.* 2001 Dec;65(6):705-10.

Grant WB, Holick MF. Benefits and requirements of vitamin D for optimal health: a review. *Altern Med Rev.* 2005 Jun;10(2):94-111.

Grant WB. Solar ultraviolet irradiance and cancer incidence and mortality. *Adv Exp Med Biol.* 2008;624:16-30.

Gray H. *Anatomy, Descriptive and Surgical.* 15th Edition. New York: Random House, 1977.

Gray-Davison F. *Ayurvedic Healing.* New York: Keats, 2002.

Griffith HW. *Healing Herbs: The Essential Guide.* Tucson: Fisher Books, 2000.

Grimshaw KE, King RM, Nordlee JA, Hefle SL, Warner JO, Hourihane JO. Presentation of allergen in different food preparations affects the nature of the allergic reaction—a case series. *Clin Exp Allergy.* 2003 Nov;33(11):1581-5.

Grob M, Reindl J, Vieths S, Wüthrich B, Ballmer-Weber BK. Heterogeneity of banana allergy: characterization of allergens in banana-allergic patients. *Ann Allergy Asthma Immunol.* 2002 Nov;89(5):513-6.

Groschwitz KR, Ahrens R, Osterfeld H, Gurish MF, Han X, Abrink M, Finkelman FD, Pejler G, Hogan SP. Mast cells regulate homeostatic intestinal epithelial migration and barrier function by a chymase/Mcpt4-dependent mechanism. *Proc Natl Acad Sci U S A.* 2009 Dec 29;106(52):22381-6.

Grzanna R, Lindmark L, Frondoza CG. Ginger—an herbal medicinal product with broad anti-inflammatory actions. *J Med Food.* 2005 Summer;8(2):125-32.

Grzybowska-Chlebowczyk U, Woś H, Sieroń AL, Wiecek S, Auguściak-Duma A, Koryciak-Komarska H, Kasznia-Kocot J. Serologic investigations in children with inflammatory bowel disease and food allergy. *Mediators Inflamm.* 2009;2009:512695.

Guandalini S. The influence of gluten: weaning recommendations for healthy children and children at risk for celiac disease. *Nestle Nutr Workshop Ser Pediatr Program.* 2007;60:139-51; discussion 151-5.

Guerin M, Huntley ME, Olaizola M. Haematococcus astaxanthin: applications for human health and nutrition. *Trends Biotechnol.* 2003 May;21(5):210-6.

Gundermann KJ, Müller J. Phytodolor—effects and efficacy of a herbal medicine. *Wien Med Wochenschr.* 2007;157(13-14):343-7.

Gupta R, Sheikh A, Strachan DP, Anderson HR (2006) Time trends in allergic disorders in the UK. *Thorax,* published online. doi: 10.1136/thx.2004.038844.

Guslandi M, Giollo P, Testoni PA. A pilot trial of Saccharomyces boulardii in ulcerative colitis. *Eur J Gastroenterol Hepatol.* 2003 Jun;15(6):697-8.

Gutmanis J. *Hawaiian Herbal Medicine.* Waipahu, HI: Island Heritage, 2001.

Guyonnet D, Woodcock A, Stefani B, Trevisan C, Hall C. Fermented milk containing Bifidobacterium lactis DN-173 010 improved self-reported digestive comfort amongst a general population of adults. A randomized, open-label, controlled, pilot study. *J Dig Dis.* 2009 Feb;10(1):61-70.

Hadjivassiliou M, Davies-Jones GA, Sanders DS, Grünewald RA. Dietary treatment of gluten ataxia. *J Neurol Neurosurg Psychiatry.* 2003 Sep;74(9):1221-4.

Hafström I, Ringertz B, Spångberg A, von Zweigbergk L, Brannemark S, Nylander I, Rönnelid J, Laasonen L, Klareskog L. A vegan diet free of gluten improves the signs and symptoms of rheumatoid arthritis: the effects on arthritis correlate with a reduction in antibodies to food antigens. *Rheumatology (Oxford).* 2001 Oct;40(10):1175-9.

Haines JL, Ter-Minassian M, Bazyk A, Gusella JF, Kim DJ, Terwedow H, Pericak-Vance MA, Rimmler JB, Haynes CS, Roses AD, Lee A, Shaner B, Menold M, Seboun E, Fitoussi RP, Gartioux C, Reyes C, Ribierre F, Gyapay G, Weissenbach J, Hauser SL, Goodkin DE, Lincoln R, Usuku K, Oksenberg JR, et al. A complete genomic screen for multiple sclerosis underscores a role for the major histocompatability complex. The Multiple Sclerosis Genetics Group. *Nat Genet.* 1996 Aug;13(4):469-71..

Halken S, Hansen KS, Jacobsen HP, Estmann A, Faelling AE, Hansen LG, Kier SR, Lassen K, Lintrup M, Mortensen S, Ibsen KK, Osterballe O, Host A. Comparison of a partially hydrolyzed infant formula with two extensively hydrolyzed formulas for allergy prevention: a prospective, randomized study. *Pediatr Allergy Immunol.* 2000 Aug;11(3):149-61.

Halpern GM, Miller AH. *Medicinal Mushrooms: Ancient Remedies for Modern Ailments.* New York: M. Evans, 2002.

Hamelmann E, Beyer K, Gruber C, Lau S, Matricardi PM, Nickel R, Niggemann B, Wahn U. Primary prevention of allergy: avoiding risk or providing protection? *Clin Exp Allergy.* 2008 Feb;38(2):233-45.

Hamilton RG. Clinical laboratory assessment of immediate-type hypersensitivity. *J Allergy Clin Immunol.* 2010 Feb;125(2 Suppl 2):S284-96.

Hammond BG, Mayhew DA, Kier LD, Mast RW, Sander WJ. Safety assessment of DHA-rich microalgae from Schizochytrium sp. *Regul Toxicol Pharmacol.* 2002 Apr;35(2 Pt 1):255-65.

Han SN, Leka LS, Lichtenstein AH, Ausman LM, Meydani SN. Effect of a therapeutic lifestyle change diet on immune functions of moderately hypercholesterolemic humans. *J Lipid Res.* 2003 Dec;44(12):2304-10.

Hansen KS, Ballmer-Weber BK, Lüttkopf D, Skov PS, Wüthrich B, Bindslev-Jensen C, Vieths S, Poulsen LK. Roasted hazelnuts—allergenic activity evaluated by double-blind, placebo-controlled food challenge. *Allergy.* 2003 Feb;58(2):132-8.

Hansen KS, Ballmer-Weber BK, Sastre J, Lidholm J, Andersson K, Oberhofer H, Lluch-Bernal M, Ostling J, Mattsson L, Schocker F, Vieths S, Poulsen LK. Component-resolved in vitro diagnosis of hazelnut allergy in Europe. *J Allergy Clin Immunol.* 2009 May;123(5):1134-41, 1141.e1-3.

Hansen KS, Khinchi MS, Skov PS, Bindslev-Jensen C, Poulsen LK, Malling HJ. Food allergy to apple and specific immunotherapy with birch pollen. *Mol Nutr Food Res.* 2004 Nov;48(6):441-8.

Hartz C, Lauer I, Del Mar San Miguel Moncin M, Cistero-Bahima A, Foetisch K, Lidholm J, Vieths S, Scheurer S. Comparison of IgE-Binding Capacity, Cross-Reactivity and Biological Potency of Allergenic Non-Specific Lipid Transfer Proteins from Peach, Cherry and Hazelnut. *Int Arch Allergy Immunol.* 2010 Jun 17;153(4):335-346.

Harvald B, Hauge M: Hereditary factors elucidated by twin studies. *In Genetics and the Epidemiology of Chronic Disease.* Edited by Neel JV, Shaw MV, Schull WJ. Washington, DC: Department of Health, Education and Welfare, 1965:64-76.

Hashem MM, Atta AH, Arbid MS, Nada SA, Asaad GF. Immunological studies on Amaranth, Sunset Yellow and Curcumin as food colouring agents in albino rats. *Food Chem Toxicol.* 2010 Jun;48(6):1581-6.

Hata K, Ishikawa K, Hori K, Konishi T. Differentiation-inducing activity of lupeol, a lupane-type triterpene from Chinese dandelion root (Hokouei-kon), on a mouse melanoma cell line. *Biol Pharm Bull.* 2000 Aug;23(8):962-7.

Hattori K, Sasai M, Yamamoto A, Taniuchi S, Kojima T, Kobayashi Y, Iwamoto H, Yaeshima T, Hayasawa H. Intestinal flora of infants with cow milk hypersensitivity fed on casein-hydrolyzed formula supplemented raffinose. *Arerugi.* 2000 Dec;49(12):1146-55.

Hawkes CP, Mulcair S, Hourihane JO. Is hospital based MMR vaccination for children with egg allergy here to stay? *Ir Med J.* 2010 Jan;103(1):17-9.

Heaney RP, Dowell MS. Absorbability of the calcium in a high-calcium mineral water. *Osteoporos Int.* 1994 Nov;4(6):323-4.

Heap GA, van Heel DA. Genetics and pathogenesis of coeliac disease. *Semin Immunol.* May 13 2009.

Helin T, Haahtela S, Haahtela T. No effect of oral treatment with an intestinal bacterial strain, Lactobacillus rhamnosus (ATCC 53103), on birch-pollen allergy: a placebo-controlled double-blind study. *Allergy.* 2002 Mar;57(3):243-6.

Hemmer W, Focke M, Marzban G, Swoboda I, Jarisch R, Laimer M. Identification of Bet v 1-related allergens in fig and other Moraceae fruits. *Clin Exp Allergy.* 2010 Apr;40(4):679-87.

Hendel B, Ferreira P. *Water & Salt: The Essence of Life.* Gaithersburg: Natural Resources, 2003.

Herbert V. Vitamin B12: Plant sources, requirements, and assay. *Am J Clin Nutr.* 1988;48:852-858.

Herman PM, Drost LM. Evaluating the clinical relevance of food sensitivity tests: a single subject experiment. *Altern Med Rev.* 2004 Jun;9(2):198-207.

Heyman M, Grasset E, Ducroc R, Desjeux JF. Antigen absorption by the jejunal epithelium of children with cow's milk allergy. *Pediatr Res.* 1988 Aug;24(2):197-202.

Hiemori M, Eguchi Y, Kimoto M, Yamasita H, Takahashi K, Takahashi K, Tsuji H. Characterization of new 18-kDa IgE-binding proteins in beer. *Biosci Biotechnol Biochem.* 2008 Apr;72(4):1095-8.

Hieta N, Hasan T, Mäkinen-Kiljunen S, Lammintausta K. Sweet lupin—a new food allergen. *Duodecim.* 2010;126(12):1393-9.

Hirose Y, Murosaki S, Yamamoto Y, Yoshikai Y, Tsuru T. Daily intake of heat-killed Lactobacillus plantarum L-137 augments acquired immunity in healthy adults. *J Nutr.* 2006 Dec;136(12):3069-73.

Hobbs C. *Medicinal Mushrooms.* Summertown, TN: Botanica Press, 2003.

Hobbs C. *Stress & Natural Healing.* Loveland, CO: Interweave Press, 1997.

Hoffmann D. *Holistic Herbal.* London: Thorsons, 1983-2002.

Hofmann AM, Scurlock AM, Jones SM, Palmer KP, Lokhnygina Y, Steele PH, Kamilaris J, Burks AW. Safety of a peanut oral immunotherapy protocol in children with peanut allergy. *J Allergy Clin Immunol.* 2009 Aug;124(2):286-91, 291.e1-6.

Holick MF. Sunlight and vitamin D for bone health and prevention of autoimmune diseases, cancers, and cardiovascular disease. *Am J Clin Nutr.* 2004 Dec;80(6 Suppl):1678S-88S.

Holick MF. The vitamin D deficiency pandemic and consequences for nonskeletal health: mechanisms of action. *Mol Aspects Med.* 2008 Dec;29(6):361-8

Holick MF. Vitamin D status: measurement, interpretation, and clinical application. *Ann Epidemiol.* 2009 Feb;19(2):73-8.

Holick MF. Vitamin D: importance in the prevention of cancers, type 1 diabetes, heart disease, and osteoporosis. *Am J Clin Nutr.* 2004 Mar;79(3):362-71.

Holladay, S.D. Prenatal Immunotoxicant Exposure and Postnatal Autoimmune Disease. *Environ Health Perspect.* 1999; 107(suppl 5):687-691.

Hönscheid A, Rink L, Haase H. T-lymphocytes: a target for stimulatory and inhibitory effects of zinc ions. *Endocr Metab Immune Disord Drug Targets.* 2009 Jun;9(2):132-44.

Hooper R, Calvert J, Thompson RL, Deetlefs ME, Burney P. Urban/rural differences in diet and atopy in South Africa. *Allergy.* 2008 Apr;63(4):425-31.

Horrobin DF. Effects of evening primrose oil in rheumatoid arthritis. *Ann Rheum Dis.* 1989 Nov;48(11):965-6.

Hospers IC, de Vries-Vrolijk K, Brand PL. Double-blind, placebo-controlled cow's milk challenge in children with alleged cow's milk allergies, performed in a general hospital: diagnosis rejected in two-thirds of the children. *Ned Tijdschr Geneeskd.* 2006 Jun 10;150(23):1292-7.

Houle CR, Leo HL, Clark NM. A developmental, community, and psychosocial approach to food allergies in children. *Curr Allergy Asthma Rep.* 2010 Sep;10(5):381-6.

Hourihane JO, Grimshaw KE, Lewis SA, Briggs RA, Trewin JB, King RM, Kilburn SA, Warner JO. Does severity of low-dose, double-blind, placebo-controlled food challenges reflect severity of allergic reactions to peanut in the community? *Clin Exp Allergy.* 2005 Sep;35(9):1227-33.

Hsu CH, Lu CM, Chang TT. Efficacy and safety of modified Mai-Men-Dong-Tang for treatment of allergic asthma. *Pediatr Allergy Immunol.* 2005;16:76–81.

Hu C, Kitts DD. Antioxidant, prooxidant, and cytotoxic activities of solvent-fractionated dandelion (Taraxacum officinale) flower extracts in vitro. *J Agric Food Chem.* 2003 Jan 1;51(1):301-10.

Hu C, Kitts DD. Dandelion (Taraxacum officinale) flower extract suppresses both reactive oxygen species and nitric oxide and prevents lipid oxidation in vitro. *Phytomedicine.* 2005 Aug;12(8):588-97.

Hu C, Kitts DD. Luteolin and luteolin-7-O-glucoside from dandelion flower suppress iNOS and COX-2 in RAW264.7 cells. *Mol Cell Biochem.* 2004 Oct;265(1-2):107-13.

Huang D, Ou B, Prior RL. The chemistry behind antioxidant capacity assays. *J Agric Food Chem.* 2005 Mar 23;53(6):1841-56.

Huang M, Wang W, Wei S. Investigation on medicinal plant resources of Glycyrrhiza uralensis in China and chemical assessment of its underground part. *Zhongguo Zhong Yao Za Zhi.* 2010 Apr;35(8):947-52.

Hun L. Bacillus coagulans significantly improved abdominal pain and bloating in patients with IBS. *Postgrad Med.* 2009 Mar;121(2):119-24.

Hunter JO. Do horses suffer from irritable bowel syndrome? *Equine Vet J.* 2009 Dec;41(9):836-40.

Hur YM, Rushton JP. Genetic and environmental contributions to prosocial behaviour in 2- to 9-year-old South Korean twins. *Biol Lett.* 2007 Dec 22;3(6):664-6.

Husby S. Dietary antigens: uptake and humoral immunity in man. *APMIS Suppl.* 1988;1:1-40.

Ibero M, Boné J, Martín B, Martínez J. Evaluation of an extensively hydrolysed casein formula (Damira 2000) in children with allergy to cow's milk proteins. *Allergol Immunopathol (Madr)*. 2010 Mar-Apr;38(2):60-8.

Iida N, Inatomi Y, Murata H, Inada A, Murata J, Lang FA, Matsuura N, Nakanishi T. A new flavone xyloside and two new flavan-3-ol glucosides from Juniperus communis var. depressa. *Chem Biodivers*. 2007 Jan;4(1):32-42.

Indrio F, Ladisa G, Mautone A, Montagna O. Effect of a fermented formula on thymus size and stool pH in healthy term infants. *Pediatr Res*. 2007 Jul;62(1):98-100.

Innis SM, Hansen JW. Plasma fatty acid responses, metabolic effects, and safety of microalgal and fungal oils rich in arachidonic and docosahexaenoic acids in adults. *Am J Clin Nutr*. 1996 Aug;64(2):159-67.

Innocenti M, Michelozzi M, Giaccherini C, Ieri F, Vincieri FF, Mulinacci N. Flavonoids and biflavonoids in Tuscan berries of Juniperus communis L.: detection and quantitation by HPLC/DAD/ESI/MS. *J Agric Food Chem*. 2007 Aug 8;55(16):6596-602.

Int J Toxicol. Final report on the safety assessment of Juniperus communis Extract, Juniperus oxycedrus Extract, Juniperus oxycedrus Tar, Juniperus phoenicea extract, and Juniperus virginiana Extract. *Int J Toxicol*. 2001;20 Suppl 2:41-56.

Ionescu JG. New insights in the pathogenesis of atopic disease. *J Med Life*. 2009 Apr-Jun;2(2):146-54.

Iribarren C, Tolstykh IV, Miller MK, Eisner MD. Asthma and the prospective risk of anaphylactic shock and other allergy diagnoses in a large integrated health care delivery system. *Ann Allergy Asthma Immunol*. 2010 May;104(5):371-7.

Ishida Y, Nakamura F, Kanzato H, Sawada D, Hirata H, Nishimura A, Kajimoto O, Fujiwara S. Clinical effects of Lactobacillus acidophilus strain L-92 on perennial allergic rhinitis: a double-blind, placebo-controlled study. *J Dairy Sci*. 2005 Feb;88(2):527-33.

Ishida Y, Nakamura F, Kanzato H, Sawada D, Yamamoto N, Kagata H, Oh-Ida M, Takeuchi H, Fujiwara S. Effect of milk fermented with Lactobacillus acidophilus strain L-92 on symptoms of Japanese cedar pollen allergy: a randomized placebo-controlled trial. *Biosci Biotechnol Biochem*. 2005 Sep;69(9):1652-60.

Ivory K, Chambers SJ, Pin C, Prieto E, Arqués JL, Nicoletti C. Oral delivery of Lactobacillus casei Shirota modifies allergen-induced immune responses in allergic rhinitis. *Clin Exp Allergy*. 2008 Aug;38(8):1282-9.

Iwańczak B, Mowszet K, Iwańczak F. Feeding disorders, ALTE syndrome, Sandifer syndrome and gastroesophageal reflux disease in the course of food hypersensitivity in 8-month old infant. *Pol Merkur Lekarski*. 2010 Jul;29(169):44-6.

Izumi K, Aihara M, Ikezawa Z. Effects of non steroidal antiinflammatory drugs (NSAIDs) on immediate-type food allergy analysis of Japanese cases from 1998 to 2009. *Arerugi*. 2009 Dec;58(12):1629-39.

Jackson PG, Lessof MH, Baker RW, Ferrett J, MacDonald DM. Intestinal permeability in patients with eczema and food allergy. *Lancet*. 1981 Jun 13;1(8233):1285-6.

Jagetia GC, Aggarwal BB. "Spicing up" of the immune system by curcumin. *J Clin Immunol*. 2007 Jan;27(1):19-35.

Jagetia GC, Nayak V, Vidyasagar MS. Evaluation of the antineoplastic activity of guduchi (Tinospora cordifolia) in cultured HeLa cells. *Cancer Lett*. 1998 May 15;127(1-2):71-82.

Jagetia GC, Rao SK. Evaluation of Cytotoxic Effects of Dichloromethane Extract of Guduchi (Tinospora cordifolia Miers ex Hook F & THOMS) on Cultured HeLa Cells. *Evid Based Complement Alternat Med*. 2006 Jun;3(2):267-72.

Janson C, Anto J, Burney P, Chinn S, de Marco R, Heinrich J, Jarvis D, Kuenzli N, Leynaert B, Luczynska C, Neukirch F, Svanes C, Sunyer J, Wjst M; European Community Respiratory Health Survey II. The European Community Respiratory Health Survey: what are the main results so far? European Community Respiratory Health Survey II. *Eur Respir J*. 2001 Sep;18(3):598-611.

Jappe U, Vieths S. Lupine, a source of new as well as hidden food allergens. *Mol Nutr Food Res*. 2010 Jan;54(1):113-26.

Jarocka-Cyrta E, Baniukiewicz A, Wasilewska J, Pawlak J, Kaczmarski M. Focal villous atrophy of the duodenum in children who have outgrown cow's milk allergy. Chromoendoscopy and magnification endoscopy evaluation. *Med Wieku Rozwoj*. 2007 Apr-Jun;11(2 Pt 1):123-7.

Järvinen KM, Amalanayagam S, Shreffler WG, Noone S, Sicherer SH, Sampson HA, Nowak-Wegrzyn A. Epinephrine treatment is infrequent and biphasic reactions are rare in food-induced reactions during oral food challenges in children. *J Allergy Clin Immunol*. 2009 Dec;124(6):1267-72.

Jazani NH, Karimzad M, Mazloomi E, Sohrabpour M, Hassan ZM, Ghasemnejad H, Roshan-Milani S, Shahabi S. Evaluation of the adjuvant activity of naloxone, an opioid receptor antagonist, in combination with heat-killed Listeria monocytogenes vaccine. *Microbes Infect*. 2010 May;12(5):382-8.

Jennings S, Prescott SL. Early dietary exposures and feeding practices: role in pathogenesis and prevention of allergic disease? *Postgrad Med J*. 2010 Feb;86(1012):94-9.

REFERENCES AND BIBLIOGRAPHY

Jensen B. *Foods that Heal.* Garden City Park, NY: Avery Publ, 1988, 1993.

Jensen B. *Nature Has a Remedy.* Los Angeles: Keats, 2001.

Jeon HJ, Kang HJ, Jung HJ, Kang YS, Lim CJ, Kim YM, Park EH. Anti-inflammatory activity of Taraxacum officinale. *J Ethnopharmacol.* 2008 Jan 4;115(1):82-8.

Jiang CY, Wang BE, Chen D. [Protective effect of compound tongfu granule on intestinal mucosal barrier in patients with cirrhosis of decompensation stage]. *Zhongguo Zhong Xi Yi Jie He Za Zhi.* 2008 Sep;28(9):784-7.

Jiang HP, Liu CA. [Protective effect of glutamine on intestinal barrier function in patients receiving chemotherapy]. *Zhonghua Wei Chang Wai Ke Za Zhi.* 2006 Jan;9(1):59-61.

Johansson G, Holmén A, Persson L, Högstedt B, Wassén C, Ottova L, Gustafsson JA. Long-term effects of a change from a mixed diet to a lacto-vegetarian diet on human urinary and faecal mutagenic activity. *Mutagenesis.* 1998 Mar;13(2):167-71.

Johansson G, Holmén A, Persson L, Högstedt B, Wassén C, Ottova L, Gustafsson JA. Dietary influence on some proposed risk factors for colon cancer: fecal and urinary mutagenic activity and the activity of some intestinal bacterial enzymes. *Cancer Detect Prev.* 1997;21(3):258-66.

Johansson G, Holmén A, Persson L, Högstedt R, Wassén C, Ottova L, Gustafsson JA. The effect of a shift from a mixed diet to a lacto-vegetarian diet on human urinary and fecal mutagenic activity. *Carcinogenesis.* 1992 Feb;13(2):153-7.

Johansson G, Ravald N. Comparison of some salivary variables between vegetarians and omnivores. *Eur J Oral Sci.* 1995 Apr;103(2 (Pt 1)):95-8.

Johari H. *Ayurvedic Massage: Traditional Indian Techniques for Balancing Body and Mind.* Rochester, VT: Healing Arts, 1996.

Johnson I.M. Gitksan medicinal plants—cultural choice and efficacy. *J Ethnobiol Ethnomed.* 2006 Jun 21;2:29.

Jones MA, Silman AJ, Whiting S, *et al.* Occurrence of rheumatoid arthritis is not increased in the first degree relatives of a population based inception cohort of inflammatory polyarthritis. *Ann Rheum Dis.* 1996;55(2): 89-93.

Jones SM, Zhong Z, Enomoto N, Schemmer P, Thurman RG. Dietary juniper berry oil minimizes hepatic reperfusion injury in the rat. *Hepatology.* 1998 Oct;28(4):1042-50.

Jorgensen VL, Nielsen SL, Espersen K, Perner A. Increased colorectal permeability in patients with severe sepsis and septic shock. *Intensive Care Med.* 2006 Nov;32(11):1790-6. Epub 2006 Sep 9.

Julkunen-Tiitto R. A chemotaxonomic survey of phenolics in leaves of northern Salicaceae species. *Phytochemistry.* 1986:25(3):663-667.

Jung HA, Yokozawa T, Kim BW, Jung JH, Choi JS. Selective inhibition of prenylated flavonoids from Sophora flavescens against BACE1 and cholinesterases. *Am J Chin Med.* 2010;38(2):415-29.

Jurakić Toncić R, Lipozencić J. Role and significance of atopy patch test. *Acta Dermatovenerol Croat.* 2010;18(1):38-55.

Jurenka JS. Anti-inflammatory properties of curcumin, a major constituent of Curcuma longa: a review of preclinical and clinical research. *Altern Med Rev.* 2009 Feb;14(2):141-153.

Kähkönen MP, Hopia AI, Vuorela HJ, Rauha JP, Pihlaja K, Kujala TS, Heinonen M. Antioxidant activity of plant extracts containing phenolic compounds. *J Agric Food Chem.* 1999 Oct;47(10):3954-62.

Kaila M, Vanto T, Valovirta E, Koivikko A, Juntunen-Backman K. Diagnosis of food allergy in Finland: survey of pediatric practices. *Pediatr Allergy Immunol.* 2000 Nov;11(4):246-9.

Kajander K, Hatakka K, Poussa T, Färkkilä M, Korpela R. A probiotic mixture alleviates symptoms in irritable bowel syndrome patients: a controlled 6-month intervention. *Aliment Pharmacol Ther.* 2005 Sep 1;22(5):387-94.

Kajander K, Krogius-Kurikka L, Rinttilä T, Karjalainen H, Palva A, Korpela R. Effects of multispecies probiotic supplementation on intestinal microbiota in irritable bowel syndrome. *Aliment Pharmacol Ther.* 2007 Aug 1;26(3):463-73.

Kajander K, Myllyluoma E, Rajilić-Stojanović M, Kyrönpalo S, Rasmussen M, Järvenpää S, Zoetendal EG, de Vos WM, Vapaatalo H, Korpela R. Clinical trial: multispecies probiotic supplementation alleviates the symptoms of irritable bowel syndrome and stabilizes intestinal microbiota. *Aliment Pharmacol Ther.* 2008 Jan 1;27(1):48-57.

Kalach N, Benhamou PH, Campeotto F, Dupont Ch. Anemia impairs small intestinal absorption measured by intestinal permeability in children. *Eur Ann Allergy Clin Immunol.* 2007 Jan;39(1):20-2.

Kalach N, Rocchiccioli F, de Boissieu D, Benhamou PH, Dupont C. Intestinal permeability in children: variation with age and reliability in the diagnosis of cow's milk allergy. *Acta Paediatr.* 2001 May;90(5):499-504.

Kalliomäki M, Salminen S, Arvilommi H, Kero P, Koskinen P, Isolauri E. Probiotics in primary prevention of atopic disease: a randomised placebo-controlled trial. *Lancet.* 2001 Apr 7;357(9262):1076-9.

Kamdar T, Bryce PJ. Immunotherapy in food allergy. Immunotherapy. 2010 May;2(3):329-38.

Kang SK, Kim JK, Ahn SH, Oh JE, Kim JH, Lim DH, Son BK. Relationship between silent gastroesophageal reflux and food sensitization in infants and young children with recurrent wheezing. *J Korean Med Sci.* 2010 Mar;25(3):425-8.

Kanny G, Grignon G, Dauca M, Guedenet JC, Moneret-Vautrin DA. Ultrastructural changes in the duodenal mucosa induced by ingested histamine in patients with chronic urticaria. *Allergy.* 1996 Dec;51(12):935-9.

Kapil A, Sharma S. Immunopotentiating compounds from Tinospora cordifolia. *J Ethnopharmacol.* 1997 Oct;58(2):89-95.

Kaptan K, Beyan C, Ural AU, Cetin T, Avcu F, Gülşen M, Finci R, Yalçin A. Helicobacter pylori—is it a novel causative agent in Vitamin B12 deficiency? *Arch Intern Med.* 2000 May 8;160(9):1349-53.

Karaman I, Sahin F, Güllüce M, Ogütçü H, Sengül M, Adigüzel A. Antimicrobial activity of aqueous and methanol extracts of Juniperus oxycedrus L. *J Ethnopharmacol.* 2003 Apr;85(2-3):231-5.

Karczewski J, Troost FJ, Konings I, Dekker J, Kleerebezem M, Brummer RJ, Wells JM. Regulation of human epithelial tight junction proteins by Lactobacillus plantarum in vivo and protective effects on the epithelial barrier. *Am J Physiol Gastrointest Liver Physiol.* 2010 Jun;298(6):G851-9.

Karkoulias K, Patouchas D, Alahiotis S, Tsiamita M, Vrodakis K, Spiropoulos K. Specific sensitization in wheat flour and contributing factors in traditional bakers. *Eur Rev Med Pharmacol Sci.* 2007 May-Jun;11(3):141-8.

Karpińska J, Mikoluć B, Motkowski R, Piotrowska-Jastrzebska J. HPLC method for simultaneous determination of retinol, alpha-tocopherol and coenzyme Q10 in human plasma. *J Pharm Biomed Anal.* 2006 Sep 18;42(2):232-6.

Kashiwada Y, Takanaka K, Tsukada H, Miwa Y, Taga T, Tanaka S, Ikeshiro Y. Sesquiterpene glucosides from anti-leukotriene B4 release fraction of Taraxacum officinale. *J Asian Nat Prod Res.* 2001;3(3):191-7.

Kattan JD, Srivastava KD, Sampson HA, Li XM. Pharmacologic and Immunologic Effects of Individual Herbs of Food Allergy Herbal Formula 2 in a Murine Model of Peanut Allergy. *J Allergy Clin Immunol.* 2006;117(2):S34.

Kattan JD, Srivastava KD, Zou ZM, Goldfarb J, Sampson HA, Li XM. Pharmacological and immunological effects of individual herbs in the Food Allergy Herbal Formula-2 (FAHF-2) on peanut allergy. *Phytother Res.* 2008 May;22(5):651-9.

Katz Y, Rajuan N, Goldberg MR, Eisenberg E, Heyman E, Cohen A, Leshno M. Early exposure to cow's milk protein is protective against IgE-mediated cow's milk protein allergy. *J Allergy Clin Immunol.* 2010 Jul;126(1):77-82.e1.

Kazansky DB. MHC restriction and allogeneic immune responses. *J Immunotoxicol.* 2008 Oct;5(4):369-84.

Kazlowska K, Hsu T, Hou CC, Yang WC, Tsai GJ. Anti-inflammatory properties of phenolic compounds and crude extract from Porphyra dentata. *J Ethnopharmacol.* 2010 Mar 2;128(1):123-30.

Keita AV, Söderholm JD. The intestinal barrier and its regulation by neuroimmune factors. *Neurogastroenterol Motil.* 2010 Jul;22(7):718-33.

Kekkonen RA, Sysi-Aho M, Seppanen-Laakso T, Julkunen I, Vapaatalo H, Oresic M, Korpela R. Effect of probiotic Lactobacillus rhamnosus GG intervention on global serum lipidomic profiles in healthy adults. *World J Gastroenterol.* 2008 May 28;14(20):3188-94.

Kelder P. *Ancient Secret of the Fountain of Youth.* New York: Doubleday, 1998.

Kelly P, Shawa T, Mwanamakondo S, Soko R, Smith G, Barclay GR, Sanderson IR. Gastric and intestinal barrier impairment in tropical enteropathy and HIV: limited impact of micronutrient supplementation during a randomised controlled trial. *BMC Gastroenterol.* 2010 Jul 6;10:72.

Keogh JB, Grieger JA, Noakes M, Clifton PM. Flow-Mediated Dilatation Is Impaired by a High-Saturated Fat Diet but Not by a High-Carbohydrate Diet. *Arterioscler Thromb Vasc Biol.* 2005 Mar 17

Kerckhoffs DA, Brouns F, Hornstra G, Mensink RP. Effects on the human serum lipoprotein profile of beta-glucan, soy protein and isoflavones, plant sterols and stanols, garlic and tocotrienols. *J Nutr.* 2002 Sep;132(9):2494-505.

Key T, Appleby P, Davey G, Allen N, Spencer E, Travis R. Mortality in British vegetarians: review and preliminary results from EPIC-Oxford. *Amer. Jour. Clin. Nutr. Suppl.* 2003;78(3): 533S-538S.

Kiefte-de Jong JC, Escher JC, Arends LR, Jaddoe VW, Hofman A, Raat H, Moll HA. Infant nutritional factors and functional constipation in childhood: the Generation R study. *Am J Gastroenterol.* 2010 Apr;105(4):940-5.

Kim BI, Kim HJ, Park JH, Park DI, Cho YK, Sohn CI, Jeon WK, Kim HS, Kim DJ. Increased intestinal permeability as a predictor of bacterial infections in patients with decompensated liver cirrhosis and hemorrhage. *J Gastroenterol Hepatol.* 2011 Mar;26(3):550-7.

Kim DC, Choi SY, Kim SH, Yun BS, Yoo ID, Reddy NR, Yoon HS, Kim KT. Isoliquiritigenin selectively inhibits H(2) histamine receptor signaling. *Mol Pharmacol.* 2006 Aug;70(2):493-500.

Kim HM, Shin HY, Lim KH, Ryu ST, Shin TY, Chae HJ, Kim HR, Lyu YS, An NH, Lim KS. Taraxacum officinale inhibits tumor necrosis factor-alpha production from rat astrocytes. *Immunopharmacol Immunotoxicol.* 2000 Aug;22(3):519-30.

Kim JH, An S, Kim JE, Choi GS, Ye YM, Park HS. Beef-induced anaphylaxis confirmed by the basophil activation test. *Allergy Asthma Immunol Res.* 2010 Jul;2(3):206-8.

Kim JY, Kim DY, Lee YS, Lee BK, Lee KH, Ro JY. DA-9601, Artemisia asiatica herbal extract, ameliorates airway inflammation of allergic asthma in mice. *Mol Cells.* 2006;22:104–12.

Kim MN, Kim N, Lee SH, Park YS, Hwang JH, Kim JW, Jeong SH, Lee DH, Kim JS, Jung HC, Song IS. The effects of probiotics on PPI-triple therapy for Helicobacter pylori eradication. Helicobacter. 2008 Aug;13(4):261-8.

Kim NI, Jo Y, Ahn SB, Son BK, Kim SH, Park YS, Kim SH, Ju JE. A case of eosinophilic esophagitis with food hypersensitivity. *J Neurogastroenterol Motil.* 2010 Jul;16(3):315-8.

Kim SJ, Jung JY, Kim HW, Park T. Anti-obesity effects of Juniperus chinensis extract are associated with increased AMP-activated protein kinase expression and phosphorylation in the visceral adipose tissue of rats. *Biol Pharm Bull.* 2008 Jul;31(7):1415-21.

Kim TE, Park SW, Noh G, Lee S. Comparison of skin prick test results between crude allergen extracts from foods and commercial allergen extracts in atopic dermatitis by double-blind placebo-controlled food challenge for milk, egg, and soybean. *Yonsei Med J.* 2002 Oct;43(5):613-20.

Kim YG, Moon JT, Lee KM, Chon NR, Park H. The effects of probiotics on symptoms of irritable bowel syndrome. *Korean J Gastroenterol.* 2006 Jun;47(6):413-9.

Kim YH, Kim KS, Han CS, Yang HC, Park SH, Ko KI, Lee SH, Kim KH, Lee NH, Kim JM, Son K. Inhibitory effects of natural plants of Jeju Island on elastase and MMP-1 expression. *Int J Cosmet Sci.* 2007 Dec;29(6):487-8.

Kimata M, Inagaki N, Nagai H. Effects of luteolin and other flavonoids on IgE-mediated allergic reactions. *Planta Med.* 2000 Feb;66(1):25-9.

Kimata M, Shichijo M, Miura T, Serizawa I, Inagaki N, Nagai H. Effects of luteolin, quercetin and baicalein on immunoglobulin E-mediated mediator release from human cultured mast cells. *Clin Exp Allergy.* 2000 Apr;30(4):501-8.

Kimber I, Dearman RJ. Factors affecting the development of food allergy. *Proc Nutr Soc.* 2002 Nov;61(4):435-9.

Kimmatkar N, Thawani V, Hingorani L, Khiyani R. Efficacy and tolerability of Boswellia serrata extract in treatment of osteoarthritis of knee—a randomized double blind placebo controlled trial. *Phytomedicine.* 2003 Jan;10(1):3-7.

Kinaciyan T, Jahn-Schmid B, Radakovics A, Zwölfer B, Schreiber C, Francis JN, Ebner C, Bohle B. Successful sublingual immunotherapy with birch pollen has limited effects on concomitant food allergy to apple and the immune response to the Bet v 1 homolog Mal d 1. *J Allergy Clin Immunol.* 2007 Apr;119(4):937-43.

Kirjavainen PV, Salminen SJ, Isolauri E. Probiotic bacteria in the management of atopic disease: underscoring the importance of viability. *J Pediatr Gastroenterol Nutr.* 2003 Feb;36(2):223-7.

Kisiel W, Barszcz B. Further sesquiterpenoids and phenolics from Taraxacum officinale. *Fitoterapia.* 2000 Jun;71(3):269-73.

Kisiel W, Michalska K. Sesquiterpenoids and phenolics from Taraxacum hondoense. *Fitoterapia.* 2005 Sep;76(6):520-4.

Kjellman NI, Björkstén B, Hattevig G, Fälth-Magnusson K. Natural history of food allergy. *Ann Allergy.* 1988 Dec;61(6 Pt 2):83-7.

Klein R, Landau MG. *Healing: The Body Betrayed.* Minneapolis: DCI:Chronimed, 1992.

Klein-Galczinsky C. Pharmacological and clinical effectiveness of a fixed phytogenic combination trembling poplar (Populus tremula), true goldenrod (Solidago virgaurea) and ash (Fraxinus excelsior) in mild to moderate rheumatic complaints. *Wien Med Wochenschr.* 1999;149(8-10):248-53.

Klemola T, Vanto T, Juntunen-Backman K, Kalimo K, Korpela R, Varjonen E. Allergy to soy formula and to extensively hydrolyzed whey formula in infants with cow's milk allergy: a prospective, randomized study with a follow-up to the age of 2 years. *J Pediatr.* 2002 Feb;140(2):219-24.

Kloss J. *Back to Eden.* Twin Oaks, WI: Lotus Press, 1939-1999.

Knutson TW, Bengtsson U, Dannaeus A, Ahlstedt S, Knutson L. Effects of luminal antigen on intestinal albumin and hyaluronan permeability and ion transport in atopic patients. *J Allergy Clin Immunol.* 1996 Jun;97(6):1225-32.

Ko J, Busse PJ, Shek L, Noone SA, Sampson HA, Li XM. Effect of Chinese Herbal Formulas on T Cell Responses in Patients with Peanut Allergy or Asthma. *J Allergy Clin Immunol* .2005;115:S34.

Ko J, Lee JI, Munoz-Furlong A, Li XM, Sicherer SH. Use of complementary and alternative medicine by food-allergic patients. *Ann Allergy Asthma Immunol.* 2006;97:365–9.

THE SCIENCE OF LEAKY GUT SYNDROME

Koo HN, Hong SH, Song BK, Kim CH, Yoo YH, Kim HM. Taraxacum officinale induces cytotoxicity through TNF-alpha and IL-1alpha secretion in Hep G2 cells. *Life Sci.* 2004 Jan 16;74(9):1149-57.

Kootstra HS, Vlieg-Boerstra BJ, Dubois AE. Assessment of the reduced allergenic properties of the Santana apple. *Ann Allergy Asthma Immunol.* 2007 Dec;99(6):522-5.

Kotzampassi K, Giamarellos-Bourboulis EJ, Voudouris A, Kazamias P, Eleftheriadis E. Benefits of a synbiotic formula (Synbiotic 2000Forte) in critically Ill trauma patients: early results of a randomized controlled trial. *World J Surg.* 2006 Oct;30(10):1848-55.

Kovács T, Mette H, Per B, Kun I, Schmelczer M, Barta J, Jean-Claude D, Nagy J. Relationship between intestinal permeability and antibodies against food antigens in IgA nephropathy. *Orr Hetil.* 1996 Jan 14;137(2):65-9.

Kovács T, Mette H, Per B, Kun L, Schmelczer M, Barta J, Jean-Claude D, Nagy J. [Relationship between intestinal permeability and antibodies against food antigens in IgA nephropathy]. *Orr Hetil.* 1996 Jan 14;137(2):65-9.

Kowalchik C, Hylton W (eds). *Rodale's Illustrated Encyclopedia of Herbs.* Emmaus, PA: 1987.

Kowalczyk E, Krzesiński P, Kura M, Niedworok J, Kowalski J, Blaszczyk J. Pharmacological effects of flavonoids from Scutellaria baicalensis. *Przegl Lek.* 2006;63(2):95-6.

Kozlowski LT, Mehta NY, Sweeney CT, Schwartz SS, Vogler GP, Jarvis MJ, West RJ. Filter ventilation and nicotine content of tobacco in cigarettes from Canada, the United Kingdom, and the United States. *Tob Control.* 1998 Winter;7(4):369-75.

Kreig M. *Black Market Medicine.* New York: Bantam, 1968.

Kristjansson I, Ardal B, Jonsson JS, Sigurdsson JA, Foldevi M, Bjorksten B (1999) Adverse reactions to food and food allergy in young children in Iceland and Sweden. *Scand J Prim Health Care.* 17: 30–34.

Krogulska A, Wasowska-Królikowska K, Dynowski J. Evaluation of bronchial hyperreactivity in children with asthma undergoing food challenges. *Pol Merkur Lekarski.* 2007 Jul;23(133):30-5.

Krogulska A, Wasowska-Królikowska K, Trzeźwińska B. Food challenges in children with asthma. *Pol Merkur Lekarski.* 2007 Jul;23(133):22-9.

Krüger P, Kanzer J, Hummel J, Fricker G, Schubert-Zsilavecz M, Abdel-Tawab M. Permeation of Boswellia extract in the Caco-2 model and possible interactions of its constituents KBA and AKBA with OATP1B3 and MRP2. *Eur J Pharm Sci.* 2009 Feb 15;36(2-3):275-84.

Kuitunen M, Kukkonen K, Juntunen-Backman K, Korpela R, Poussa T, Tuure T, Haahtela T, Savilahti E. Probiotics prevent IgE-associated allergy until age 5 years in cesarean-delivered children but not in the total cohort. *J Allergy Clin Immunol.* 2009 Feb;123(2):335-41.

Kuitunen M, Savilahti E, Sarnesto A. Human alpha-lactalbumin and bovine beta-lactoglobulin absorption in infants. *Allergy.* 1994 May;49(5):354-60.

Kuitunen M, Savilahti E. Mucosal IgA, mucosal cow's milk antibodies, serum cow's milk antibodies and gastrointestinal permeability in infants. *Pediatr Allergy Immunol.* 1995 Feb;6(1):30-5.

Kukkonen K, Kuitunen M, Haahtela T, Korpela R, Poussa T, Savilahti E. High intestinal IgA associates with reduced risk of IgE-associated allergic diseases. *Pediatr Allergy Immunol.* 2010 Feb;21(1 Pt 1):67-73.

Kukkonen K, Savilahti E, Haahtela T, Juntunen-Backman K, Korpela R, Poussa T, Tuure T, Kuitunen M. Probiotics and prebiotic galacto-oligosaccharides in the prevention of allergic diseases: a randomized, double-blind, placebo-controlled trial. *J Allergy Clin Immunol.* 2007 Jan;119(1):192-8.

Kulka M. The potential of natural products as effective treatments for allergic inflammation: implications for allergic rhinitis. *Curr Top Med Chem.* 2009;9(17):1611-24.

Kull I, Bergström A, Lilja G, Pershagen G, Wickman M. Fish consumption during the first year of life and development of allergic diseases during childhood. *Allergy.* 2006 Aug;61(8):1009-15.

Kull I, Melen E, Alm J, Hallberg J, Svartengren M, van Hage M, Pershagen G, Wickman M, Bergström A. Breast-feeding in relation to asthma, lung function, and sensitization in young schoolchildren. *J Allergy Clin Immunol.* 2010 May;125(5):1013-9.

Kumar R, Singh BP, Srivastava P, Sridhara S, Arora N, Gaur SN. Relevance of serum IgE estimation in allergic bronchial asthma with special reference to food allergy. *Asian Pac J Allergy Immunol.* 2006 Dec;24(4):191-9.

Kummeling I, Mills EN, Clausen M, Dubakiene R, Pérez CF, Fernández-Rivas M, Knulst AC, Kowalski ML, Lidholm J, Le TM, Metzler C, Mustakov T, Popov T, Potts J, van Ree R, Sakellariou A, Töndury B, Tzannis K, Burney P. The EuroPrevall surveys on the prevalence of food allergies in children and adults: background and study methodology. *Allergy.* 2009 Oct;64(10):1493-7.

Kung HC, Hoyert DL, Xu J, Murphy SL. Deaths: Final Data for 2005. *National Vital Statistics Reports.* 2008;56(10). http://www.cdc.gov/nchs/data/ nvsr/nvsr56/nvsr56_10.pdf. Accessed: 2008 Jun.

Kunisawa J, Kiyono H. Aberrant interaction of the gut immune system with environmental factors in the development of food allergies. *Curr Allergy Asthma Rep.* 2010 May;10(3):215-21.

Kusano M, Zai H, Hosaka H, Shimoyama Y, Nagoshi A, Maeda M, Kawamura O, Mori M. New frontiers in gut nutrient sensor research: monosodium L-glutamate added to a high-energy, high-protein liquid diet promotes gastric emptying: a possible therapy for patients with functional dyspepsia. *J Pharmacol Sci.* 2010 Jan;112(1):33-6.

Kusunoki T, Miyanomae T, Inoue Y, Itoh M, Yoshioka T, Okafuji I, Nishikomori R, Heike T, Nakahata T. Changes in food allergen sensitization rates of Japanese allergic children during the last 15 years. *Arerugi.* 2004 Jul;53(7):683-8.

Kusunoki T, Morimoto T, Nishikomori R, Yasumi T, Heike T, Mukaida K, Fujii T, Nakahata T. Breastfeeding and the prevalence of allergic diseases in schoolchildren: Does reverse causation matter? *Pediatr Allergy Immunol.* 2010 Feb;21(1 Pt 1):60-6.

Kuvaeva IB. Permeability of the gastronintestinal tract for macromolecules in health and disease. *Hum Physiol.* 1979 Mar-Apr;4(2):272-83.

Kuznetsova TA, Shevchenko NM, Zviagintseva TN, Besednova NN. Biological activity of fucoidans from brown algae and the prospects of their use in medicine]. *Antibiot Khimioter.* 2004;49(5):24-30..

Lad V. *Ayurveda: The Science of Self-Healing.* Twin Lakes, WI: Lotus Press.

Lamaison JL, Carnat A, Petitjean-Freytet C. Tannin content and inhibiting activity of elastase in Rosaceae. *Ann Pharm Fr.* 1990;48(6):335-40.

Lambert GP, Broussard LJ, Mason BL, Mauermann WJ, Gisolfi CV. Gastrointestinal permeability during exercise: effects of aspirin and energy-containing beverages. *J Appl Physiol.* 2001 Jun;90(6):2075-80.

Lambert GP, Lang J, Bull A, Pfeifer PC, Eckerson J, Moore G, Lanspa S, O'Brien J. Fluid restriction during running increases GI permeability. *Int J Sports Med.* 2008 Mar;29(3):194-8. Epub 2007 Jul 5.

Lappe FM. *Diet for a Small Planet.* New York: Ballantine, 1971.

Lau BH, Riesen SK, Truong KP, Lau EW, Rohdewald P, Barreta RA. Pycnogenol as an adjunct in the management of childhood asthma. *J Asthma.* 2004;41(8):825-32.

Laubereau B, Filipiak-Pittroff B, von Berg A, Grübl A, Reinhardt D, Wichmann HE, Koletzko S; GINI Study Group. Caesarean section and gastrointestinal symptoms, atopic dermatitis, and sensitisation during the first year of life. *Arch Dis Child.* 2004 Nov;89(11):993-7.

Laudat A, Arnaud P, Napoly A, Brion F. The intestinal permeability test applied to the diagnosis of food allergy in paediatrics. West Indian Med J. 1994 Sep;43(3):87-8.

Laugesen M, Elliott R. Ischaemic heart disease, Type 1 diabetes, and cow milk A1 beta-casein. *N Z Med J.* 2003 Jan 24;116(1168):U295.

Laurière M, Pecquet C, Bouchez-Mahiout I, Snégaroff J, Bayrou O, Raison-Peyron N, Vigan M. Hydrolysed wheat proteins present in cosmetics can induce immediate hypersensitivities. *Contact Dermatitis.* 2006 May;54(5):283-9.

LaValle JB. *The Cox-2 Connection.* Rochester, VT: Healing Arts, 2001.

Lean G. US study links more than 200 diseases to pollution. *London Independent.* 2004 Nov 14.

Lee BJ, Park HS. Common whelk (Buccinum undatum) allergy: identification of IgE-binding components and effects of heating and digestive enzymes. *J Korean Med Sci.* 2004 Dec;19(6):793-9.

Lee CK, Cheng YS. Diterpenoids from the leaves of Juniperus chinensis var. kaizuka. *J Nat Prod.* 2001 Apr;64(4):511-4.

Lee JH, Noh J, Noh G, Kim HS, Mun SH, Choi WS, Cho S, Lee S. Allergen-specific B cell subset responses in cow's milk allergy of late eczematous reactions in atopic dermatitis. *Cell Immunol.* 2010;262(1):44-51.

Lee JY, Kim CJ. Determination of allergenic egg proteins in food by protein-, mass spectrometry-, and DNA-based methods. *J AOAC Int.* 2010 Mar-Apr;93(2):462-77.

Lee YS, Kim SH, Jung SH, Kim JK, Pan CH, Lim SS. Aldose reductase inhibitory compounds from Glycyrrhiza uralensis. *Biol Pharm Bull.* 2010;33(5):917-21.

Leffler DA, Schuppan D. Update on serologic testing in celiac disease. *Am J Gastroenterol.* 2010 Dec;105(12):2520-4.

Lehmann B. The vitamin D3 pathway in human skin and its role for regulation of biological processes. *Photochem Photobiol.* 2005 Nov-Dec;81(6):1246-51.

Lehto M, Airaksinen L, Puustinen A, Tillander S, Hannula S, Nyman T, Toskala E, Alenius H, Lauerma A. Thaumatin-like protein and baker's respiratory allergy. *Ann Allergy Asthma Immunol.* 2010 Feb;104(2):139-46.

Lehto M, Airaksinen L, Puustinen A, Tillander S, Hannula S, Nyman T, Toskala E, Alenius H, Lauerma A. Thaumatin-like protein and baker's respiratory allergy. *Ann Allergy Asthma Immunol.* 2010 Feb;104(2):139-46.

Leitzmann C. Vegetarian diets: what are the advantages? *Forum Nutr.* 2005;(57):147-56.

Leu YL, Shi LS, Damu AG. Chemical constituents of Taraxacum formosanum. Chem *Pharm Bull.* 2003 May;51(5):599-601.

Leu YL, Wang YL, Huang SC, Shi LS. Chemical constituents from roots of Taraxacum formosanum. *Chem Pharm Bull*. 2005 Jul;53(7):853-5.

Leung DY, Sampson HA, Yunginger JW, Burks AW Jr, Schneider LC, Wortel CH, Davis FM, Hyun JD, Shanahan WR Jr; Avon Longitudinal Study of Parents and Children Study Team. Effect of anti-IgE therapy in patients with peanut allergy. *N Engl J Med*. 2003 Mar 13;348(11):986-93.

Leung DY, Shanahan WR Jr, Li XM, Sampson HA. New approaches for the treatment of anaphylaxis. *Novartis Found Symp*. 2004;257:248-60; discussion 260-4, 276-85.

Lewerin C, Jacobsson S, Lindstedt G, Nilsson-Ehle H. Serum biomarkers for atrophic gastritis and antibodies against Helicobacter pylori in the elderly: Implications for vitamin B12, folic acid and iron status and response to oral vitamin therapy. *Scand J Gastroenterol*. 2008;43(9):1050-6.

Lewis SA, Grimshaw KE, Warner JO, Hourihane JO. The promiscuity of immunoglobulin E binding to peanut allergens, as determined by Western blotting, correlates with the severity of clinical symptoms. *Clin Exp Allergy*. 2005 Jun;35(6):767-73.

Lewis WH, Elvin-Lewis MPF. *Medical Botany: Plants Affecting Man's Health*. New York: Wiley, 1977.

Lewontin R. *The Genetic Basis of Evolutionary Change*. New York: Columbia Univ Press, 1974.

Leyel CF. *Culpeper's English Physician & Complete Herbal*. Hollywood, CA: Wilshire, 1971.

Leynadier F. Mast cells and basophils in asthma. Ann Biol Clin (Paris). 1989;47(6):351-6.

Li H, Tan G, Jiang X, Qiao H, Pan S, Jiang H, Kanwar JR, Sun X. Therapeutic effects of matrine on primary and metastatic breast cancer. *Am J Chin Med*. 2010;38(6):1115-30.

Li S, Li W, Wang Y, Asada Y, Koike K. Prenylflavonoids from Glycyrrhiza uralensis and their protein tyrosine phosphatase-1B inhibitory activities. *Bioorg Med Chem Lett*. 2010 Sep 15;20(18):5398-401.

Li XM, Huang CK, Zhang TF, Teper AA, Srivastava K, Schofield BH, Sampson HA. The chinese herbal medicine formula MSSM-002 suppresses allergic airway hyperreactivity and modulates TH1/TH2 responses in a murine model of allergic asthma. *J Allergy Clin Immunol*. 2000;106:660–8.

Li XM, Schofield BH, Huang CK, Kleiner GA, Sampson HA. A Murine Model of IgE Mediated Cow Milk Hypersensitivity. *J Allergy Clin Immunol*. 1999;103:206–14.

Li XM, Serebrisky D, Lee SY, Huang CK, Bardina L, Schofield BH, Stanley JS, Burks AW, Bannon GA, Sampson HA. A murine model of peanut anaphylaxis: T- and B-cell responses to a major peanut allergen mimic human responses. *J Allergy Clin Immunol*. 2000;106:150–8.

Li XM, Zhang TF, Huang CK, Srivastava K, Teper AA, Zhang L, Schofield BH, Sampson HA. Food Allergy Herbal Formula-1 (FAHF-1) blocks peanut-induced anaphylaxis in a murine model. *J Allergy Clin Immunol*. 2001;108:639–46.

Li XM, Zhang TF, Sampson H, Zou ZM, Beyer K, Wen MC, Schofield B. The potential use of Chinese herbal medicines in treating allergic asthma. *Ann Allergy Asthma Immunol*. 2004;93:S35–S44.

Li XM. Beyond allergen avoidance: update on developing therapies for peanut allergy. *Curr Opin Allergy Clin Immunol*. 2005;5:287–92.

Lidén M, Kristjánsson G, Valtysdottir S, Venge P, Hällgren R. Cow's milk protein sensitivity assessed by the mucosal patch technique is related to irritable bowel syndrome in patients with primary Sjögren's syndrome. *Clin Exp Allergy*. 2008 Jun;38(6):929-35.

Lidén M, Kristjánsson G, Valtysdottir S, Venge P, Hällgren R. Self-reported food intolerance and mucosal reactivity after rectal food protein challenge in patients with rheumatoid arthritis. *Scand J Rheumatol*. 2010 Aug;39(4):292-8.

Lied GA, Lillestol K, Valeur J, Berstad A. Intestinal B cell-activating factor: an indicator of non-IgE-mediated hypersensitivity reactions to food? *Aliment Pharmacol Ther*. 2010 Jul;32(1):66-73.

Lillestol K, Berstad A, Lind R, Florvaag E, Arslan Lied G, Tangen T. Anxiety and depression in patients with self-reported food hypersensitivity. *Gen Hosp Psychiatry*. 2010 Jan-Feb;32(1):42-8.

Lillestol K, Helgeland L, Arslan Lied G, Florvaag E, Valeur J, Lind R, Berstad A. Indications of 'atopic bowel' in patients with self-reported food hypersensitivity. *Aliment Pharmacol Ther*. 2010 May;31(10):1112-22.

Lim JP, Song YC, Kim JW, Ku CH, Eun JS, Leem KH, Kim DK. Free radical scavengers from the heartwood of Juniperus chinensis. *Arch Pharm Res*. 2002 Aug;25(4):449-52.

Lindfors K, Blomqvist T, Juuti-Uusitalo K, Stenman S, Venäläinen J, Mäki M, Kaukinen K. Live probiotic Bifido-bacterium lactis bacteria inhibit the toxic effects induced by wheat gliadin in epithelial cell culture. Clin Exp Immunol. 2008 Jun;152(3):552-8. doi: 10.1111/j.1365-2249.2008.03635.x.

Ling WH, Hänninen O. Shifting from a conventional diet to an uncooked vegan diet reversibly alters fecal hydrolytic activities in humans. *J Nutr*. 1992 Apr;122(4):924-30.

Lininger S, Gaby A, Austin S, Brown D, Wright J, Duncan A. *The Natural Pharmacy*. New York: Three Rivers, 1999.

Linsalata M, Russo F, Berloco P, Caruso ML, Matteo GD, Cifone MG, Simone CD, Ierardi E, Di Leo A. The influence of Lactobacillus brevis on ornithine decarboxylase activity and polyamine profiles in

REFERENCES AND BIBLIOGRAPHY

Helicobacter pylori-infected gastric mucosa. Helicobacter. 2004 Apr;9(2):165-72. Madden JA, Plummer SF, Tang J, Garaiova I, Plummer NT, Herbison M, Hunter JO, Shimada T, Cheng L, Shirakawa T. Effect of probiotics on preventing disruption of the intestinal microflora following antibiotic therapy: a double-blind, placebo-controlled pilot study. Int Immunopharmacol. 2005 Jun;5(6):1091-7.

Lipozencić J, Wolf R. The diagnostic value of atopy patch testing and prick testing in atopic dermatitis: facts and controversies. Clin Dermatol. 2010 Jan-Feb;28(1):38-44.

Lipski E. Digestive Wellness. Los Angeles, CA: Keats, 2000.

Liu GM, Cao MJ, Huang YY, Cai QF, Weng WY, Su WJ. Comparative study of in vitro digestibility of major allergen tropomyosin and other food proteins of Chinese mitten crab (Eriocheir sinensis). J Sci Food Agric. 2010 Aug 15;90(10):1614-20.

Liu HY, Giday Z, Moore BF. Possible pathogenetic mechanisms producing bovine milk protein inducible malabsorption: a hypothesis. Ann Allergy. 1977 Jul;39(1):1-7.

Liu JY, Hu JH, Zhu QG, Li FQ, Wang J, Sun HJ. Effect of matrine on the expression of substance P receptor and inflammatory cytokines production in human skin keratinocytes and fibroblasts. Int Immunopharmacol. 2007 Jun;7(6):816-23.

Liu X, Beaty TH, Deindl P, Huang SK, Lau S, Sommerfeld C, Fallin MD, Kao WH, Wahn U, Nickel R. Associations between specific serum IgE response and 6 variants within the genes IL4, IL13, and IL4RA in German children: the German Multicenter Atopy Study. J Allergy Clin Immunol. 2004 Mar;113(3):489-95.

Liu XJ, Cao MA, Li WH, Shen CS, Yan SQ, Yuan CS. Alkaloids from Sophora flavescens Aition. Fitoterapia. 2010 Sep;81(6):524-7.

Lloyd JU. American Materia Medica, Therapeutics and Pharmacognosy. Portland, OR: Eclectic Medical Publications, 1989-1983.

Lloyd-Still JD, Powers CA, Hoffman DR, Boyd-Trull K, Lester LA, Benisek DC, Arterburn LM. Bioavailability and safety of a high dose of docosahexaenoic acid triacylglycerol of algal origin in cystic fibrosis patients: a randomized, controlled study. Nutrition. 2006 Jan;22(1):36-46.

Loizzo MR, Saab AM, Tundis R, Statti GA, Menichini F, Lampronti I, Gambari R, Cinatl J, Doerr HW. Phytochemical analysis and in vitro antiviral activities of the essential oils of seven Lebanon species. Chem Biodivers. 2008 Mar;5(3):461-70.

Lomax AR, Calder PC. Probiotics, immune function, infection and inflammation: a review of the evidence from studies conducted in humans. Curr Pharm Des. 2009;15(13):1428-518.

Longo G, Barbi E, Berti I, Meneghetti R, Pittalis A, Ronfani L, Ventura A. Specific oral tolerance induction in children with very severe cow's milk-induced reactions. J Allergy Clin Immunol. 2008 Feb;121(2):343-7.

López N, de Barros-Mazón S, Vilela MM, Silva CM, Ribeiro JD. Genetic and environmental influences on atopic immune response in early life. J Investig Allergol Clin Immunol. 1999 Nov-Dec;9(6):392-8.

Lopez-Garcia E, Schulze MB, Meigs JB, Manson JE, Rifai N, Stampfer MJ, Willett WC, Hu FB. Consumption of trans fatty acids is related to plasma biomarkers of inflammation and endothelial dysfunction. J Nutr. 2005 Mar;135(3):562-6.

Lorea Baroja M, Kirjavainen PV, Hekmat S, Reid G. Anti-inflammatory effects of probiotic yogurt in inflammatory bowel disease patients. Clin Exp Immunol. 2007 Sep;149(3):470-9.

Lovchik MA, Fráter G, Goeke A, Hug W. Total synthesis of junionone, a natural monoterpenoid from Juniperus communis L., and determination of the absolute configuration of the naturally occurring enantiomer by ROA spectroscopy. Chem Biodivers. 2008 Jan;5(1):126-39.

Lu MK, Shih YW, Chang Chien TT, Fang LH, Huang HC, Chen PS. α-Solanine inhibits human melanoma cell migration and invasion by reducing matrix metalloproteinase-2/9 activities. Biol Pharm Bull. 2010;33(10):1685-91.

Ludvigsson JF, Olén O, Bell M, Ekbom A, Montgomery SM. Coeliac disease and risk of sepsis. Gut. 2008 Aug;57(8):1074-80.

Lykken DT, Tellegen A, DeRubeis R: Volunteer bias in twin research: the rule of two-thirds. Soc Biol 1978, 25(1): 1-9. Phillips DI: Twin studies in medical research: can they tell us whether diseases are genetically determined? Lancet 1993;341(8851): 1008-1009.

Mabey R, ed. The New Age Herbalist. New York: Simon & Schuster, 1941.

Macdonald TT, Monteleone G. Immunity, inflammation, and allergy in the gut. Science. 2005 Mar 25;307(5717):1920-5. Review. PubMed PMID: 15790845.

Maciorkowska E, Kaczmarski M, Andrzej K. Endoscopic evaluation of upper gastrointestinal tract mucosa in children with food hypersensitivity. Med Wieku Rozwoj. 2000 Jan-Mar;4(1):37-48.

Maeda N, Inomata N, Morita A, Kirino M, Ikezawa Z. Correlation of oral allergy syndrome due to plant-derived foods with pollen sensitization in Japan. Ann Allergy Asthma Immunol. 2010 Mar;104(3):205-10.

Maes HH, Silberg JL, Neale MC, Eaves LJ. Genetic and cultural transmission of antisocial behavior: an extended twin parent model. *Twin Res Hum Genet.* 2007 Feb;10(1):136-50.

Maes M, Kubera M, Leunis JC. The gut-brain barrier in major depression: intestinal mucosal dysfunction with an increased translocation of LPS from gram negative enterobacteria (leaky gut) plays a role in the inflammatory pathophysiology of depression. *Neuro Endocrinol Lett.* 2008 Feb;29(1):117-24.

Mahady GB, Pendland SL, Stoia A, Hamill FA, Fabricant D, Dietz BM, Chadwick LR. In vitro susceptibility of Helicobacter pylori to botanical extracts used traditionally for the treatment of gastrointestinal disorders. *Phytother Res.* 2005 Nov;19(11):988-91.

Mai XM, Kull I, Wickman M, Bergström A. Antibiotic use in early life and development of allergic diseases: respiratory infection as the explanation. *Clin Exp Allergy.* 2010 Aug;40(8):1230-7.

Majamaa H, Isolauri E. Probiotics: a novel approach in the management of food allergy. *J Allergy Clin Immunol.* 1997 Feb;99(2):179-85.

Maki KC, Gibson GR, Dickmann RS, Kendall CW, Oliver Chen CY, Costabile A, Comelli EM, McKay DL, Almeida NG, Jenkins D, Zello GA, Blumberg JB. Digestive and physiologic effects of a wheat bran extract, arabino-xylan-oligosaccharide, in breakfast cereal. Nutrition. 2012 Jul 6.

Makrides M, Neumann M, Gibson R. Effect of maternal docosahexaenoic acid (DHA) supplementation on breast milk composition. *Europ Jrnl of Clin Nutr.* 1996;50:352-357.

Maliakal PP, Wanwimolruk S. Effect of herbal teas on hepatic drug metabolizing enzymes in rats. *J Pharm Pharmacol.* 2001 Oct;53(10):1323-9.

Mälkönen T, Alanko K, Jolanki R, Luukkonen R, Aalto-Korte K, Lauerma A, Susitaival P. Long-term follow-up study of occupational hand eczema. Br J Dermatol. 2010 Aug 13.

Månsson HL. Fatty acids in bovine milk fat. *Food Nutr Res.* 2008;52. doi: 10.3402/fnr.v52i0.1821.

Manz F. Hydration and disease. *J Am Coll Nutr.* 2007 Oct;26(5 Suppl):535S-541S.

Marcucci F, Duse M, Frati F, Incorvaia C, Marseglia GL, La Rosa M. The future of sublingual immunotherapy. *Int J Immunopathol Pharmacol.* 2009 Oct-Dec;22(4 Suppl):31-3.

Margioris AN. Fatty acids and postprandial inflammation. *Curr Opin Clin Nutr Metab Care.* 2009 Mar;12(2):129-37.

Martinez M. Docosahexaenoic acid therapy in docosahexaenoic acid-deficient patients with disorders of peroxisomal biogenesis. *Versicherungsmedizin.* 1996;31 Suppl:145-152

Martínez-Augustin O, Boza JJ, Del Pino JI, Lucena J, Martínez-Valverde A, Gil A. Dietary nucleotides might influence the humoral immune response against cow's milk proteins in preterm neonates. *Biol Neonate.* 1997;71(4):215-23.

Martin-Venegas R, Roig-Perez S, Ferrer R, Moreno JJ. Arachidonic acid cascade and epithelial barrier function during Caco-2 cell differentiation. J Lipid Res. 2006 Apr;3.

Massey DG, Chien YK, Fournier-Massey G. Mamane: scientific therapy for asthma? *Hawaii Med J.* 1994;53:350-1. 363.

Massicot JG, Cohen SG. Epidemiologic and socioeconomic aspects of allergic diseases. *J Allergy Clin Immunol.* 1986 Nov;78(5 Pt 2):954-8.

Matheson MC, Haydn Walters E, Burgess JA, Jenkins MA, Giles GG, Hopper JL, Abramson MJ, Dharmage SC. Childhood immunization and atopic disease into middle-age—a prospective cohort study. *Pediatr Allergy Immunol.* 2010 Mar;21(2 Pt 1):301-6.

Matricardi PM, Bockelbrink A, Beyer K, Keil T, Niggemann B, Grüber C, Wahn U, Lau S. Primary versus secondary immunoglobulin E sensitization to soy and wheat in the Multi-Centre Allergy Study cohort. *Clin Exp Allergy.* 2008 Mar;38(3):493-500.

Matsuda T, Maruyama T, Iizuka H, Kondo A, Tamai T, Kurohane K, Imai Y. Phthalate esters reveal skin-sensitizing activity of phenethyl isothiocyanate in mice. *Food Chem Toxicol.* 2010 Jun;48(6):1704-8.

Maxton DG, Bjarnason I, Reynolds AP, Catt SD, Peters TJ, Menzies IS. Lactulose, 51Cr-labelled ethylenediaminetetra-acetate, L-rhamnose and polyethyleneglycol 400 [corrected] as probe markers for assessment in vivo of human intestinal permeability. *Clin Sci (Lond).* 1986 Jul;71(1):71-80.

Mayes MD. Epidemiologic studies of environmental agents and systemic autoimmune diseases. *Environ Health Perspect.* 1999 Oct;107 Suppl 5:743-8.

McAlindon TE. Nutraceuticals: do they work and when should we use them? *Best Pract Res Clin Rheumatol.* 2006 Feb;20(1):99-115.

McBride C, McBride-Henry K, Wissen K. Parenting a child with medically diagnosed severe food allergies in New Zealand: The experience of being unsupported in keeping their children healthy and safe. *Contemp Nurse.* 2010 Apr;35(1):77-87.

McConnaughey E. *Sea Vegetables.* Happy Camp, CA: Naturegraph, 1985.

McCune LM, Johns T. Antioxidant activity in medicinal plants associated with the symptoms of diabetes mellitus used by the indigenous peoples of the North American boreal forest. *J Ethnopharmacol.* 2002 Oct;82(2-3):197-205.

REFERENCES AND BIBLIOGRAPHY

McDougall J, McDougall M. *The McDougal Plan.* Clinton, NJ: New Win, 1983.

McKenzie H, Main J, Pennington CR, Parratt D. Antibody to selected strains of Saccharomyces cerevisiae (baker's and brewer's yeast) and Candida albicans in Crohn's disease. *Gut.* 1990 May;31(5):536-8.

McLachlan CN. beta-casein A1, ischaemic heart disease mortality, and other illnesses. *Med Hypotheses.* 2001 Feb;56(2):262-72.

McLean S, Sheikh A. Does avoidance of peanuts in early life reduce the risk of peanut allergy? *BMJ.* 2010 Mar 11;340:c424. doi: 10.1136/bmj.c424.

McNally ME, Atkinson SA, Cole DE. Contribution of sulfate and sulfoesters to total sulfur intake in infants fed human milk. *J Nutr.* 1991 Aug;121(8):1250-4.

Meglio P, Bartone E, Plantamura M, Arabito E, Giampietro PG. A protocol for oral desensitization in children with IgE-mediated cow's milk allergy. Allergy. 2004 Sep;59(9):980-7.

Mehra PN, Puri HS. Studies on Gaduchi satwa. *Indian J Pharm.* 1969;31:180-2.

Meier B, Shao Y, Julkunen-Tiitto R, Bettschart A, Sticher O. A chemotaxonomic survey of phenolic compounds in Swiss willow species. *Planta Med.* 1992;58:A698.

Meier B, Sticher O, Julkunen-Tiitto R. Pharmaceutical aspects of the use of willows in herbal remedies. *Planta Med.* 1988;54(6):559-560.

Melcion C, Verroust P, Baud L, Ardaillou N, Morel-Maroger L, Ardaillou R. Protective effect of procyanidolic oligomers on the heterologous phase of glomerulonephritis induced by anti-glomerular basement membrane antibodies. *C R Seances Acad Sci III.* 1982 Dec 6;295(12):721-6.

Melzig MF. Goldenrod—a classical exponent in the urological phytotherapy. *Wien Med Wochenschr.* 2004 Nov;154(21-22):523-7.

Merchant RE and Andre CA. 2001. A review of recent clinical trials of the nutritional supplement Chlorella pyrenoidosa in the treatment of fibromyalgia, hypertension, and ulcerative colitis. *Altern Ther Health Med.* May-Jun;7(3):79-91.

Metsälä J, Lundqvist A, Kaila M, Gissler M, Klaukka T, Virtanen SM. Maternal and perinatal characteristics and the risk of cow's milk allergy in infants up to 2 years of age: a case-control study nested in the Finnish population. *Am J Epidemiol.* 2010 Jun 15;171(12):1310-6.

Meyer A, Kirsch H, Domergue F, Abbadi A, Sperling P, Bauer J, Cirpus P, Zank TK, Moreau H, Roscoe TJ, Zahringer U, Heinz E. Novel fatty acid elongases and their use for the reconstitution of docosahexaenoic acid biosynthesis. *J Lipid Res.* 2004 Oct;45(10):1899-909.

Miceli N, Trovato A, Dugo P, Cacciola F, Donato P, Marino A, Bellinghieri V, La Barbera TM, Güvenç A, Taviano MF. Comparative Analysis of Flavonoid Profile, Antioxidant and Antimicrobial Activity of the Berries of Juniperus communis L. var. communis and Juniperus communis L. var. saxatilis Pall. *J Agric Food Chem.* 2009 Jul 6.

Michaelsen KF. Probiotics, breastfeeding and atopic eczema. *Acta Derm Venereol Suppl (Stockh).* 2005 Nov;(215):21-4.

Michalska K, Kisiel W. Sesquiterpene lactones from Taraxacum obovatum. *Planta Med.* 2003 Feb;69(2):181-3.

Michetti P, Dorta G, Wiesel PH, Brassart D, Verdu E, Herranz M, Felley C, Porta N, Rouvet M, Blum AL, Corthésy-Theulaz I. Effect of whey-based culture supernatant of Lactobacillus acidophilus (johnsonii) La1 on Helicobacter pylori infection in humans. *Digestion.* 1999;60(3):203-9.

Mikoluc B, Motkowski R, Karpinska J, Piotrowska-Jastrzebska J. Plasma levels of vitamins A and E, coenzyme Q10, and anti-ox-LDL antibody titer in children treated with an elimination diet due to food hypersensitivity. *Int J Vitam Nutr Res.* 2009 Sep;79(5-6):328-36.

Miller GT. *Living in the Environment.* Belmont, CA: Wadsworth, 1996.

Miller K. Cholesterol and In-Hospital Mortality in Elderly Patients. *Am Family Phys.* 2004 May.

Mindell E, Hopkins V. *Prescription Alternatives.* New Canaan, CT: Keats, 1998.

Miranda H, Outeiro TF. The sour side of neurodegenerative disorders: the effects of protein glycation. J Pathol. 2010 May;221(1):13-25.

Mitchell AE, Hong YJ, Koh E, Barrett DM, Bryant DE, Denison RF, Kaffka S. Ten-year comparison of the influence of organic and conventional crop management practices on the content of flavonoids in tomatoes. *J Agric Food Chem.* 2007 Jul 25;55(15):6154-9.

Mittag D, Akkerdaas J, Ballmer-Weber BK, Vogel L, Wensing M, Becker WM, Koppelman SJ, Knulst AC, Helbling A, Hefle SL, Van Ree R, Vieths S. Ara h 8, a Bet v 1-homologous allergen from peanut, is a major allergen in patients with combined birch pollen and peanut allergy. *J Allergy Clin Immunol.* 2004 Dec;114(6):1410-7.

Mittag D, Vieths S, Vogel L, Becker WM, Rihs HP, Helbling A, Wüthrich B, Ballmer-Weber BK. Soybean allergy in patients allergic to birch pollen: clinical investigation and molecular characterization of allergens. *J Allergy Clin Immunol.* 2004 Jan;113(1):148-54.

Miyazawa T, Itahashi K, Imai T. Management of neonatal cow's milk allergy in high-risk neonates. *Pediatr Int.* 2009 Aug;51(4):544-7.

213

Molkhou P, Dupont C. Ketotifen in prevention and therapy of food allergy. *Ann Allergy.* 1987 Nov;59(5 Pt 2):187-93.

Monarca S. Zerbini I, Simonati C, Gelatti U. Drinking water hardness and chronic degenerative diseases. Part II. Cardiovascular diseases. *Ann. Ig.* 2003;15:41-56.

Moneret-Vautrin DA, Kanny G, Thévenin F. Asthma caused by food allergy. *Rev Med Interne.* 1996;17(7):551-7.

Moneret-Vautrin DA, Morisset M. Adult food allergy. *Curr Allergy Asthma Rep.* 2005 Jan;5(1):80-5.

Monks H, Gowland MH, Mackenzie H, Erlewyn-Lajeunesse M, King R, Lucas JS, Roberts G. How do teenagers manage their food allergies? *Clin Exp Allergy.* 2010 Aug 2.

Moorhead KJ, Morgan HC. *Spirulina: Nature's Superfood.* Kailua-Kona, HI: Nutrex, 1995.

Morel AF, Dias GO, Porto C, Simionatto E, Stuker CZ, Dalcol II. Antimicrobial activity of extractives of Solidago microglossa. *Fitoterapia.* 2006 Sep;77(6):453-5.

Morgan CB, Hughes J, McCants M, Lehrer SB. Food specific skin-test reactivity in atopic subjects. *Clin Exp Allergy.* 1989 Jul;19(4):431-5.

Mori F, Bianchi I, Pucci N, Azzari C, De Martino M, Novembre E. CD4+CD25+Foxp3+ T regulatory cells are not involved in oral desensitization. *Int J Immunopathol Pharmacol.* 2010 Jan-Mar;23(1):359-61.

Morisset M, Moneret-Vautrin DA, Guenard L, Cuny JM, Frentz P, Hatahet R, Hanss Ch, Beaudouin E, Petit N, Kanny G. Oral desensitization in children with milk and egg allergies obtains recovery in a significant proportion of cases. A randomized study in 60 children with cow's milk allergy and 90 children with egg allergy. *Eur Ann Allergy Clin Immunol.* 2007 Jan;39(1):12-9.

Morisset M, Moneret-Vautrin DA, Kanny G, Guénard L, Beaudouin E, Flabbée J, Hatahet R. Thresholds of clinical reactivity to milk, egg, peanut and sesame in immunoglobulin E-dependent allergies: evaluation by double-blind or single-blind placebo-controlled oral challenges. *Clin Exp Allergy.* 2003 Aug;33(8):1046-51.

Morisset M, Moneret-Vautrin DA, Kanny G; Allergo-Vigilance Network. Prevalence of peanut sensitization in a population of 4,737 subjects—an Allergo-Vigilance Network enquiry carried out in 2002. *Eur Ann Allergy Clin Immunol.* 2005 Feb;37(2):54-7.

Morisset M, Moneret-Vautrin DA, Maadi F, Frémont S, Guénard L, Croizier A, Kanny G. Prospective study of mustard allergy: first study with double-blind placebo-controlled food challenge trials (24 cases). *Allergy.* 2003 Apr;58(4):295-9.

Morris AJ, Howden CW, Robertson C, Duncan A, Torley H, Sturrock RD, Russell RI. Increased intestinal permeability in ankylosing spondylitis—primary lesion or drug effect? *Gut.* 1991 Dec;32(12):1470-2.

Moujir L, Seca AM, Silva AM, Barreto MC. Cytotoxic activity of diterpenes and extracts of Juniperus brevifolia. *Planta Med.* 2008 Jun;74(7):751-3.

Moussaieff A, Shein NA, Tsenter J, Grigoriadis S, Simeonidou C, Alexandrovich AG, Trembovler V, Ben-Neriah Y, Schmitz ML, Fiebich BL, Munoz E, Mechoulam R, Shohami E. Incensole acetate: a novel neuroprotective agent isolated from Boswellia carterii. *J Cereb Blood Flow Metab.* 2008 Jul;28(7):1341-52.

Mozaffarian D, Aro A, Willett WC. Health effects of trans-fatty acids: experimental and observational evidence. *Eur J Clin Nutr.* 2009 May;63 Suppl 2:S5-21.

Mrowietz-Ruckstuhl B. Bacteriological stool examinations. *Dtsch Arztebl Int.* 2010 Jan;107(3):40; author reply 40-1.

Mullin GE, Swift KM, Lipski L, Turnbull LK, Rampertab SD. Testing for food reactions: the good, the bad, and the ugly. *Nutr Clin Pract.* 2010 Apr;25(2):192-8.

Murray M, Pizzorno J. *Encyclopedia of Natural Medicine.* 2nd Edition. Roseville, CA: Prima Publishing, 1998.

Na HJ, Koo HN, Lee GG, Yoo SJ, Park JH, Lyu YS, Kim HM. Juniper oil inhibits the heat shock-induced apoptosis via preventing the caspase-3 activation in human astrocytes CCF-STTG1 cells. *Clin Chim Acta.* 2001 Dec;314(1-2):215-20.

Nadkarni AK, Nadkarni KM. *Indian Materia Medica.* (Vols 1 and 2). Bombay, India: Popular Pradashan, 1908, 1976.

Nagel G, Weinmayr G, Kleiner A, Garcia-Marcos L, Strachan DP; ISAAC Phase Two Study Group. Effect of diet on asthma and allergic sensitisation in the International Study on Allergies and Asthma in Childhood (ISAAC) Phase Two. *Thorax.* 2010 Jun;65(6):516-22.

Naghii MR, Samman S. The role of boron in nutrition and metabolism. *Prog Food Nutr Sci.* 1993 Oct-Dec;17(4):331-49.

Nair PK, Rodriguez S, Ramachandran R, Alamo A, Melnick SJ, Escalon E, Garcia PI Jr, Wnuk SF, Ramachandran C. Immune stimulating properties of a novel polysaccharide from the medicinal plant Tinospora cordifolia. *Int Immunopharmacol.* 2004 Dec 15;4(13):1645-59.

Nakano T, Shimojo N, Morita Y, Arima T, Tomiita M, Kohno Y. Sensitization to casein and beta-lactoglobulin (BLG) in children with cow's milk allergy (CMA). *Arerugi.* 2010 Feb;59(2):117-22.

REFERENCES AND BIBLIOGRAPHY

Napoli, J.E., Brand-Miller, J.C., Conway, P. (2003) Bifidogenic effects of feeding infant formula containing galactooligosaccharides in healthy formula-fed infants. *Asia Pac J Clin Nutr.* 12(Suppl): S60

Nariya M, Shukla V, Jain S, Ravishankar B. Comparison of enteroprotective efficacy of triphala formulations (Indian Herbal Drug) on methotrexate-induced small intestinal damage in rats. *Phytother Res.* 2009 Aug;23(8):1092-8.

Naruszewicz M, Johansson ML, Zapolska-Downar D, Bukowska H. Effect of Lactobacillus plantarum 299v on cardiovascular disease risk factors in smokers. *Am J Clin Nutr.* 2002 Dec;76(6):1249-55.

Nchito M, Friis H, Michaelsen KF, Mubila L, Olsen A. Iron supplementation increases small intestine permeability in primary schoolchildren in Lusaka, Zambia. *Trans R Soc Trop Med Hyg.* 2006 Aug;100(8):791-4.

NDL, BHNRC, ARS, USDA. *Oxygen Radical Absorbance Capacity (ORAC) of Selected Foods - 2007.* Beltsville, MD: USDA-ARS. 2007.

Nehra V. New clinical issues in celiac disease. *Gastroenterol Clin North Am.* 1998 Jun;27(2):453-65.

Neilan NA, Dowling PJ, Taylor DL, Ryan P, Schurman JV, Friesen CA. Useful biomarkers in pediatric eosinophilic duodenitis and their existence: a case-control, single-blind, observational pilot study. *J Pediatr Gastroenterol Nutr.* 2010 Apr;50(4):377-84.

Nentwich I, Michková E, Nevoral J, Urbanek R, Szépfalusi Z. Cow's milk-specific cellular and humoral immune responses and atopy skin symptoms in infants from atopic families fed a partially (pHF) or extensively (eHF) hydrolyzed infant formula. *Allergy.* 2001 Dec;56(12):1144-56.

Nermes M, Karvonen H, Sarkkinen E, Isolauri E. Safety of barley starch syrup in patients with allergy to cereals. *Br J Nutr.* 2009 Jan;101(2):165-8.

Newall CA, Anderson LA, Philpson JD. *Herbal Medicine: A Guide for Healthcare Professionals.* London: Pharmaceutical Press, 1996.

Newmark T, Schulick P. *Beyond Aspirin.* Prescott, AZ: Holm, 2000.

Neyestani TR, Shariatzadeh N, Gharavi A, Kalayi A, Khalaji N. Physiological dose of lycopene suppressed oxidative stress and enhanced serum levels of immunoglobulin M in patients with Type 2 diabetes mellitus: a possible role in the prevention of long-term complications. *J Endocrinol Invest.* 2007 Nov;30(10):833-8.

Nicholls SJ, Lundman P, Harmer JA, Cutri B, Griffiths KA, Rye KA, Barter PJ, Celermajer DS. Consumption of saturated fat impairs the anti-inflammatory properties of high-density lipoproteins and endothelial function. *J Am Coll Cardiol.* 2006 Aug 15;48(4):715-20.

Nicolaou N, Poorafshar M, Murray C, Simpson A, Winell H, Kerry G, Härlin A, Woodcock A, Ahlstedt S, Custovic A. Allergy or tolerance in children sensitized to peanut: prevalence and differentiation using component-resolved diagnostics. *J Allergy Clin Immunol.* 2010 Jan;125(1):191-7.e1-13.

Niederau C, Göpfert E. The effect of chelidonium- and turmeric root extract on upper abdominal pain due to functional disorders of the biliary system. Results from a placebo-controlled double-blind study. *Med Klin.* 1999 Aug 15;94(8):425-30.

Niederberger V, Horak F, Vrtala S, Spitzauer S, Krauth MT, Valent P, Reisinger J, Pelzmann M, Hayek B, Kronqvist M, Gafvelin G, Grönlund H, Purohit A, Suck R, Fiebig H, Cromwell O, Pauli G, van Hage-Hamsten M, Valenta R. Vaccination with genetically engineered allergens prevents progression of allergic disease. *Proc Natl Acad Sci U S A.* 2004 Oct 5;101 Suppl 2:14677-82.

Niedzielin K, Kordecki H, Birkenfeld B. A controlled, double-blind, randomized study on the efficacy of Lactobacillus plantarum 299V in patients with irritable bowel syndrome. *Eur J Gastroenterol Hepatol.* 2001 Oct;13(10):1143-7.

Nielsen RG, Bindslev-Jensen C, Kruse-Andersen S, Husby S. Severe gastroesophageal reflux disease and cow milk hypersensitivity in infants and children: disease association and evaluation of a new challenge procedure. *J Pediatr Gastroenterol Nutr.* 2004 Oct;39(4):383-91.

Nielsen WW, Lindsey K. When there is no school nurse—are teachers prepared for students with peanut allergies? *School Nurse News.* 2010 Jan;27(1):12-5.

Niggemann B, Binder C, Dupont C, Hadji S, Arvola T, Isolauri E. Prospective, controlled, multi-center study on the effect of an amino-acid-based formula in infants with cow's milk allergy/intolerance and atopic dermatitis. *Pediatr Allergy Immunol.* 2001 Apr;12(2):78-82.

Niggemann B, Celik-Bilgili S, Ziegert M, Reibel S, Sommerfeld C, Wahn U. Specific IgE levels do not indicate persistence or transience of food allergy in children with atopic dermatitis. *J Investig Allergol Clin Immunol.* 2004;14(2):98-103.

Niggemann B, von Berg A, Bollrath C, Berdel D, Schauer U, Rieger C, Haschke-Becher E, Wahn U. Safety and efficacy of a new extensively hydrolyzed formula for infants with cow's milk protein allergy. *Pediatr Allergy Immunol.* 2008 Jun;19(4):348-54.

Nobaek S, Johansson ML, Molin G, Ahrné S, Jeppsson B. Alteration of intestinal microflora is associated with reduction in abdominal bloating and pain in patients with irritable bowel syndrome. *Am J Gastroenterol.* 2000 May;95(5):1231-8.

Nodake Y, Fukomoto S, Fukasawa M, Sakakibara R, Yamasaki N. Reduction of the immunogenicity of beta-lactoglobulin from cow's milk by conjugation with a dextran derivative. *Biosci Biotechnol Biochem.* 2010;74(4):721-6.

Noh J, Lee JH, Noh G, Bang SY, Kim HS, Choi WS, Cho S, Lee SS. Characterisation of allergen-specific responses of IL-10-producing regulatory B cells (Br1) in Cow Milk Allergy. *Cell Immunol.* 2010;264(2):143-9.

Noorbakhsh R, Mortazavi SA, Sankian M, Shahidi F, Assarehzadegan MA, Varasteh A. Cloning, expression, characterization, and computational approach for cross-reactivity prediction of manganese superoxide dismutase allergen from pistachio nut. *Allergol Int.* 2010 Sep;59(3):295-304.

Nowak-Wegrzyn A, Fiocchi A. Is oral immunotherapy the cure for food allergies? *Curr Opin Allergy Clin Immunol.* 2010 Jun;10(3):214-9.

Nowak-Wegrzyn A, Muraro A. Food protein-induced enterocolitis syndrome. *Curr Opin Allergy Clin Immunol.* 2009 Aug;9(4):371-7.

Nowak-Wegrzyn A, Sampson HA, Wood RA, Sicherer SH. Food protein-induced enterocolitis syndrome caused by solid food proteins. *Pediatrics.* 2003 Apr;111(4 Pt 1):829-35.

Nuñez YO, Salabarria IS, Collado IG, Hernández-Galán R. Sesquiterpenes from the wood of Juniperus lucayana. *Phytochemistry.* 2007 Oct;68(19):2409-14.

O'Connor J., Bensky D. (ed). *Shanghai College of Traditional Chinese Medicine: Acupuncture: A Comprehensive Text.* Seattle: Eastland Press, 1981.

O'Connor MI. Warming strengthens an herbivore-plant interaction. *Ecology.* 2009 Feb;90(2):388-98.

Odamaki T, Xiao JZ, Iwabuchi N, Sakamoto M, Takahashi N, Kondo S, Miyaji K, Iwatsuki K, Togashi H, Enomoto T, Benno Y. Influence of Bifidobacterium longum BB536 intake on faecal microbiota in individuals with Japanese cedar pollinosis during the pollen season. *J Med Microbiol.* 2007 Oct;56(Pt 10):1301-8.

Oehme FW (ed.). *Toxicity of heavy metals in the environment. Part 1.* New York: M.Dekker, 1979.

Oh CK, Lücker PW, Wetzelsberger N, Kuhlmann F. The determination of magnesium, calcium, sodium and potassium in assorted foods with special attention to the loss of electrolytes after various forms of food preparations. *Mag.-Bull.* 1986;8:297-302.

Oh JW, Pyun BY, Choung JT, Ahn KM, Kim CH, Song SW, Son JA, Lee SY, Lee SI. Epidemiological change of atopic dermatitis and food allergy in school-aged children in Korea between 1995 and 2000. *J Korean Med Sci.* 2004 Oct;19(5):716-23.

Oh SY, Chung J, Kim MK, Kwon SO, Cho BH. Antioxidant nutrient intakes and corresponding biomarkers associated with the risk of atopic dermatitis in young children. *Eur J Clin Nutr.* 2010 Mar;64(3):245-52.

Okasaka M, Takaishi Y, Kashiwada Y, Kodzhimatov OK, Ashurmetov O, Lin AJ, Consentino LM, Lee KH.Terpenoids from Juniperus polycarpus var. seravschanica. *Phytochemistry.* 2006 Dec;67(24):2635-40.

Oldak E, Kurzatkowska B, Stasiak-Barmuta A. Natural course of sensitization in children: follow-up study from birth to 6 years of age, I. Evaluation of total serum IgE and specific IgE antibodies with regard to atopic family history. *Rocz Akad Med Bialymst.* 2000;45:87-95.

Olguin F, Araya M, Hirsch S, Brunser O, Ayala V, Rivera R, Gotteland M. Prebiotic ingestion does not improve gastrointestinal barrier function in burn patients. *Burns.* 2005 Jun;31(4):482-8.

O'Mahony L, McCarthy J, Kelly P, Hurley G, Luo F, Chen K, O'Sullivan GC, Kiely B, Collins JK, Shanahan F, Quigley EM. Lactobacillus and bifidobacterium in irritable bowel syndrome: symptom responses and relationship to cytokine profiles. *Gastroenterology.* 2005 Mar;128(3):541-51.

O'Neil C, Helbling AA, Lehrer SB. Allergic reactions to fish. *Clin Rev Allergy.* 1993 Summer;11(2):183-200.

O'Neil C, Helbling AA, Lehrer SB. Allergic reactions to fish. *Clin Rev Allergy.* 1993;11(2):183-200.

Orhan F, Karakas T, Cakir M, Aksoy A, Baki A, Gedik Y. Prevalence of immunoglobulin E-mediated food allergy in 6-9-year-old urban schoolchildren in the eastern Black Sea region of Turkey. *Clin Exp Allergy.* 2009 Jul;39(7):1027-35.

Ortiz-Andrellucchi A, Sánchez-Villegas A, Rodríguez-Gallego C, Lemes A, Molero T, Soria A, Peña-Quintana L, Santana M, Ramírez O, García J, Cabrera F, Cobo J, Serra-Majem L. Immunomodulatory effects of the intake of fermented milk with Lactobacillus casei DN114001 in lactating mothers and their children. *Br J Nutr.* 2008 Oct;100(4):834-45.

Osguthorpe JD. Immunotherapy. *Curr Opin Otolaryngol Head Neck Surg.* 2010 Jun;18(3):206-12.

Ostlund RE Jr, Racette SB, Stenson WF. Inhibition of cholesterol absorption by phytosterol-replete wheat germ compared with phytosterol-depleted wheat germ. *Am J Clin Nutr.* 2003 Jun;77(6):1385-9.

216

REFERENCES AND BIBLIOGRAPHY

Otto SJ, van Houwelingen AC, Hornstra G. The effect of supplementation with docosahexaenoic and arachidonic acid derived from single cell oils on plasma and erythrocyte fatty acids of pregnant women in the second trimester. *Prostaglandins Leukot Essent Fatty Acids*. 2000 Nov;63(5):323-8.

Ou CC, Tsao SM, Lin MC, Yin MC. Protective action on human LDL against oxidation and glycation by four organosulfur compounds derived from garlic. *Lipids*. 2003 Mar;38(3):219-24.

Ouwehand AC, Nermes M, Collado MC, Rautonen N, Salminen S, Isolauri E. Specific probiotics alleviate allergic rhinitis during the birch pollen season. *World J Gastroenterol*. 2009 Jul 14;15(26):3261-8.

Ouwehand AC, Tiihonen K, Saarinen M, Putaala H, Rautonen N. Influence of a combination of Lactobacillus acidophilus NCFM and lactitol on healthy elderly: intestinal and immune parameters. *Br J Nutr*. 2009 Feb;101(3):367-75.

Ozdemir O. Any benefits of probiotics in allergic disorders? *Allergy Asthma Proc*. 2010 Mar;31(2):103-11.

Paajanen L, Tuure T, Poussa T, Korpela R. No difference in symptoms during challenges with homogenized and unhomogenized cow's milk in subjects with subjective hypersensitivity to homogenized milk. *J Dairy Res*. 2003 May;70(2):175-9.

Paganelli R, Pallone F, Montano S, Le Moli S, Matricardi PM, Fais S, Paoluzi P, D'Amelio R, Aiuti F. Isotypic analysis of antibody response to a food antigen in inflammatory bowel disease. *Int Arch Allergy Appl Immunol*. 1985;78(1):81-5.

Pahud JJ, Schwarz K. Research and development of infant formulae with reduced allergenic properties. *Ann Allergy*. 1984 Dec;53(6 Pt 2):609-14.

Pak CH, Oleneva VA, Agadzhanov SA. Dietetic aspects of preventing urolithiasis in patients with gout and uric acid diathesis. *Vopr Pitan*. 1985 Jan-Feb;(1):21-4.

Palacin A, Bartra J, Muñoz R, Diaz-Perales A, Valero A, Salcedo G. Anaphylaxis to wheat flour-derived foodstuffs and the lipid transfer protein syndrome: a potential role of wheat lipid transfer protein Tri a 14. *Int Arch Allergy Immunol*. 2010;152(2):178-83.

Paller AS, Nimmagadda S, Schachner L, Mallory SB, Kahn T, Willis I, Eichenfield LF. Fluocinolone acetonide 0.01% in peanut oil: therapy for childhood atopic dermatitis, even in patients who are peanut sensitive. *J Am Acad Dermatol*. 2003 Apr;48(4):569-77.

Palmer DJ, Gold MS, Makrides M. Effect of cooked and raw egg consumption on ovalbumin content of human milk: a randomized, double-blind, cross-over trial. *Clin Exp Allergy*. 2005 Feb;35(2):173-8.

Panzani R, Ariano R, Mistrello G. Cypress pollen does not cross-react to plant-derived foods. *Eur Ann Allergy Clin Immunol*. 2010 Jun;42(3):125-6.

Parcell S. Sulfur in human nutrition and applications in medicine. *Altern Med Rev*. 2002 Feb;7(1):22-44.

Pastorello EA, Farioli L, Conti A, Pravettoni V, Bonomi S, Iametti S, Fortunato D, Scibilia J, Bindslev-Jensen C, Ballmer-Weber B, Robino AM, Ortolani C. Wheat IgE-mediated food allergy in European patients: alpha-amylase inhibitors, lipid transfer proteins and low-molecular-weight glutenins. Allergenic molecules recognized by double-blind, placebo-controlled food challenge. Int Arch Allergy Immunol. 2007;144(1):10-22.

Pastorello EA, Farioli L, Pravettoni V, Robino AM, Scibilia J, Fortunato D, Conti A, Borgonovo L, Bengtsson A, Ortolani C. Lipid transfer protein and vicilin are important walnut allergens in patients not allergic to pollen. *J Allergy Clin Immunol*. 2004 Oct;114(4):908-14.

Pastorello EA, Farioli L, Pravettoni V, Scibilia J, Conti A, Fortunato D, Borgonovo L, Bonomi S, Primavesi L, Ballmer-Weber B. Maize food allergy: lipid-transfer proteins, endochitinases, and alpha-zein precursor are relevant maize allergens in double-blind placebo-controlled maize-challenge-positive patients. *Anal Bioanal Chem*. 2009 Sep;395(1):93-102.

Pastorello EA, Pompei C, Pravettoni V, Farioli L, Calamari AM, Scibilia J, Robino AM, Conti A, Iametti S, Fortunato D, Bonomi S, Ortolani C. Lipid-transfer protein is the major maize allergen maintaining IgE-binding activity after cooking at 100 degrees C, as demonstrated in anaphylactic patients and patients with positive double-blind, placebo-controlled food challenge results. *J Allergy Clin Immunol*. 2003 Oct;112(4):775-83.

Pastorello EA, Vieths S, Pravettoni V, Farioli L, Trambaioli C, Fortunato D, Lüttkopf D, Calamari M, Ansaloni R, Scibilia J, Ballmer-Weber BK, Poulsen LK, Wütrich B, Hansen KS, Robino AM, Ortolani C, Conti A. Identification of hazelnut major allergens in sensitive patients with positive double-blind, placebo-controlled food challenge results. *J Allergy Clin Immunol*. 2002 Mar;109(3):563-70.

Patriarca G, Nucera E, Pollastrini E, Roncallo C, De Pasquale T, Lombardo C, Pedone C, Gasbarrini G, Buonomo A, Schiavino D. Oral specific desensitization in food-allergic children. *Dig Dis Sci*. 2007 Jul;52(7):1662-72.

Patriarca G, Nucera E, Roncallo C, Pollastrini E, Bartolozzi F, De Pasquale T, Buonomo A, Gasbarrini G, Di Campli C, Schiavino D. Oral desensitizing treatment in food allergy: clinical and immunological results. *Aliment Pharmacol Ther*. 2003 Feb;17(3):459-65.

Patwardhan B, Gautam M. Botanical immunodrugs: scope and opportunities. *Drug Discov Today*. 2005 Apr 1;10(7):495-502.

Payment P, Franco E, Richardson L, Siemiatyck, J. Gastrointestinal health effects associated with the consumption of drinking water produced by point-of-use domestic reverse-osmosis filtration units. *Appl. Environ. Microbiol.* 1991;57:945-948.

Peeters KA, Koppelman SJ, van Hoffen E, van der Tas CW, den Hartog Jager CF, Penninks AH, Hefle SL, Bruijnzeel-Koomen CA, Knol EF, Knulst AC. Does skin prick test reactivity to purified allergens correlate with clinical severity of peanut allergy? *Clin Exp Allergy*. 2007 Jan;37(1):108-15.

Pehowich DJ, Gomes AV, Barnes JA. Fatty acid composition and possible health effects of coconut constituents. *West Indian Med J*. 2000 Jun;49(2):128-33.

Peña AS, Crusius JB. Food allergy, coeliac disease and chronic inflammatory bowel disease in man. *Vet Q*. 1998;20 Suppl 3:S49-52.

Peng X, You ZY, Huang XK, Zhang CQ, He GZ, Xie WG, Quan ZF, Wang SL. [Analysis of the therapeutic effect and the safety of glutamine granules per os in patients with severe burns and trauma]. Zhonghua Shao Shang Za Zhi. 2004 Aug;20(4):206-9.

Pepeljnjak S, Kosalec I, Kalodera Z, Blazević N. Antimicrobial activity of juniper berry essential oil (Juniperus communis L., Cupressaceae). *Acta Pharm*. 2005 Dec;55(4):417-22.

Pereira B, Venter C, Grundy J, Clayton CB, Arshad SH, Dean T (2005) Prevalence of sensitization to food allergens, reported adverse reaction to foods, food avoidance, and food hypersensitivity among teenagers. *J Allergy Clin Immunol*. 116: 884–892.

Perez-Galvez A, Martin HD, Sies H, Stahl W. Incorporation of carotenoids from paprika oleoresin into human chylomicrons. *Br J Nutr*. 2003 Jun;89(6):787-93.

Perez-Pena R. Secrets of the Mummy's Medicine Chest. *NY Times*. 2005 Sept 10.

Permaul P, Stutius LM, Sheehan WJ, Rangsithienchai P, Walter JE, Twarog FJ, Young MC, Scott JE, Schneider LC, Phipatanakul W. Sesame allergy: role of specific IgE and skin-prick testing in predicting food challenge results. *Allergy Asthma Proc*. 2009 Nov-Dec;30(6):643-8.

Perrier C, Thierry AC, Mercenier A, Corthésy B. Allergen-specific antibody and cytokine responses, mast cell reactivity and intestinal permeability upon oral challenge of sensitized and tolerized mice. *Clin Exp Allergy*. 2010 Jan;40(1):153-62.

Pessi T, Sütas Y, Hurme M, Isolauri E. Interleukin-10 generation in atopic children following oral Lactobacillus rhamnosus GG. *Clin Exp Allergy*. 2000 Dec;30(12):1804-8.

Peterson CG, Hansson T, Skott A, Bengtsson U, Ahlstedt S, Magnussons J. Detection of local mast-cell activity in patients with food hypersensitivity. *J Investig Allergol Clin Immunol*. 2007;17(5):314-20.

Petlevski R, Hadzija M, Slijepcević M, Juretić D, Petrik J. Glutathione S-transferases and malondialdehyde in the liver of NOD mice on short-term treatment with plant mixture extract P-9801091. *Phytother Res*. 2003 Apr;17(4):311-4.

Petlevski R, Hadzija M, Slijepcević M, Juretić D. Toxicological assessment of P-9801091 plant mixture extract after chronic administration in CBA/HZg mice—a biochemical and histological study. *Coll Antropol*. 2008 Jun;32(2):577-81.

Pfefferle PI, Sel S, Ege MJ, Büchele G, Blümer N, Krauss-Etschmann S, Herzum I, Albers CE, Lauener RP, Roponen M, Hirvonen MR, Vuitton DA, Riedler J, Brunekreef B, Dalphin JC, Braun-Fahrländer C, Pekkanen J, von Mutius E, Renz H; PASTURE Study Group. Cord blood allergen-specific IgE is associated with reduced IFN-gamma production by cord blood cells: the Protection against Allergy-Study in Rural Environments (PASTURE) Study. *J Allergy Clin Immunol*. 2008 Oct;122(4):711-6.

Pfundstein B, El Desouky SK, Hull WE, Haubner R, Erben G, Owen RW. Polyphenolic compounds in the fruits of Egyptian medicinal plants (Terminalia bellerica, Terminalia chebula and Terminalia horrida): characterization, quantitation and determination of antioxidant capacities. *Phytochemistry*. 2010 Jul;71(10):1132-48.

Pharmacopoeia of the People's Republic of China. English. Beijing: Chemical Industry Press; 2005. The State Pharmacopoeia Commission of The People's Republic of China.Nusem D, Panasoff J. Beer anaphylaxis. *Isr Med Assoc J*. 2009 Jun;11(6):380-1.

Physicians' Desk Reference. Montvale, NJ: Thomson, 2003-2008

Phytochemical investigation of juniper rufescens Juniperus oxycedrus L. leaves and fruits. *Georgian Med News*. 2009 Mar;(168):107-11.

Piboonpocanun S, Boonchoo S, Pariyaprasert W, Visitsunthorn N, Jirapongsananuruk O. Determination of storage conditions for shrimp extracts: analysis of specific IgE-allergen profiles. *Asian Pac J Allergy Immunol*. 2010 Mar;28(1):47-52.

Pierce SK, Klinman NR. Antibody-specific immunoregulation. *J Exp Med*. 1977 Aug 1;146(2):509-19.

Piirainen L, Haahtela S, Helin T, Korpela R, Haahtela T, Vaarala O. Effect of Lactobacillus rhamnosus GG on rBet v1 and rMal d1 specific IgA in the saliva of patients with birch pollen allergy. *Ann Allergy Asthma Immunol.* 2008 Apr;100(4):338-42.

Pike MG, Heddle RJ, Boulton P, Turner MW, Atherton DJ. Increased intestinal permeability in atopic eczema. *J Invest Dermatol.* 1986 Feb;86(2):101-4.

Pitt-Rivers R, Trotter WR. *The Thyroid Gland.* London: Butterworth Publ, 1954.

Plein K, Hotz J. Therapeutic effects of Saccharomyces boulardii on mild residual symptoms in a stable phase of Crohn's disease with special respect to chronic diarrhea—a pilot study. *Z Gastroenterol.* 1993 Feb;31(2):129-34.

Plohmann B, Bader G, Hiller K, Franz G. Immunomodulatory and antitumoral effects of triterpenoid saponins. *Pharmazie.* 1997 Dec;52(12):953-7.

Poblocka-Olech L, Krauze-Baranowska M. SPE-HPTLC of procyanidins from the barks of different species and clones of Salix. *J Pharm Biomed Anal.* 2008 Nov 4;48(3):965-8.

Pochard P, Vickery B, Berin MC, Grishin A, Sampson HA, Caplan M, Bottomly K. Targeting Toll-like receptors on dendritic cells modifies the T(H)2 response to peanut allergens in vitro. *J Allergy Clin Immunol.* 2010 Jul;126(1):92-7.e5.

Pohjavuori E, Viljanen M, Korpela R, Kuitunen M, Tiittanen M, Vaarala O, Savilahti E. Lactobacillus GG effect in increasing IFN-gamma production in infants with cow's milk allergy. *J Allergy Clin Immunol.* 2004 Jul;114(1):131-6.

Polimeno L, Loiacono M, Pesetti B, Mallamaci R, Mastrodonato M, Azzarone A, Annoscia E, Gatti F, Amoruso A, Ventura MT. Anisakiasis, an underestimated infection: effect on intestinal permeability of Anisakis simplex-sensitized patients. *Foodborne Pathog Dis.* 2010 Jul;7(7):809-14.

Pollini F, Capristo C, Boner AL. Upper respiratory tract infections and atopy. *Int J Immunopathol Pharmacol.* 2010 Jan-Mar;23(1 Suppl):32-7.

Ponsonby AL, McMichael A, van der Mei I. Ultraviolet radiation and autoimmune disease: insights from epidemiological research. *Toxicology.* 2002 Dec 27;181-182:71-8.

Potterton D. (Ed.) *Culpeper's Color Herbal.* New York: Sterling, 1983.

Poulos LM, Waters AM, Correll PK, Loblay RH, Marks GB. Trends in hospitalizations for anaphylaxis, angioedema, and urticaria in Australia, 1993-1994 to 2004-2005. *J Allergy Clin Immunol.* 2007 Oct;120(4):878-84.

Prescott SL, Wickens K, Westcott L, Jung W, Currie H, Black PN, Stanley TV, Mitchell EA, Fitzharris P, Siebers R, Wu L, Crane J; Probiotic Study Group. Supplementation with Lactobacillus rhamnosus or Bifidobacterium lactis probiotics in pregnancy increases cord blood interferon-gamma and breast milk transforming growth factor-beta and immunoglobin A detection. *Clin Exp Allergy.* 2008 Oct;38(10):1606-14.

Prieto A, Razzak E, Lindo DP, Alvarez-Perea A, Rueda M, Baeza ML. Recurrent anaphylaxis due to lupin flour: primary sensitization through inhalation. *J Investig Allergol Clin Immunol.* 2010;20(1):76-9.

Prioult G, Fliss I, Pecquet S. Effect of probiotic bacteria on induction and maintenance of oral tolerance to beta-lactoglobulin in gnotobiotic mice. *Clin Diagn Lab Immunol.* 2003 Sep;10(5):787-92.

Proujansky R, Winter HS, Walker WA. Gastrointestinal syndromes associated with food sensitivity. *Adv Pediatr.* 1988;35:219-37.

Prucksunand C, Indrasukhsri B, Leethochawalit M, Hungspreugs K. Phase II clinical trial on effect of the long turmeric (Curcuma longa Linn) on healing of peptic ulcer. *Southeast Asian J Trop Med Public Health.* 2001 Mar;32(1):208-15.

Prussin C, Lee J, Foster B. Eosinophilic gastrointestinal disease and peanut allergy are alternatively associated with IL-5+ and IL-5(-) T(H)2 responses. *J Allergy Clin Immunol.* 2009 Dec;124(6):1326-32.e6.

Pruthi S, Thapa MM. Infectious and inflammatory disorders. *Magn Reson Imaging Clin N Am.* 2009 Aug;17(3):423-38, v.

Pulcini JM, Sease KK, Marshall GD. Disparity between the presence and absence of food allergy action plans in one school district. *Allergy Asthma Proc.* 2010 Mar;31(2):141-6.

Pustisek N, Jaklin-Kekez A, Frkanec R, Sikanić-Dugić N, Misak Z, Jadresin O, Kolacek S. Our experiences with the use of atopy patch test in the diagnosis of cow's milk hypersensitivity. *Acta Dermatovenerol Croat.* 2010;18(1):14-20. Kim JH, Kim JE, Choi GS, Hwang EK, An S, Ye YM, Park HS. A case of occupational rhinitis caused by rice powder in the grain industry. *Allergy Asthma Immunol Res.* 2010 Apr;2(2):141-3.

Pyle GG, Paaso B, Anderson BE, Allen DD, Marti T, Li Q, Siegel M, Khosla C, Gray GM. Effect of pretreatment of food gluten with prolyl endopeptidase on gluten-induced malabsorption in celiac sprue. *Clin Gastroenterol Hepatol.* 2005 Jul;3(7):687-94.

Qin HL, Zheng JJ, Tong DN, Chen WX, Fan XB, Hang XM, Jiang YQ. Effect of Lactobacillus plantarum enteral feeding on the gut permeability and septic complications in the patients with acute pancreatitis. Eur J Clin Nutr. 2008 Jul;62(7):923-30.

Qu C, Srivastava K, Ko J, Zhang TF, Sampson HA, Li XM. Induction of tolerance after establishment of peanut allergy by the food allergy herbal formula-2 is associated with up-regulation of interferon-gamma. Clin Exp Allergy. 2007 Jun;37(6):846-55.

Quan ZF, Yang C, Li N, Li JS. Effect of glutamine on change in early postoperative intestinal permeability and its relation to systemic inflammatory response. World J Gastroenterol. 2004 Jul 1;10(13):1992-4.

Rabbani GH, Teka T, Saha SK, Zaman B, Majid N, Khatun M, Wahed MA, Fuchs GJ. Green banana and pectin improve small intestinal permeability and reduce fluid loss in Bangladeshi children with persistent diarrhea. Dig Dis Sci. 2004 Mar;49(3):475-84.

Rafter J, Bennett M, Caderni G, Clune Y, Hughes R, Karlsson PC, Klinder A, O'Riordan M, O'Sullivan GC, Pool-Zobel B, Rechkemmer G, Roller M, Rowland I, Salvadori M, Thijs H, Van Loo J, Watzl B, Collins JK. Dietary synbiotics reduce cancer risk factors in polypectomized and colon cancer patients. Am J Clin Nutr. 2007 Feb;85(2):488-96.

Raherison C, Pénard-Morand C, Moreau D, Caillaud D, Charpin D, Kopferschmitt C, Lavaud F, Taytard A, Maesano IA. Smoking exposure and allergic sensitization in children according to maternal allergies. Ann Allergy Asthma Immunol. 2008 Apr;100(4):351-7.

Rahman MM, Bhattacharya A, Fernandes G. Docosahexaenoic acid is more potent inhibitor of osteoclast differentiation in RAW 264.7 cells than eicosapentaenoic acid. J Cell Physiol. 2008 Jan;214(1):201-9.

Railey MD, Burks AW. Therapeutic approaches for the treatment of food allergy. Expert Opin Pharmacother. 2010 May;11(7):1045-8.

Raimondi F, Indrio F, Crivaro V, Araimo G, Capasso L, Paludetto R. Neonatal hyperbilirubinemia increases intestinal protein permeability and the prevalence of cow's milk protein intolerance. Acta Paediatr. 2008 Jun;97(6):751-3.

Raithel M, Weidenhiller M, Abel R, Baenkler HW, Hahn EG. Colorectal mucosal histamine release by mucosa oxygenation in comparison with other established clinical tests in patients with gastrointestinally mediated allergy. World J Gastroenterol. 2006 Aug 7;12(29):4699-705.

Ramagopalan SV, Dyment DA, Guimond C, Orton SM, Yee IM, Ebers GC, Sadovnick AD. Childhood cow's milk allergy and the risk of multiple sclerosis: a population based study. J Neurol Sci. 2010 Apr 15;291(1-2):86-8.

Rampton DS, Murdoch RD, Sladen GE. Rectal mucosal histamine release in ulcerative colitis. Clin Sci (Lond). 1980 Nov;59(5):389-91.

Rancé F, Abbal M, Lauwers-Cancès V. Improved screening for peanut allergy by the combined use of skin prick tests and specific IgE assays. J Allergy Clin Immunol. 2002 Jun;109(6):1027-33.

Rancé F, Bidat E, Bourrier T, Sabouraud D. Cashew allergy: observations of 42 children without associated peanut allergy. Allergy. 2003 Dec;58(12):1311-4.

Rance F, Kanny G, Dutau G, Moneret-Vautrin DA. Food allergens in children. Arch Pediatr. 1999;6(Suppl 1):61S-66S.

Randal Bollinger R, Barbas AS, Bush EL, Lin SS, Parker W. Biofilms in the large bowel suggest an apparent function of the human vermiform appendix. J Theor Biol. 2007 Dec 21;249(4):826-31.

Rao SK, Rao PS, Rao BN. Preliminary investigation of the radiosensitizing activity of guduchi (Tinospora cordifolia) in tumor-bearing mice. Phytother Res. 2008 Nov;22(11):1482-9.

Rapin JR, Wiernsperger N. Possible links between intestinal permeablity and food processing: A potential therapeutic niche for glutamine. Clinics (Sao Paulo). 2010 Jun;65(6):635-43.

Rappoport J. Both sides of the pharmaceutical death coin. Townsend Letter for Doctors and Patients. 2006 Oct.

Rauha JP, Remes S, Heinonen M, Hopia A, Kähkönen M, Kujala T, Pihlaja K, Vuorela H, Vuorela P. Antimicrobial effects of Finnish plant extracts containing flavonoids and other phenolic compounds. Int J Food Microbiol. 2000 May 25;56(1):3-12.

Rauma A. Antioxidant status in vegetarians versus omnivores. Nutrition. 2003;16(2): 111-119.

Rautava S, Isolauri E. Cow's milk allergy in infants with atopic eczema is associated with aberrant production of interleukin-4 during oral cow's milk challenge. J Pediatr Gastroenterol Nutr. 2004 Nov;39(5):529-35.

Reger D, Goode S, Mercer E. Chemistry: Principles & Practice. Fort Worth, TX: Harcourt Brace, 1993.

Reha CM, Ebru A. Specific immunotherapy is effective in the prevention of new sensitivities. Allergol Immunopathol (Madr). 2007 Mar-Apr;35(2):44-51.

Reichling J, Schmökel H, Fitzi J, Bucher S, Saller R. Dietary support with Boswellia resin in canine inflammatory joint and spinal disease. Schweiz Arch Tierheilkd. 2004 Feb;146(2):71-9.

Reuter A, Lidholm J, Andersson K, Ostling J, Lundberg M, Scheurer S, Enrique E, Cistero-Bahima A, San Miguel-Moncin M, Ballmer-Weber BK, Vieths S. A critical assessment of allergen component-based in vitro diagnosis in cherry allergy across Europe. Clin Exp Allergy. 2006 Jun;36(6):815-23.

Rimbaud L, Heraud F, La Vieille S, Leblanc JC, Crepet A. Quantitative risk assessment relating to adventitious presence of allergens in food: a probabilistic model applied to peanut in chocolate. *Risk Anal.* 2010 Jan;30(1):7-19.

Rinne M, Kalliomaki M, Arvilommi H, Salminen S, Isolauri E. Effect of probiotics and breastfeeding on the bifidobacterium and lactobacillus/enterococcus microbiota and humoral immune responses. *J Pediatr.* 2005 Aug;147(2):186-91.

Río ME, Zago Beatriz L, Garcia H, Winter L. The nutritional status change the effectiveness of a dietary supplement of lactic bacteria on the emerging of respiratory tract diseases in children. *Arch Latinoam Nutr.* 2002 Mar;52(1):29-34.

Robert AM, Groult N, Six C, Robert L. The effect of procyanidolic oligomers on mesenchymal cells in culture II—Attachment of elastic fibers to the cells. *Pathol Biol.* 1990 Jun;38(6):601-7.

Robert AM, Groult N, Six C, Robert L. The effect of procyanidolic oligomers on mesenchymal cells in culture II—Attachment of elastic fibers to the cells. *Pathol Biol.* 1990 Jun;38(6):601-7.

Roberts G, Lack G. Diagnosing peanut allergy with skin prick and specific IgE testing. *J Allergy Clin Immunol.* 2005 Jun;115(6):1291-6.

Rodriguez J, Crespo JF, Burks W, Rivas-Plata C, Fernandez-Anaya S, Vives R, Daroca P. Randomized, double-blind, crossover challenge study in 53 subjects reporting adverse reactions to melon (Cucumis melo). *J Allergy Clin Immunol.* 2000 Nov;106(5):968-72.

Rodriguez-Fragoso L, Reyes-Esparza J, Burchiel SW, Herrera-Ruiz D, Torres E. Risks and benefits of commonly used herbal medicines in Mexico. *Toxicol Appl Pharmacol.* 2008 Feb 15;227(1):125-35.

Rodríguez-Ortiz PG, Muñoz-Mendoza D, Arias-Cruz A, González-Díaz SN, Herrera-Castro D, Vidaurri-Ojeda AC. Epidemiological characteristics of patients with food allergy assisted at Regional Center of Allergies and Clinical Immunology of Monterrey. *Rev Alerg Mex.* 2009 Nov-Dec;56(6):185-91.

Roduit C, Scholtens S, de Jongste JC, Wijga AH, Gerritsen J, Postma DS, Brunekreef B, Hoekstra MO, Aalberse R, Smit HA. Asthma at 8 years of age in children born by caesarean section. *Thorax.* 2009 Feb;64(2):107-13.

Roessler A, Friedrich U, Vogelsang H, Bauer A, Kaatz M, Hipler UC, Schmidt I, Jahreis G. The immune system in healthy adults and patients with atopic dermatitis seems to be affected differently by a probiotic intervention. *Clin Exp Allergy.* 2008 Jan;38(1):93-102.

Rollins NC, Filteau SM, Coutsoudis A, Tomkins AM. Feeding mode, intestinal permeability, and neopterin excretion: a longitudinal study in infants of HIV-infected South African women. *J Acquir Immune Defic Syndr.* 2001 Oct 1;28(2):132-9.

Romeo J, Wärnberg J, Nova E, Díaz LE, González-Gross M, Marcos A. Changes in the immune system after moderate beer consumption. *Ann Nutr Metab.* 2007;51(4):359-66.

Rona RJ, Keil T, Summers C, Gislason D, Zuidmeer L, Sodergren E, Sigurdardottir ST, Lindner T, Goldhahn K, Dahlstrom J, McBride D, Madsen C. The prevalence of food allergy: a meta-analysis. *J Allergy Clin Immunol.* 2007 Sep;120(3):638-46.

Ronteltap A, van Schaik J, Wensing M, Rynja FJ, Knulst AC, de Vries JH. Sensory testing of recipes masking peanut or hazelnut for double-blind placebo-controlled food challenges. Allergy. 2004 Apr;59(4):457-60. Clark S, Bock SA, Gaeta TJ, Brenner BE, Cydulka RK, Camargo CA; Multicenter Airway Research Collaboration-8 Investigators. Multicenter study of emergency department visits for food allergies. *J Allergy Clin Immunol.* 2004 Feb;113(2):347-52.

Ros E, Mataix J. Fatty acid composition of nuts—implications for cardiovascular health. *Br J Nutr.* 2006 Nov;96 Suppl 2:S29-35.

Rosenfeldt V, Benfeldt E, Valerius NH, Paerregaard A, Michaelsen KF. Effect of probiotics on gastrointestinal symptoms and small intestinal permeability in children with atopic dermatitis. *J Pediatr.* 2004 Nov;145(5):612-6.

Roy SK, Behrens RH, Haider R, Akramuzzaman SM, Mahalanabis D, Wahed MA, Tomkins AM. Impact of zinc supplementation on intestinal permeability in Bangladeshi children with acute diarrhoea and persistent diarrhoea syndrome. *J Pediatr Gastroenterol Nutr.* 1992 Oct;15(3):289-96.

Rozycki VR, Baigorria CM, Freyre MR, Bernard CM, Zannier MS, Charpentier M. Nutrient content in vegetable species from the Argentine Chaco. *Arch Latinoam Nutr.* 1997 Sep;47(3):265-70.

Rubin E., Farber JL. *Pathology.* 3rd Ed. Philadelphia: Lippincott-Raven, 1999.

Rudders SA, Espinola JA, Camargo CA Jr. North-south differences in US emergency department visits for acute allergic reactions. *Ann Allergy Asthma Immunol.* 2010 May;104(5):413-6.

Saarinen KM, Juntunen-Backman K, Järvenpää AL, Klemetti P, Kuitunen P, Lope L, Renlund M, Siivola M, Vaarala O, Savilahti E. Breast-feeding and the development of cows' milk protein allergy. *Adv Exp Med Biol.* 2000;478:121-30.

Saggioro A. Probiotics in the treatment of irritable bowel syndrome. *J Clin Gastroenterol.* 2004 Jul;38(6 Suppl):S104-6.

Sahagún-Flores JE, López-Peña LS, de la Cruz-Ramírez Jaimes J, García-Bravo MS, Peregrina-Gómez R, de Alba-García JE. Eradication of Helicobacter pylori: triple treatment scheme plus Lactobacillus vs. triple treatment alone. Cir Cir. 2007 Sep-Oct;75(5):333-6.

Sahin-Yilmaz A, Nocon CC, Corey JP. Immunoglobulin E-mediated food allergies among adults with allergic rhinitis. Otolaryngol Head Neck Surg. 2010 Sep;143(3):379-85.

Salem N, Wegher B, Mena P, Uauy R. Arachidonic and docosahexaenoic acids are biosynthesized from their 18-carbon precursors in human infants. Proc Natl Acad Sci. 1996;93:49-54.

Salido S, Altarejos J, Nogueras M, Sánchez A, Pannecouque C, Witvrouw M, De Clercq E. Chemical studies of essential oils of Juniperus oxycedrus ssp. badia. J Ethnopharmacol. 2002 Jun;81(1):129-34.

Salim AS. Sulfhydryl-containing agents in the treatment of gastric bleeding induced by nonsteroidal anti-inflammatory drugs. Can J Surg. 1993 Feb;36(1):53-8.

Salim, A.S., Role of oxygen-derived free radical scavengers in the management of recurrent attacks of ulcerative colitis: A new approach. J. Lab Clin Med. 1992;119:740-747.

Salmi H, Kuitunen M, Viljanen M, Lapatto R. Cow's milk allergy is associated with changes in urinary organic acid concentrations. Pediatr Allergy Immunol. 2010 Mar;21(2 Pt 2):e401-6.

Salminen S, Isolauri E, Salminen E. Clinical uses of probiotics for stabilizing the gut mucosal barrier: successful strains and future challenges. Antonie Van Leeuwenhoek. 1996 Oct;70(2-4):347-58.

Salom IL, Silvis SE, Doscherholmen A. Effect of cimetidine on the absorption of vitamin B12. Scand J Gastroenterol. 1982;17:129-31.

Salpietro CD, Gangemi S, Briuglia S, Meo A, Merlino MV, Muscolino G, Bisignano G, Trombetta D, Saija A. The almond milk: a new approach to the management of cow-milk allergy/intolerance in infants. Minerva Pediatr. 2005 Aug;57(4):173-80.

Samoylenko V, Dunbar DC, Gafur MA, Khan SI, Ross SA, Mossa JS, El-Feraly FS, Tekwani BL, Bosselaers J, Muhammad I. Antiparasitic, nematicidal and antifouling constituents from Juniperus berries. Phytother Res. 2008 Dec;22(12):1570-6.

Sancho AI, Hoffmann-Sommergruber K, Alessandri S, Conti A, Giuffrida MG, Shewry P, Jensen BM, Skov P, Vieths S. Authentication of food allergen quality by physicochemical and immunological methods. Clin Exp Allergy. 2010 Jul;40(7):973-86.

Sandin A, Annus T, Björkstén B, Nilsson L, Riikjärv MA, van Hage-Hamsten M, Bråbäck L. Prevalence of self-reported food allergy and IgE antibodies to food allergens in Swedish and Estonian schoolchildren. Eur J Clin Nutr. 2005 Mar;59(3):399-403.

Sandler NG, Wand H, Roque A, Law M, Nason MC, Nixon DE, Pedersen C, Ruxrungtham K, Lewin SR, Emery S, Neaton JD, Brenchley JM, Deeks SG, Sereti I, Douek DC; INSIGHT SMART Study Group. Plasma levels of soluble CD14 independently predict mortality in HIV infection. J Infect Dis. 2011 Mar 15;203(6):780-90. Epub 2011 Jan 20.

Santos A, Dias A, Pinheiro JA. Predictive factors for the persistence of cow's milk allergy. Pediatr Allergy Immunol. 2010 Apr 27.

Sanz Ortega J, Martorell Aragonés A, Michavila Gómez A, Nieto García A; Grupo de Trabajo para el Estudio de la Alergia Alimentaria. Incidence of IgE-mediated allergy to cow's milk proteins in the first year of life. An Esp Pediatr. 2001 Jun;54(6):536-9.

Sato S, Tachimoto H, Shukuya A, Kurosaka N, Yanagida N, Utsunomiya T, Iguchi M, Komata T, Imai T, Tomikawa M, Ebisawa M. Basophil activation marker CD203c is useful in the diagnosis of hen's egg and cow's milk allergies in children. Int Arch Allergy Immunol. 2010;152 Suppl 1:54-61.

Sato Y, Akiyama H, Matsuoka H, Sakata K, Nakamura R, Ishikawa S, Inakuma T, Totsuka M, Sugita-Konishi Y, Ebisawa M, Teshima R. Dietary carotenoids inhibit oral sensitization and the development of food allergy. J Agric Food Chem. 2010 Jun 23;58(12):7180-6.

Satyanarayana S, Sushruta K, Sarma GS, Srinivas N, Subba Raju GV. Antioxidant activity of the aqueous extracts of spicy food additives—evaluation and comparison with ascorbic acid in in-vitro systems. J Herb Pharmacother. 2004;4(2):1-10.

Savage JH, Kaeding AJ, Matsui EC, Wood RA. The natural history of soy allergy. J Allergy Clin Immunol. 2010 Mar;125(3):683-6.

Savilahti EM, Karinen S, Salo HM, Klemetti P, Saarinen KM, Klemola T, Kuitunen M, Hautaniemi S, Savilahti E, Vaarala O. Combined T regulatory cell and Th2 expression profile identifies children with cow's milk allergy. Clin Immunol. 2010 Jul;136(1):16-20.

Savilahti EM, Rantanen V, Lin JS, Karinen S, Saarinen KM, Goldis M, Mäkelä MJ, Hautaniemi S, Savilahti E, Sampson HA. Early recovery from cow's milk allergy is associated with decreasing IgE and increasing IgG4 binding to cow's milk epitopes. J Allergy Clin Immunol. 2010 Jun;125(6):1315-1321.e9.

Savilahti EM, Rantanen V, Lin JS, Karinen S, Saarinen KM, Goldis M, Mäkelä MJ, Hautaniemi S, Savilahti E, Sampson HA. Early recovery from cow's milk allergy is associated with decreasing IgE and increasing IgG4 binding to cow's milk epitopes. J Allergy Clin Immunol. 2010 Jun;125(6):1315-1321.e9.

Sazanova NE, Varnacheva LN, Novikova AV, Pletneva NB. Immunological aspects of food intolerance in children during first years of life. *Pediatriia*. 1992;(3):14-8. Russian.

Scadding G, Bjarnason I, Brostoff J, Levi AJ, Peters TJ. Intestinal permeability to 51Cr-labelled ethylenediaminetetraacetate in food-intolerant subjects. *Digestion*. 1989;42(2):104-9.

Scalabrin DM, Johnston WH, Hoffman DR, P'Pool VL, Harris CL, Mitmesser SH. Growth and tolerance of healthy term infants receiving hydrolyzed infant formulas supplemented with Lactobacillus rhamnosus GG: randomized, double-blind, controlled trial. *Clin Pediatr (Phila)*. 2009 Sep;48(7):734-44.

Schabelman E, Witting M. The Relationship of Radiocontrast, Iodine, and Seafood Allergies: A Medical Myth Exposed. *J Emerg Med*. 2009 Dec 31.

Schade RP, Meijer Y, Pasmans SG, Knulst AC, Kimpen JL, Bruijnzeel-Koomen CA. Double blind placebo controlled cow's milk provocation for the diagnosis of cow's milk allergy in infants and children. *Ned Tijdschr Geneeskd*. 2002 Sep 14;146(37):1739-42.

Schauenberg P, Paris F. *Guide to Medicinal Plants*. New Canaan, CT: Keats Publ, 1977.

Schauss AG, Wu X, Prior RL, Ou B, Huang D, Owens J, Agarwal A, Jensen GS, Hart AN, Shanbrom E. Antioxidant capacity and other bioactivities of the freeze-dried Amazonian palm berry, Euterpe oleraceae mart. (acai). *J Agric Food Chem*. 2006 Nov 1;54(22):8604-10.

Schempp H, Weiser D, Elstner EF. Biochemical model reactions indicative of inflammatory processes. Activities of extracts from Fraxinus excelsior and Populus tremula. *Arzneimittelforschung*. 2000 Apr;50(4):362-72.

Schepetkin IA, Faulkner CL, Nelson-Overton LK, Wiley JA, Quinn MT. Macrophage immunomodulatory activity of polysaccharides isolated from Juniperus scopolorum. *Int Immunopharmacol*. 2005 Dec;5(13-14):1783-99.

Schilcher H, Leuschner F. The potential nephrotoxic effects of essential juniper oil. *Arzneimittelforschung*. 1997 Jul;47(7):855-8.

Schillaci D, Arizza V, Dayton T, Camarda L, Di Stefano V. In vitro anti-biofilm activity of Boswellia spp. oleogum resin essential oils. *Lett Appl Microbiol*. 2008 Nov;47(5):433-8.

Schmid B, Kötter I, Heide L. Pharmacokinetics of salicin after oral administration of a standardised willow bark extract. *Eur J Clin Pharmacol*. 2001 Aug;57(5):387-91.

Schmitt DA, Maleki SJ (2004) Comparing the effects of boiling, frying and roasting on the allergenicity of peanuts. *J Allergy Clin Immunol*. 113: S155.

Schnappinger M, Sausenthaler S, Linseisen J, Hauner H, Heinrich J. Fish consumption, allergic sensitisation and allergic diseases in adults. *Ann Nutr Metab*. 2009;54(1):67-74.

Schneider I, Gibbons S, Bucar F. Inhibitory activity of Juniperus communis on 12(S)-HETE production in human platelets. *Planta Med*. 2004 May;70(5):471-4.

Schönfeld P. Phytanic Acid toxicity: implications for the permeability of the inner mitochondrial membrane to ions. *Toxicol Mech Methods*. 2004;14(1-2):47-52.

Schottner M, Gansser D, Spiteller G. Lignans from the roots of Urtica dioica and their metabolites bind to human sex hormone binding globulin (SHBG). *Planta Med*. 1997;63:529–532.

Schouten B, van Esch BC, Hofman GA, Boon L, Knippels LM, Willemsen LE, Garssen J. Oligosaccharide-induced whey-specific CD25(+) regulatory T-cells are involved in the suppression of cow milk allergy in mice. *J Nutr*. 2010 Apr;140(4):835-41.

Schouten B, van Esch BC, van Thuijl AO, Blokhuis BR, Groot Kormelink T, Hofman GA, Moro GE, Boehm G, Arslanoglu S, Sprikkelman AB, Willemsen LE, Knippels LM, Redegeld FA, Garssen J. Contribution of IgE and immunoglobulin free light chain in the allergic reaction to cow's milk proteins. *J Allergy Clin Immunol*. 2010 Jun;125(6):1308-14.

Schroecksnadel S, Jenny M, Fuchs D. Sensitivity to sulphite additives. *Clin Exp Allergy*. 2010 Apr;40(4):688-9.

Schulick P. *Ginger: Common Spice & Wonder Drug*. Brattleboro, VT: Herbal Free Perss, 1996.

Schumacher P. *Biophysical Therapy Of Allergies*. Stuttgart: Thieme, 2005.

Schütz K, Carle R, Schieber A. Taraxacum—a review on its phytochemical and pharmacological profile. *J Ethnopharmacol*. 2006 Oct 11;107(3):313-23.

Schwab D, Hahn EG, Raithel M. Enhanced histamine metabolism: a comparative analysis of collagenous colitis and food allergy with respect to the role of diet and NSAID use. *Inflamm Res*. 2003 Apr;52(4):142-7.

Schwab D, Müller S, Aigner T, Neureiter D, Kirchner T, Hahn EG, Raithel M. Functional and morphologic characterization of eosinophils in the lower intestinal mucosa of patients with food allergy. *Am J Gastroenterol*. 2003 Jul;98(7):1525-34.

Schwelberger HG. Histamine intolerance: a metabolic disease? *Inflamm Res*. 2010 Mar;59 Suppl 2:S219-21.

Scibilia J, Pastorello EA, Zisa G, Ottolenghi A, Ballmer-Weber B, Pravettoni V, Scovena E, Robino A, Ortolani C. Maize food allergy: a double-blind placebo-controlled study. *Clin Exp Allergy*. 2008 Dec;38(12):1943-9.

Scott-Taylor TH, O'B Hourihane J, Strobel S. Correlation of allergen-specific IgG subclass antibodies and T lymphocyte cytokine responses in children with multiple food allergies. *Pediatr Allergy Immunol.* 2010 Sep;21(6):935-44.

Scurlock AM, Jones SM. An update on immunotherapy for food allergy. *Curr Opin Allergy Clin Immunol.* 2010 Dec;10(6):587-93.

Sealey-Voyksner JA, Khosla C, Voyksner RD, Jorgenson JW. Novel aspects of quantitation of immunogenic wheat gluten peptides by liquid chromatography-mass spectrometry/mass spectrometry. *J Chromatogr A.* 2010 Jun 18;1217(25):4167-83.

Seca AM, Silva AM, Bazzocchi IL, Jimenez IA. Diterpene constituents of leaves from Juniperus brevifolia. *Phytochemistry.* 2008 Jan;69(2):498-505.

Seca AM, Silva AM. The chemical composition of hexane extract from bark of Juniperus brevifolia. *Nat Prod Res.* 2008;22(11):975-83.

Senna G, Gani F, Leo G, Schiappoli M. Alternative tests in the diagnosis of food allergies. *Recenti Prog Med.* 2002 May;93(5):327-34.

Seo K, Jung S, Park M, Song Y, Choung S. Effects of leucocyanidines on activities of metabolizing enzymes and antioxidant enzymes. *Biol Pharm Bull.* 2001 May;24(5):592-3.

Seo SW, Koo HN, An HJ, Kwon KB, Lim BC, Seo EA, Ryu DG, Moon G, Kim HY, Kim HM, Hong SH. Taraxacum officinale protects against cholecystokinin-induced acute pancreatitis in rats. *World J Gastroenterol.* 2005 Jan 28;11(4):597-9.

Seppo L, Korpela R, Lönnerdal B, Metsäniitty L, Juntunen-Backman K, Klemola T, Paganus A, Vanto T. A follow-up study of nutrient intake, nutritional status, and growth in infants with cow milk allergy fed either a soy formula or an extensively hydrolyzed whey formula. *Am J Clin Nutr.* 2005 Jul;82(1):140-5.

Settipane RA, Siri D, Bellanti JA. Egg allergy and influenza vaccination. *Allergy Asthma Proc.* 2009 Nov-Dec;30(6):660-5.

Shahani KM, Meshbesher BF, Mangalampalli V. *Cultivate Health From Within.* Danbury, CT: Vital Health Publ, 2005.

Shakib F, Brown HM, Phelps A, Redhead R. Study of IgG sub-class antibodies in patients with milk intolerance. *Clin Allergy.* 1986 Sep;16(5):451-8.

Shao J, Sheng J, Dong W, Li YZ, Yu SC. Effects of feeding intervention on development of eczema in atopy high-risk infants: an 18-month follow-up study. *Zhonghua Er Ke Za Zhi.* 2006 Sep;44(9):684-7. Chinese.

Sharma P, Sharma BC, Puri V, Sarin SK. An open-label randomized controlled trial of lactulose and probiotics in the treatment of minimal hepatic encephalopathy. *Eur J Gastroent Hepatol.* 2008 Jun;20(6):506-11.

Sharma SC, Sharma S, Gulati OP. Pycnogenol inhibits the release of histamine from mast cells. *Phytother Res.* 2003 Jan;17(1):66-9.

Sharnan J, Kumar L, Singh S. Comparison of results of skin prick tests, enzyme-linked immunosorbent assays and food challenges in children with respiratory allergy. *J Trop Pediatr.* 2001 Dec;47(6):367-8.

Shaw J, Roberts G, Grimshaw K, White S, Hourihane J. Lupin allergy in peanut-allergic children and teenagers. *Allergy.* 2008 Mar;63(3):370-3.

Shawcross DL, Wright G, Olde Damink SW, Jalan R. Role of ammonia and inflammation in minimal hepatic encephalopathy. *Metab Brain Dis.* 2007 Mar;22(1):125-38.

Shea-Donohue T, Stiltz J, Zhao A, Notari L. Mast Cells. *Curr Gastroenterol Rep.* 2010 Aug 14.

Sheth SS, Waserman S, Kagan R, Alizadehfar R, Primeau MN, Elliot S, St Pierre Y, Wickett R, Joseph L, Harada L, Dufresne C, Allen M, Allen M, Godefroy SB, Clarke AE. Role of food labels in accidental exposures in food-allergic individuals in Canada. *Ann Allergy Asthma Immunol.* 2010 Jan;104(1):60-5.

Shi S, Zhao Y, Zhou H, Zhang Y, Jiang X, Huang K. Identification of antioxidants from Taraxacum mongolicum by high-performance liquid chromatography-diode array detection-radical-scavenging detection-electrospray ionization mass spectrometry and nuclear magnetic resonance experiments. *J Chromatogr A.* 2008 Oct 31;1209(1-2):145-52

Shi S, Zhou H, Zhang Y, Huang K, Liu S. Chemical constituents from Neo-Taraxacum siphonathum. *Zhongguo Zhong Yao Za Zhi.* 2009 Apr;34(8):1002-4.

Shi SY, Zhou CX, Xu Y, Tao QF, Bai H, Lu FS, Lin WY, Chen HY, Zheng W, Wang LW, Wu YH, Zeng S, Huang KX, Zhao Y, Li XK, Qu J. Studies on chemical constituents from herbs of Taraxacum mongolicum. *Zhongguo Zhong Yao Za Zhi.* 2008 May;33(10):1147-57.

Shibata H, Nabe T, Yamamura H, Kohno S. l-Ephedrine is a major constituent of Mao-Bushi-Saishin-To, one of the formulas of Chinese medicine, which shows immediate inhibition after oral administration of passive cutaneous anaphylaxis in rats. *Inflamm Res.* 2000 Aug;49(8):398-403.

Shimoi T, Ushiyama H, Kan K, Saito K, Kamata K, Hirokado M. Survey of glycoalkaloids content in the various potatoes. Shokuhin Eiseigaku Zasshi. 2007 Jun;48(3):77-82.

Shishehbor F, Behroo L, Ghafouriyan Broujerdnia M, Namjoyan F, Latifi SM. Quercetin effectively quells peanut-induced anaphylactic reactions in the peanut sensitized rats. *Iran J Allergy Asthma Immunol.* 2010 Mar;9(1):27-34.

Shoaf, K., Muvey, G.L., Armstrong, G.D., Hutkins, R.W. (2006) Prebiotic galactooligosaccharides reduce adherence of enteropathogenic Escherichia coli to tissue culture cells. *Infect Immun.* Dec;74(12):6920-8.

Sicherer SH, Muñoz-Furlong A, Godbold JH, Sampson HA. US prevalence of self-reported peanut, tree nut, and sesame allergy: 11-year follow-up. *J Allergy Clin Immunol.* 2010 Jun;125(6):1322-6.

Sicherer SH, Munoz-Furlong A, Sampson HA (2003) Prevalence of peanut and tree nut allergy in the United States determined by means of a random digit dial telephone survey: a 5-year follow-up study. *J Allergy Clin Immunol.* 112: 1203–1207.

Sicherer SH, Noone SA, Koerner CB, Christie L, Burks AW, Sampson HA. Hypoallergenicity and efficacy of an amino acid-based formula in children with cow's milk and multiple food hypersensitivities. *J Pediatr.* 2001 May;138(5):688-93.

Sicherer SH, Sampson HA. Food allergy. *J Allergy Clin Immunol.* 2010 Feb;125(2 Suppl 2):S116-25.

Sicherer SH, Wood RA, Stablein D, Burks AW, Liu AH, Jones SM, Fleischer DM, Leung DY, Grishin A, Mayer L, Shreffler W, Lindblad R, Sampson HA. Immunologic features of infants with milk or egg allergy enrolled in an observational study (Consortium of Food Allergy Research) of food allergy. *J Allergy Clin Immunol.* 2010 May;125(5):1077-1083.e8.

Sigstedt SC, Hooten CJ, Callewaert MC, Jenkins AR, Romero AE, Pullin MJ, Kornienko A, Lowrey TK, Slambrouck SV, Steelant WF. Evaluation of aqueous extracts of Taraxacum officinale on growth and invasion of breast and prostate cancer cells. *Int J Oncol.* 2008 May;32(5):1085-90.

Silman AJ, MacGregor AJ, Thomson W, Holligan S, Carthy D, Farhan A, Ollier WE. Twin concordance rates for rheumatoid arthritis: results from a nationwide study. *Br J Rheumatol.* 1993 Oct;32(10):903-7.

Silva MF, Kamphorst AO, Hayashi EA, Bellio M, Carvalho CR, Faria AM, Sabino KC, Coelho MG, Nobrega A, Tavares D, Silva AC. Innate profiles of cytokines implicated on oral tolerance correlate with low- or high-suppression of humoral response. *Immunology.* 2010 Jul;130(3):447-57.

Simeone D, Miele E, Boccia G, Marino A, Troncone R, Staiano A. Prevalence of atopy in children with chronic constipation. *Arch Dis Child.* 2008 Dec;93(12):1044-7.

Simonte SJ, Ma S, Mofidi S, Sicherer SH. Relevance of casual contact with peanut butter in children with peanut allergy. *J Allergy Clin Immunol.* 2003 Jul;112(1):180-2.

Simopoulos AP. Essential fatty acids in health and chronic disease. *Am J Clin Nutr.* 1999 Sep;70(3 Suppl):560S-569S.

Simpson AB, Yousef E, Hossain J. Association between peanut allergy and asthma morbidity. *J Pediatr.* 2010 May;156(5):777-81, 781.e1.

Singer P, Shapiro H, Theilla M, Anbar R, Singer J, Cohen J. Anti-inflammatory properties of omega-3 fatty acids in critical illness: novel mechanisms and an integrative perspective. *Intensive Care Med.* 2008 Sep;34(9):1580-92.

Singh S, Khajuria A, Taneja SC, Johri RK, Singh J, Qazi GN. Boswellic acids: A leukotriene inhibitor also effective through topical application in inflammatory disorders. *Phytomedicine.* 2008 Jun;15(6-7):400-7.

Sirvent S, Palomares O, Vereda A, Villalba M, Cuesta-Herranz J, Rodríguez R. nsLTP and profilin are allergens in mustard seeds: cloning, sequencing and recombinant production of Sin a 3 and Sin a 4. *Clin Exp Allergy.* 2009 Dec;39(12):1929-36.

Skamstrup Hansen K, Vieths S, Vestergaard H, Skov PS, Bindslev-Jensen C, Poulsen LK. Seasonal variation in food allergy to apple. *J Chromatogr B Biomed Sci Appl.* 2001 May 25;756(1-2):19-32.

Skripak JM, Nash SD, Rowley H, Brereton NH, Oh S, Hamilton RG, Matsui EC, Burks AW, Wood RA. A randomized, double-blind, placebo-controlled study of milk oral immunotherapy for cow's milk allergy. *J Allergy Clin Immunol.* 2008 Dec;122(6):1154-60.

Sletten GB, Halvorsen R, Egaas E, Halstensen TS. Changes in humoral responses to beta-lactoglobulin in tolerant patients suggest a particular role for IgG4 in delayed, non-IgE-mediated cow's milk allergy. *Pediatr Allergy Immunol.* 2006 Sep;17(6):435-43.

Smecuol E, Hwang HJ, Sugai E, Corso L, Cherñavsky AC, Bellavite FP, González A, Vodánovich F, Moreno ML, Vázquez H, Lozano G, Niveloni S, Mazure R, Meddings J, Mauriño E, Bai JC. Exploratory, randomized, double-blind, placebo-controlled study on the effects of Bifidobacterium infantis natren life start strain super strain in active celiac disease. J Clin Gastroenterol. 2013 Feb;47(2):139-47. doi: 10.1097/MCG.0b013e31827759ac.

Smith J. *Genetic Roulette: The Documented Health Risks of Genetically Engineered Foods.* White River Jct, Vermont: Chelsea Green, 2007.

Smith K, Warholak T, Armstrong E, Leib M, Rehfeld R, Malone D. Evaluation of risk factors and health outcomes among persons with asthma. *J Asthma.* 2009 Apr;46(3):234-7.

Smith S, Sullivan K. Examining the influence of biological and psychological factors on cognitive performance in chronic fatigue syndrome: a randomized, double-blind, placebo-controlled, crossover study. *Int
J Behav Med.* 2003;10(2):162-73.

Sofic E, Denisova N, Youdim K, Vatrenjak-Velagic V, De Filippo C, Mehmedagic A, Causevic A, Cao G,
Joseph JA, Prior RL. Antioxidant and pro-oxidant capacity of catecholamines and related compounds.
Effects of hydrogen peroxide on glutathione and sphingomyelinase activity in pheochromocytoma
PC12 cells: potential relevance to age-related diseases. *J Neural Transm.* 2001;108(5):541-57.

Soleo L, Colosio C, Alinovi R, Guarneri D, Russo A, Lovreglio P, Vimercati L, Birindelli S, Cortesi I, Flore
C, Carta P, Colombi A, Parrinello G, Ambrosi L. Immunologic effects of exposure to low levels of in-
organic mercury. *Med Lav.* 2002 May-Jun;93(3):225-32. Italian.

Sompamit K, Kukongviriyapan U, Nakmareong S, Pannangpetch P, Kukongviriyapan V. Curcumin improves vascular function and alleviates oxidative stress in non-lethal lipopolysaccharide-induced en-
dotoxaemia in mice. *Eur J Pharmacol.* 2009 Aug 15;616(1-3):192-9.

Song HY, Jiang CH, Yang JR, Chen QH, Huang J, Huang YH, Liang LX. [The change of intestinal mucosa
barrier in chronic severe hepatitis B patients and clinical intervention]. *Zhonghua Gan Zang Bing Za Zhi.*
2009 Oct;17(10):754-8.

Soyland Wasenius AK, Halvorsen R. Oral provocation tests for adverse reactions to food. *Tidsskr Nor
Laegeforen.* 2003 Jun 26;123(13-14):1829-30.

Spence A. *Basic Human Anatomy.* Menlo Park, CA: Benjamin/Commings, 1986.

Spiller G. *The Super Pyramid.* New York: HRS Press, 1993.

Srivastava K, Zou ZM, Sampson HA, Dansky H, Li XM. Direct Modulation of Airway Reactivity by the
Chinese Anti-Asthma Herbal Formula ASHMI. *J Allergy Clin Immunol.* 2005;115:S7.

Srivastava KD, Kattan JD, Zou ZM, Li JH, Zhang L, Wallenstein S, Goldfarb J, Sampson HA, Li XM. The
Chinese herbal medicine formula FAHF-2 completely blocks anaphylactic reactions in a murine model
of peanut allergy. *J Allergy Clin Immunol.* 2005;115:171–8.

Srivastava KD, Qu C, Zhang T, Goldfarb J, Sampson HA, Li XM. Food Allergy Herbal Formula-2 silences
peanut-induced anaphylaxis for a prolonged posttreatment period via IFN-gamma-producing CD8+ T
cells. *J Allergy Clin Immunol.* 2009 Feb;123(2):443-51.

Srivastava KD, Zhang TF, Qu C, Sampson HA, Li XM. Silencing Peanut Allergy: A Chinese Herbal Formula, FAHF-2, Completely Blocks Peanut-induced Anaphylaxis for up to 6 Months Following Therapy in a Murine Model Of Peanut Allergy. *J Allergy Clin Immunol.* 2006;117:S328.

Staden U, Rolinck-Werninghaus C, Brewe F, Wahn U, Niggemann B, Beyer K. Specific oral tolerance
induction in food allergy in children: efficacy and clinical patterns of reaction. *Allergy.* 2007
Nov;62(11):1261-9.

Stahl SM. Selective histamine H1 antagonism: novel hypnotic and pharmacologic actions challenge classical
notions of antihistamines. *CNS Spectr.* 2008 Dec;13(12):1027-38.

Stenberg JA, Hambäck PA, Ericson L. Herbivore-induced "rent rise" in the host plant may drive a diet
breadth enlargement in the tenant. *Ecology.* 2008 Jan;89(1):126-33.

Stengler M. *The Natural Physician's Healing Therapies.* Stamford, CT: Bottom Line Books, 2008.

Stenman SM, Venäläinen JI, Lindfors K, Auriola S, Mauriala T, Kaukovirta-Norja A, Jantunen A, Laurila K,
Qiao SW, Sollid LM, Männisto PT, Kaukinen K, Mäki M. Enzymatic detoxification of gluten by ger-
minating wheat proteases: implications for new treatment of celiac disease. Ann Med. 2009;41(5):390-
400. doi: 10.1080/07853890902878138.

Stirapongsasuti P, Tanglertsampan C, Aunhachoke K, Sangasapaviliya A. Anaphylactic reaction to phuk-
waan-ban in a patient with latex allergy. *J Med Assoc Thai.* 2010 May;93(5):616-9.

Stratiki Z, Costalos C, Sevastiadou S, Kastanidou O, Skouroliakou M, Giakoumatou A, Petrohilou V. The
effect of a bifidobacter supplemented bovine milk on intestinal permeability of preterm infants. *Early
Hum Dev.* 2007 Sep;83(9):575-9.

Strinnholm A, Brulin C, Lindh V. Experiences of double-blind, placebo-controlled food challenges
(DBPCFC): a qualitative analysis of mothers' experiences. *J Child Health Care.* 2010 Jun;14(2):179-88.

Stutius LM, Sheehan WJ, Rangsithienchai P, Bharmanee A, Scott JE, Young MC, Dioun AF, Schneider LC,
Phipatanakul W. Characterizing the relationship between sesame, coconut, and nut allergy in children.
Pediatr Allergy Immunol. 2010 Dec;21(8):1114-8.

Sugawara G, Nagino M, Nishio H, Ebata T, Takagi K, Asahara T, Nomoto K, Nimura Y. Perioperative
synbiotic treatment to prevent postoperative infectious complications in biliary cancer surgery: a randomized controlled trial. *Ann Surg.* 2006 Nov;244(5):706-14.

Suh KY. Food allergy and atopic dermatitis: separating fact from fiction. *Semin Cutan Med Surg.* 2010
Jun;29(2):72-8.

REFERENCES AND BIBLIOGRAPHY

Sumantran VN, Kulkarni AA, Harsulkar A, Wele A, Koppikar SJ, Chandwaskar R, Gaire V, Dalvi M, Wagh UV. Hyaluronidase and collagenase inhibitory activities of the herbal formulation Triphala guggulu. *J Biosci.* 2007 Jun;32(4):755-61.

Sumiyoshi M, Sakanaka M, Kimura Y. Effects of Red Ginseng extract on allergic reactions to food in Balb/c mice. *J Ethnopharmacol.* 2010 Aug 14.

Sundqvist T, Lindström F, Magnusson KE, Sköldstam L, Stjernström I, Tagesson C. Influence of fasting on intestinal permeability and disease activity in patients with rheumatoid arthritis. *Scand J Rheumatol.* 1982;11(1):33-8.

Sung JH, Lee JO, Son JK, Park NS, Kim MR, Kim JG, Moon DC. Cytotoxic constituents from Solidago virga-aurea var. gigantea MIQ. *Arch Pharm Res.* 1999 Dec;22(6):633-7.

Suomalainen H, Isolauri E. New concepts of allergy to cow's milk. *Ann Med.* 1994 Aug;26(4):289-96.

Sütas Y, Kekki OM, Isolauri E. Late onset reactions to oral food challenge are linked to low serum inter-leukin-10 concentrations in patients with atopic dermatitis and food allergy. *Clin Exp Allergy.* 2000 Aug;30(8):1121-8.

Svendsen AJ, Holm NV, Kyvik K, *et al.* Relative importance of genetic effects in rheumatoid arthritis: historical cohort study of Danish nationwide twin population. *BMJ* 2002;324(7332): 264-266.

Sweeney B, Vora M, Ulbricht C, Basch E. Evidence-based systematic review of dandelion (Taraxacum officinale) by natural standard research collaboration. *J Herb Pharmacother.* 2005;5(1):79-93.

Swiderska-Kielbik S, Krakowiak A, Wiszniewska M, Dudek W, Walusiak-Skorupa J, Krawczyk-Szulc P, Michowicz A, Palczyński C. Health hazards associated with occupational exposure to birds. *Med Pr.* 2010;61(2):213-22.

Szyf M, McGowan P, Meaney MJ. The social environment and the epigenome. *Environ Mol Mutagen.* 2008 Jan;49(1):46-60.

Takada Y, Ichikawa H, Badmaev V, Aggarwal BB. Acetyl-11-keto-beta-boswellic acid potentiates apoptosis, inhibits invasion, and abolishes osteoclastogenesis by suppressing NF-kappa B and NF-kappa B-regulated gene expression. *J Immunol.* 2006 Mar 1;176(5):3127-40.

Takahashi N, Eisenhuth G, Lee I, Schachtele C, Laible N, Binion S. Nonspecific antibacterial factors in milk from cows immunized with human oral bacterial pathogens. *J Dairy Sci.* 1992 Jul;75(7):1810-20.

Takasaki M, Konoshima T, Tokuda H, Masuda K, Arai Y, Shiojima K, Ageta H. Anti-carcinogenic activity of Taraxacum plant. I. *Biol Pharm Bull.* 1999 Jun;22(6):602-5.

Tamura M, Shikina T, Morihana T, Hayama M, Kajimoto O, Sakamoto A, Kajimoto Y, Watanabe O, Nonaka C, Shida K, Nanno M. Effects of probiotics on allergic rhinitis induced by Japanese cedar pollen: randomized double-blind, placebo-controlled clinical trial. *Int Arch Allergy Imml.* 2007;143(1):75-82.

Tapiero H, Ba GN, Couvreur P, Tew KD. Polyunsaturated fatty acids (PUFA) and eicosanoids in human health and pathologies. *Biomed Pharmacother.* 2002 Jul;56(5):215-22.

Tapsell LC, Hemphill I, Cobiac L, Patch CS, Sullivan DR, Fenech M, Roodenrys S, Keogh JB, Clifton PM, Williams PG, Fazio VA, Inge KE. Health benefits of herbs and spices: the past, the present, the future. *Med J Aust.* 2006 Aug 21;185(4 Suppl):S4-24.

Tasli L, Mat C, De Simone C, Yazici H. Lactobacilli lozenges in the management of oral ulcers of Behçet's syndrome. *Clin Exp Rheumatol.* 2006 Sep-Oct;24(5 Suppl 42):S83-6.

Taussig SJ, Batkin S. Bromelain, the enzyme complex of pineapple (Ananas comosus) and its clinical application. An update. *J Ethnopharmacol.* 1988 Feb-Mar;22(2):191-203.

Taylor AL, Dunstan JA, Prescott SL. Probiotic supplementation for the first 6 months of life fails to reduce the risk of atopic dermatitis and increases the risk of allergen sensitization in high-risk children: a randomized controlled trial. *J Allergy Clin Immunol.* 2007 Jan;119(1):184-91.

Taylor AL, Hale J, Wiltschut J, Lehmann H, Dunstan JA, Prescott SL. Effects of probiotic supplementation for the first 6 months of life on allergen- and vaccine-specific immune responses. *Clin Exp Allergy.* 2006 Oct;36(10):1227-35.

Taylor RB, Lindquist N, Kubanek J, Hay ME. Intraspecific variation in palatability and defensive chemistry of brown seaweeds: effects on herbivore fitness. *Oecologia.* 2003 Aug;136(3):412-23.

Taylor SL, Moneret-Vautrin DA, Crevel RW, Sheffield D, Morisset M, Dumont P, Remington BC, Baumert JL. Threshold dose for peanut: Risk characterization based upon diagnostic oral challenge of a series of 286 peanut-allergic individuals. *Food Chem Toxicol.* 2010 Mar;48(3):814-9.

Teitelbaum J. *From Fatigue to Fantastic.* New York: Avery, 2001.

Ten Bruggencate SJ, Bovee-Oudenhoven IM, Lettink-Wissink ML, Katan MB, van der Meer R. Dietary fructooligosaccharides affect intestinal barrier function in healthy men. *J Nutr.* 2006 Jan;136(1):70-4.

Terheggen-Lagro SW, Khouw IM, Schaafsma A, Wauters EA. Safety of a new extensively hydrolysed formula in children with cow's milk protein allergy: a double blind crossover study. *BMC Pediatr.* 2002 Oct 14;2:10.

Terracciano L, Bouygue GR, Sarratud T, Veglia F, Martelli A, Fiocchi A. Impact of dietary regimen on the duration of cow's milk allergy: a random allocation study. *Clin Exp Allergy*. 2010 Apr;40(4):637-42.

Tham KW, Zuraimi MS, Koh D, Chew FT, Ooi PL. Associations between home dampness and presence of molds with asthma and allergic symptoms among young children in the tropics. *Pediatr Allergy Immunol*. 2007 Aug;18(5):418-24.

Thampithak A, Jaisin Y, Meesarapee B, Chongthammakun S, Piyachaturawat P, Govitrapong P, Supavilai P, Sanvarinda Y. Transcriptional regulation of iNOS and COX-2 by a novel compound from Curcuma comosa in lipopolysaccharide-induced microglial activation. *Neurosci Lett*. 2009 Sep 22;462(2):171-5.

Theler B, Brockow K, Ballmer-Weber BK. Clinical presentation and diagnosis of meat allergy in Switzerland and Southern Germany. *Swiss Med Wkly*. 2009 May 2;139(17-18):264-70.

Theofilopoulos AN, Kono DH: The genes of systemic autoimmunity. *Proc Assoc Am Physicians*. 1999;111(3): 228-240.

Thomas, R.G., Gebhardt, S.E. 2008. Nutritive value of pomegranate fruit and juice. *Maryland Dietetic Association Annual Meeting, USDA-ARS*. 2008 April 11.

Thompson RL, Miles LM, Lunn J, Devereux G, Dearman RJ, Strid J, Buttriss JL. Peanut sensitisation and allergy: influence of early life exposure to peanuts. *Br J Nutr*. 2010 May;103(9):1278-86.

Thompson T, Lee AR, Grace T. Gluten contamination of grains, seeds, and flours in the United States: a pilot study. J Am Diet Assoc. 2010 Jun;110(6):937-40.

Tierra L. *The Herbs of Life*. Freedom, CA: Crossing Press, 1992.

Tierra M. *The Way of Herbs*. New York: Pocket Books, 1990.

Tisserand R. *The Art of Aromatherapy*. New York: Inner Traditions, 1979.

Tiwari M. *Ayurveda: A Life of Balance*. Rochester, VT: Healing Arts, 1995.

Tlaskalová-Hogenová H, Stepánková R, Hudcovic T, Tucková L, Cukrowska B, Lodinová-Zádníková R, Kozáková H, Rossmann P, Bártová J, Sokol D, Funda DP, Borovská D, Reháková Z, Sinkora J, Hofman J, Drastich P, Kokesová A. Commensal bacteria (normal microflora), mucosal immunity and chronic inflammatory and autoimmune diseases. *Immunol Lett*. 2004 May 15;93(2-3):97-108.

Todd GR, Acerini CL, Ross-Russell R, Zahra S, Warner JT, McCance D. Survey of adrenal crisis associated with inhaled corticosteroids in the United Kingdom. *Arch Dis Child*. 2002 Dec;87(6):457-61.

Tomicić S, Norrman G, Fälth-Magnusson K, Jenmalm MC, Devenney I, Böttcher MF. High levels of IgG4 antibodies to foods during infancy are associated with tolerance to corresponding foods later in life. *Pediatr Allergy Immunol*. 2009 Feb;20(1):35-41.

Tonkal AM, Morsy TA. An update review on Commiphora molmol and related species. *J Egypt Soc Parasitol*. 2008 Dec;38(3):763-96.

Topçu G, Erenler R, Cakmak O, Johansson CB, Celik C, Chai HB, Pezzuto JM. Diterpenes from the berries of Juniperus excelsa. *Phytochemistry*. 1999 Apr;50(7):1195-9.

Tordesillas L, Pacios LF, Palacín A, Cuesta-Herranz J, Madero M, Díaz-Perales A. Characterization of IgE epitopes of Cuc m 2, the major melon allergen, and their role in cross-reactivity with pollen profilins. *Clin Exp Allergy*. 2010 Jan;40(1):174-81.

Towers GH. FAHF-1 purporting to block peanut-induced anaphylaxis. *J Allergy Clin Immunol*. 2003 May;111(5):1140; author reply 1140-1.

Towle A. *Modern Biology*. Austin: Harcourt Brace, 1993.

Trojanová I, Rada V, Kokoska L, Vlková E. The bifidogenic effect of Taraxacum officinale root. *Fitoterapia*. 2004 Dec;75(7-8):760-3.

Troncone R, Caputo N, Florio G, Finelli E. Increased intestinal sugar permeability after challenge in children with cow's milk allergy or intolerance. *Allergy*. 1994 Mar;49(3):142-6.

Truswell AS. The A2 milk case: a critical review. *Euro J Clin Nutr*. 2005:59;623–631.

Tsai JC, Tsai S, Chang WC. Comparison of two Chinese medical herbs, Huangbai and Qianniuzi, on influence of short circuit current across the rat intestinal epithelia. *J Ethnopharmacol*. 2004 Jul;93(1):21-5.

Tsong T. Deciphering the language of cells. *Trends in Biochem Sci*. 1989;14:89-92.

Tsuchiya J, Barreto R, Okura R, Kawakita S, Fesce E, Marotta F. Single-blind follow-up study on the effectiveness of a symbiotic preparation in irritable bowel syndrome. *Chin J Dig Dis*. 2004;5(4):169-74.

Tulk HM, Robinson LE. Modifying the n-6/n-3 polyunsaturated fatty acid ratio of a high-saturated fat challenge does not acutely attenuate postprandial changes in inflammatory markers in men with metabolic syndrome. *Metabolism*. 2009 Jul 20.

Tursi A, Brandimarte G, Giorgetti GM, Elisei W. Mesalazine and/or Lactobacillus casei in maintaining long-term remission of symptomatic uncomplicated diverticular disease of the colon. *Hepatogastroenterology*. 2008 May-Jun;55(84):916-20.

U.S. Food and Drug Administration CfDEaR. *Guidance for Industry Botanical Drug Products*. 2000

Ueno H, Yoshioka K, Matsumoto T. Usefulness of the skin index in predicting the outcome of oral challenges in children. *J Investig Allergol Clin Immunol*. 2007;17(4):207-10.

REFERENCES AND BIBLIOGRAPHY

Ueno M, Adachi A, Fukumoto T, Nishitani N, Fujiwara N, Matsuo H, Kohno K, Morita E. Analysis of causative allergen of the patient with baker's asthma and wheat-dependent exercise-induced anaphylaxis (WDEIA). *Arerugi*. 2010 May;59(5):552-7.

Ukabam SO, Mann RJ, Cooper BT. Small intestinal permeability to sugars in patients with atopic eczema. *Br J Dermatol*. 1984 Jun;110(6):649-52.

Unsel M, Ardeniz O, Mete N, Ersoy R, Sin AZ, Gulbahar O, Kokuludag A. Food allergy due to olive. J Investig Allergol Clin Immunol. 2009;19(6):497-9. García BE, Gamboa PM, Asturias JA, López-Hoyos M, Sanz ML, Caballero MT, García JM, Labrador M, Lahoz C, Longo Areso N, Martínez Quesada J, Mayorga L, Monteseirín FJ; Clinical Immunology Committee; Spanish Society of Allergology and Clinical Immunology. Guidelines on the clinical usefulness of determination of specific immunoglobulin E to foods. *J Investig Allergol Clin Immunol*. 2009;19(6):423-32.

Unsel M, Sin AZ, Ardeniz O, Erdem N, Ersoy R, Gulbahar O, Mete N, Kokuludağ A. New onset egg allergy in an adult. *J Investig Allergol Clin Immunol*. 2007;17(1):55-8.

Untersmayr E, Vestergaard H, Malling HJ, Jensen LB, Platzer MH, Boltz-Nitulescu G, Scheiner O, Skov PS, Jensen-Jarolim E, Poulsen LK. Incomplete digestion of codfish represents a risk factor for anaphylaxis in patients with allergy. *J Allergy Clin Immunol*. 2007 Mar;119(3):711-7.

Upadhyay AK, Kumar K, Kumar A, Mishra HS. Tinospora cordifolia (Willd.) Hook. f. and Thoms. (Guduchi) - validation of the Ayurvedic pharmacology through experimental and clinical studies. *Int J Ayurveda Res*. 2010 Apr;1(2):112-21.

Vally H, Thompson PJ, Misso NL. Changes in bronchial hyperresponsiveness following high- and low-sulphite wine challenges in wine-sensitive asthmatic patients. *Clin Exp Allergy*. 2007 Jul;37(7):1062-6.

van Beelen VA, Roeleveld J, Mooibroek H, Sijtsma L, Bino RJ, Bosch D, Rietjens IM, Alink GM. A comparative study on the effect of algal and fish oil on viability and cell proliferation of Caco-2 cells. *Food Chem Toxicol*. 2007 May;45(5):716-24.

van der Hulst RR, van Kreel BK, von Meyenfeldt MF, Brummer RJ, Arends JW, Deutz NE, Soeters PB. Glutamine and the preservation of gut integrity. *Lancet*. 1993 May 29;341(8857):1363-5.

van Elburg RM, Uil JJ, de Monchy JG, Heymans HS. Intestinal permeability in pediatric gastroenterology. *Scand J Gastroenterol Suppl*. 1992;194:19-24.

van Kampen V, Merget R, Rabstein S, Sander I, Bruening T, Broding HC, Keller C, Muesken H, Overlack A, Schultze-Werninghaus G, Walusiak J, Raulf-Heimsoth M. Comparison of wheat and rye flour solutions for skin prick testing: a multi-centre study (Stad 1). *Clin Exp Allergy*. 2009 Dec;39(12):1896-902.

van Nieuwenhoven MA, Brouns F, Brummer RJ. The effect of physical exercise on parameters of gastrointestinal function. *Neurogastroenterol Motil*. 1999 Dec;11(6):431-9.

van Odijk J, Peterson CG, Ahlstedt S, Bengtsson U, Borres MP, Hulthén L, Magnusson J, Hansson T. Measurements of eosinophil activation before and after food challenges in adults with food hypersensitivity. *Int Arch Allergy Immunol*. 2006;140(4):334-41.

Vanderhoof JA. Probiotics in allergy management. *J Pediatr Gastroenterol Nutr*. 2008 Nov;47 Suppl 2:S38-40.

Vanto T, Helppilä S, Juntunen-Backman K, Kalimo K, Klemola T, Korpela R, Koskinen P. Prediction of the development of tolerance to milk in children with cow's milk hypersensitivity. *J Pediatr*. 2004 Feb;144(2):218-22.

Vassallo MF, Banerji A, Rudders SA, Clark S, Mullins RJ, Camargo CA Jr. Season of birth and food allergy in children. *Ann Allergy Asthma Immunol*. 2010 Apr;104(4):307-13.

Vendt N, Grünberg H, Tuure T, Malminiemi O, Wuolijoki E, Tillmann V, Sepp E, Korpela R. Growth during the first 6 months of life in infants using formula enriched with Lactobacillus rhamnosus GG: double-blind, randomized trial. *J Hum Nutr Diet*. 2006 Feb;19(1):51-8.

Venkatachalam KV. Human 3'-phosphoadenosine 5'-phosphosulfate (PAPS) synthase: biochemistry, molecular biology and genetic deficiency. *IUBMB Life*. 2003 Jan;55(1):1-11.

Venter C, Hasan Arshad S, Grundy J, Pereira B, Bernie Clayton C, Voigt K, Higgins B, Dean T. Time trends in the prevalence of peanut allergy: three cohorts of children from the same geographical location in the UK. *Allergy*. 2010 Jan;65(1):103-8.

Venter C, Meyer R. Session 1: Allergic disease: The challenges of managing food hypersensitivity. *Proc Nutr Soc*. 2010 Feb;69(1):11-24.

Venter C, Pereira B, Grundy J, Clayton CB, Arshad SH, Dean T (2006a) Prevalence of sensitization reported and objectively assessed food hypersensitivity amongst six-year-old children: A population-based study. *Pediatr Allergy Immunol*. 17: 356–363.

Venter C, Pereira B, Grundy J, Clayton CB, Roberts G, Higgins B, Dean T (2006b) Incidence of parentally reported and clinically diagnosed food hypersensitivity in the first year of life. *J Allergy Clin Immunol*. 117: 1118–1124.

Ventura MT, Polimeno L, Amoruso AC, Gatti F, Annoscia E, Marinaro M, Di Leo E, Matino MG, Buquic-chio R, Bonini S, Tursi A, Francavilla A. Intestinal permeability in patients with adverse reactions to food. *Dig Liver Dis.* 2006 Oct;38(10):732-6.

Venturi A, Gionchetti P, Rizzello F, Johansson R, Zucconi E, Brigidi P, Matteuzzi D, Campieri M. Impact on the composition of the faecal flora by a new probiotic preparation: preliminary data on mainte-nance treatment of patients with ulcerative colitis. *Aliment Pharmacol Ther.* 1999 Aug;13(8):1103-8.

Verhasselt V. Oral tolerance in neonates: from basics to potential prevention of allergic disease. *Mucosal Immunol.* 2010 Jul;3(4):326-33.

Verstege A, Mehl A, Rolinck-Werninghaus C, Staden U, Nocon M, Beyer K, Niggemann B. The predictive value of the skin prick test weal size for the outcome of oral food challenges. Clin Exp Allergy. 2005 Sep;35(9):1220-6. Rolinck-Werninghaus C, Staden U, Mehl A, Hamelmann E, Beyer K, Niggemann B. Specific oral tolerance induction with food in children: transient or persistent effect on food allergy? *Allergy.* 2005 Oct;60(10):1320-2.

Vidgren HM, Agren JJ, Schwab U, Rissanen T, Hanninen O, Uusitupa MI. Incorporation of n-3 fatty acids into plasma lipid fractions, and erythrocyte membranes and platelets during dietary supplementation with fish, fish oil, and docosahexaenoic acid-rich oil among healthy young men. *Lipids.* 1997 Jul;32(7):697-705.

Vila R, Mundina M, Tomi F, Furlán R, Zacchino S, Casanova J, Cañigueral S. Composition and antifungal activity of the essential oil of Solidago chilensis. *Planta Med.* 2002 Feb;68(2):164-7.

Viljanen M, Kuitunen M, Haahtela T, Juntunen-Backman K, Korpela R, Savilahti E. Probiotic effects on faecal inflammatory markers and on faecal IgA in food allergic atopic eczema/dermatitis syndrome in-fants. *Pediatr Allergy Immunol.* 2005 Feb;16(1):65-71.

Viljanen M, Savilahti E, Haahtela T, Juntunen-Backman K, Korpela R, Poussa T, Tuure T, Kuitunen M. Probiotics in the treatment of atopic eczema/dermatitis syndrome in infants: a double-blind placebo-controlled trial. *Allergy.* 2005 Apr;60(4):494-500.

Vinson JA, Proch J, Bose P. MegaNatural((R)) Gold Grapeseed Extract: In Vitro Antioxidant and In Vivo Human Supplementation Studies. *J Med Food.* 2001 Spring;4(1):17-26.

Visness CM, London SJ, Daniels JL, Kaufman JS, Yeatts KB, Siega-Riz AM, Liu AH, Calatroni A, Zeldin DC. Association of obesity with IgE levels and allergy symptoms in children and adolescents: results from the National Health and Nutrition Examination Survey 2005-2006. *J Allergy Clin Immunol.* 2009 May;123(5):1163-9, 1169.e1-4.

Vlieg-Boerstra BJ, Dubois AE, van der Heide S, Bijleveld CM, Wolt-Plompen SA, Oude Elberink JN, Kukler J, Jansen DF, Venter C, Duiverman EJ. Ready-to-use introduction schedules for first exposure to allergenic foods in children at home. Allergy. 2008 Jul;63(7):903-9.

Vlieg-Boerstra BJ, van der Heide S, Bijleveld CM, Kukler J, Duiverman EJ, Dubois AE. Placebo reactions in double-blind, placebo-controlled food challenges in children. *Allergy.* 2007 Aug;62(8):905-12.

Vlieg-Boerstra BJ, van der Heide S, Bijleveld CM, Kukler J, Duiverman EJ, Wolt-Plompen SA, Dubois AE. Dietary assessment in children adhering to a food allergen avoidance diet for allergy prevention. *Eur J Clin Nutr.* 2006 Dec;60(12):1384-90.

Vojdani A. Antibodies as predictors of complex autoimmune diseases. *Int J Immunopathol Pharmacol.* 2008 Apr-Jun;21(2):267-78.

von Berg A, Filipiak-Pittroff B, Krämer U, Link E, Bollrath C, Brockow I, Koletzko S, Grübl A, Heinrich J, Wichmann HE, Bauer CP, Reinhardt D, Berdel D; GINIplus study group. Preventive effect of hydro-lyzed infant formulas persists until age 6 years: long-term results from the German Infant Nutritional Intervention Study (GINI). *J Allergy Clin Immunol.* 2008 Jun;121(6):1442-7.

von Berg A, Koletzko S, Grübl A, Filipiak-Pittroff B, Wichmann HE, Bauer CP, Reinhardt D, Berdel D; German Infant Nutritional Intervention Study Group. The effect of hydrolyzed cow's milk formula for allergy prevention in the first year of life: the German Infant Nutritional Intervention Study, a ran-domized double-blind trial. J Allergy Clin Immunol. 2003 Mar;111(3):533-40.

von Kruedener S, Schneider W, Elstner EF. A combination of Populus tremula, Solidago virgaurea and Fraxinus excelsior as an anti-inflammatory and antirheumatic drug. A short review. *Arzneimittelforschung.* 1995 Feb;45(2):169-71.

Vulevic J, Drakoularakou A, Yaqoob P, Tzortzis G and Gibson GR; Modulation of the fecal microflora profile and immune function by a novel trans-galactooligosaccharide mixture (B-GOS) in healthy eld-erly volunteers. *Am J Clin Nutr.* 1988 88;1438-1446.

Waddell L. Food allergies in children: the difference between cow's milk protein allergy and food intolerance. *J Fam Health Care.* 2010;20(3):104.

Wahler D, Gronover CS, Richter C, Foucu F, Twyman RM, Moerschbacher BM, Fischer R, Muth J, Prufer D. Polyphenoloxidase silencing affects latex coagulation in Taraxacum spp. *Plant Physiol.* 2009 Jul 15.

Wahn U, Warner J, Simons FE, de Benedictis FM, Diepgen TL, Naspitz CK, de Longueville M, Bauchau V; EPAAC Study Group. IgE antibody responses in young children with atopic dermatitis. *Pediatr Allergy Immunol.* 2008 Jun;19(4):332-6.

Wainstein BK, Yee A, Jelley D, Ziegler M, Ziegler JB. Combining skin prick, immediate skin application and specific-IgE testing in the diagnosis of peanut allergy in children. Pediatr Allergy Immunol. 2007 May;18(3):231-9. Nolan RC, Richmond P, Prescott SL, Mallon DF, Gong G, Franzmann AM, Naidoo R, Loh RK. Skin prick testing predicts peanut challenge outcome in previously allergic or sensitized children with low serum peanut-specific IgE antibody concentration. *Pediatr Allergy Immunol.* 2007 May;18(3):224-30.

Walker S, Wing A. Allergies in children. *J Fam Health Care.* 2010;20(1):24-6.

Walker WA. Antigen absorption from the small intestine and gastrointestinal disease. *Pediatr Clin North Am.* 1975 Nov;22(4):731-46.

Walker WA. Antigen handling by the small intestine. *Clin Gastroenterol.* 1986 Jan;15(1):1-20.

Walle UK, Walle T. Transport of the cooked-food mutagen 2-amino-1-methyl-6-phenylimidazo- 4,5-b pyridine (PhIP) across the human intestinal Caco-2 cell monolayer: role of efflux pumps. *Carcinogenesis.* 1999 Nov;20(11):2153-7.

Walsh SJ, Rau LM: Autoimmune diseases: a leading cause of death among young and middle-aged women in the United States. *Am J Public Health* 2000, 90(9): 1463-1466.

Walton GE, Lu C, Trogh I, Arnaut F, Gibson GR. A randomised, double-blind, placebo controlled cross-over study to determine the gastrointestinal effects of consumption of arabinoxylanoligosaccharides enriched bread in healthy volunteers. Nutr J. 2012 Jun 1;11(1):36.

Wan KS, Yang W, Wu WF. A survey of serum specific-IgE to common allergens in primary school children of Taipei City. *Asian Pac J Allergy Immunol.* 2010 Mar;28(1):1-6.

Wang J, Lin J, Bardina L, Goldis M, Nowak-Wegrzyn A, Shreffler WG, Sampson HA. Correlation of IgE/IgG4 milk epitopes and affinity of milk-specific IgE antibodies with different phenotypes of clinical milk allergy. *J Allergy Clin Immunol.* 2010 Mar;125(3):695-702, 702.e1-702.e6.

Wang J, Patil SP, Yang N, Ko J, Lee J, Noone S, Sampson HA, Li XM. Safety, tolerability, and immunologic effects of a food allergy herbal formula in food allergic individuals: a randomized, double-blinded, placebo-controlled, dose escalation, phase 1 study. *Ann Allergy Asthma Immunol.* 2010 Jul;105(1):75-84.

Wang J. Management of the patient with multiple food allergies. *Curr Allergy Asthma Rep.* 2010 Jul;10(4):271-7.

Wang KY, Li SN, Liu CS, Perng DS, Su YC, Wu DC, Jan CM, Lai CH, Wang TN, Wang WM. Effects of ingesting Lactobacillus- and Bifidobacterium-containing yogurt in subjects with colonized Helicobacter pylori. *Am J Clin Nutr.* 2004 Sep;80(3):737-41.

Wang WS, Li EW, Jia ZJ. Terpenes from Juniperus przewalskii and their antitumor activities. *Pharmazie.* 2002 May;57(5):343-5.

Wang YM, Huan GX. *Utilization of Classical Formulas.* Beijing, China: Chinese Medicine and Pharmacology Publishing Co, 1998.

Waring G, Levy D. Challenging adverse reactions in children with food allergies. *Paediatr Nurs.* 2010 Jul;22(6):16-22.

Waser M, Michels KB, Bieli C, Flöistrup H, Pershagen G, von Mutius E, Ege M, Riedler J, Schram-Bijkerk D, Brunekreef B, van Hage M, Lauener R, Braun-Fahrländer C; PARSIFAL Study team. Inverse association of farm milk consumption with asthma and allergy in rural and suburban populations across Europe. *Clin Exp Allergy.* 2007 May;37(5):661-70.

Watkins BA, Hannon K, Ferruzzi M, Li Y. Dietary PUFA and flavonoids as deterrents for environmental pollutants. *J Nutr Biochem.* 2007 Mar;18(3):196-205.

Watzl B, Bub A, Blockhaus M, Herbert BM, Lührmann PM, Neuhäuser-Berthold M, Rechkemmer G. Prolonged tomato juice consumption has no effect on cell-mediated immunity of well-nourished elderly men and women. *J Nutr.* 2000 Jul;130(7):1719-23.

Webber CM, England RW. Oral allergy syndrome: a clinical, diagnostic, and therapeutic challenge. *Ann Allergy Asthma Immunol.* 2010 Feb;104(2):101-8; quiz 109-10, 117.

Webster D, Taschereau P, Belland RJ, Sand C, Rennie RP. Antifungal activity of medicinal plant extracts; preliminary screening studies. *J Ethnopharmacol.* 2008 Jan 4;115(1):140-6.

Wedge DE, Tabanca N, Sampson BJ, Werle C, Demirci B, Baser KH, Nan P, Duan J, Liu Z. Antifungal and insecticidal activity of two Juniperus essential oils. *Nat Prod Commun.* 2009 Jan;4(1):123-7.

Wei A, Shibamoto T. Antioxidant activities and volatile constituents of various essential oils. *J Agric Food Chem.* 2007 Mar 7;55(5):1737-42.

Weiner MA. *Secrets of Fijian Medicine.* Berkeley, CA: Univ. of Calif., 1969.

Weiss RF. *Herbal Medicine.* Gothenburg, Sweden: Beaconsfield, 1988.

Wen MC, Huang CK, Srivastava KD, Zhang TF, Schofield B, Sampson HA, Li XM. Ku–Shen (Sophora flavescens Ait), a single Chinese herb, abrogates airway hyperreactivity in a murine model of asthma. *J Allergy Clin Immunol.* 2004;113:218.

Wen MC, Taper A, Srivastava KD, Huang CK, Schofield B, Li XM. Immunology of T cells by the Chinese Herbal Medicine Ling Zhi (Ganoderma lucidum) *J Allergy Clin Immunol.* 2003;111:S320.

Wen MC, Wei CH, Hu ZQ, Srivastava K, Ko J, Xi ST, Mu DZ, Du JB, Li GH, Wallenstein S, Sampson H, Kattan M, Li XM. Efficacy and tolerability of anti-asthma herbal medicine intervention in adult patients with moderate-severe allergic asthma. *J Allergy Clin Immunol.* 2005;116:517–24.

Wensing M, Penninks AH, Hefle SL, Akkerdaas JH, van Ree R, Koppelman SJ, Bruijnzeel-Koomen CA, Knulst AC. The range of minimum provoking doses in hazelnut-allergic patients as determined by double-blind, placebo-controlled food challenges. *Clin Exp Allergy.* 2002 Dec;32(12):1757-62.

Werbach M. *Nutritional Influences on Illness.* Tarzana, CA: Third Line Press, 1996.

West CE, Hammarström ML, Hernell O. Probiotics during weaning reduce the incidence of eczema. *Pediatr Allergy Immunol.* 2009 Aug;20(5):430-7.

West R. Risk of death in meat and non-meat eaters. *BMJ.* 1994 Oct 8;309(6959):955.

Westerholm-Ormio M, Vaarala O, Tiittanen M, Savilahti E. Infiltration of Foxp3- and Toll-like receptor-4-positive cells in the intestines of children with food allergy. *J Pediatr Gastroenterol Nutr.* 2010 Apr;50(4):367-76.

Wheeler JG, Shema SJ, Bogle ML, Shirrell MA, Burks AW, Pittler A, Helm RM. Immune and clinical impact of Lactobacillus acidophilus on asthma. *Ann Allergy Asthma Immunol.* 1997 Sep;79(3):229-33.

Whitfield KE, Wiggins SA, Belue R, Brandon DT. Genetic and environmental influences on forced expiratory volume in African Americans: the Carolina African-American Twin Study of Aging. *Ethn Dis.* 2004 Spring;14(2):206-11.

WHO. *Guidelines for Drinking-water Quality.* 2nd ed, vol. 2. Geneva: World Health Organization, 1996.

WHO. Health effects of the removal of substances occurring naturally in drinking water, with special reference to demineralized and desalinated water. Report on a working group (Brussels, 20-23 March 1978). *EURO Reports and Studies.* 1979;16.

WHO. How trace elements in water contribute to health. *WHO Chronicle.* 1978;32:382-385.

WHO. *INFOSAN Food Allergies. Information Note No. 3.* Geneva, Switzerland: World Health Organization, 2006.

Whorwell PJ, Altringer L, Morel J, Bond Y, Charbonneau D, O'Mahony L, Kiely B, Shanahan F, Quigley EM. Efficacy of an encapsulated probiotic Bifidobacterium infantis 35624 in women with irritable bowel syndrome. *Am J Gastroenterol.* 2006 Jul;101(7):1581-90.

Wildt S, Munck LK, Vinter-Jensen L, Hanse BF, Nordgaard-Lassen I, Christensen S, Avnstroem S, Rasmussen SN, Rumessen JJ. Probiotic treatment of collagenous colitis: a randomized, double-blind, placebo-controlled trial with Lactobacillus acidophilus and Bifidobacterium animalis subsp. *Lactis. Inflamm Bowel Dis.* 2006 May;12(5):395-401.

Willard T, Jones K. *Reishi Mushroom: Herb of Spiritual Potency and Medical Wonder.* Issaquah, Washington: Sylvan Press, 1990.

Willard T. *Edible and Medicinal Plants of the Rocky Mountains and Neighbouring Territories.* Calgary: 1992.

Willemsen LE, Koetsier MA, Balvers M, Beermann C, Stahl B, van Tol EA. Polyunsaturated fatty acids support epithelial barrier integrity and reduce IL-4 mediated permeability in vitro. *Eur J Nutr.* 2008 Jun;47(4):183-91.

Wilson D, Evans M, Guthrie N, Sharma P, Baisley J, Schonlau F, Burki C. A randomized, double-blind, placebo-controlled exploratory study to evaluate the potential of pycnogenol for improving allergic rhinitis symptoms. *Phytother Res.* 2010 Aug;24(8):1115-9.

Wilson K, McDowall L, Hodge D, Chetcuti P, Cartledge P. Cow's milk protein allergy. *Community Pract.* 2010 May;83(5):40-1.

Wilson L. *Nutritional Balancing and Hair Mineral Analysis.* Prescott, AZ: LD Wilson, 1998.

Winchester AM. *Biology and its Relation to Mankind.* New York: Van Nostrand Reinhold, 1969.

Wittenberg JS. *The Rebellious Body.* New York: Insight, 1996.

Wöhrl S, Hemmer W, Focke M, Rappersberger K, Jarisch R. Histamine intolerance-like symptoms in healthy volunteers after oral provocation with liquid histamine. *Allergy Asthma Proc.* 2004 Sep-Oct;25(5):305-11.

Wolvers DA, van Herpen-Broekmans WM, Logman MH, van der Wielen RP, Albers R. Effect of a mixture of micronutrients, but not of bovine colostrum concentrate, on immune function parameters in healthy volunteers: a randomized placebo-controlled study. *Nutr J.* 2006 Nov 21;5:28.

Wood M. *The Book of Herbal Wisdom.* Berkeley, CA: North Atlantic, 1997.

Wood RA, Kraynak J. *Food Allergies for Dummies.* Hoboken, NJ: Wiley Publ, 2007.

Woods RK, Abramson M, Bailey M, Walters EH (2001) International prevalences of reported food allergies and intolerances. Comparisons arising from the European Community Respiratory Health Survey (ECRHS) 1991–1994. *Eur J Clin Nutr* 55: 298–304.

Woods RK, Abramson M, Bailey M, Walters EH. International prevalences of reported food allergies and intolerances. Comparisons arising from the European Community Respiratory Health Survey (ECRHS) 1991-1994. *Eur J Clin Nutr.* 2001 Apr;55(4):298-304.

Woods RK, Abramson M, Raven JM, Bailey M, Weiner JM, Walters EH (1998) Reported food intolerance and respiratory symptoms in young adults. *Eur Respir J.* 11: 151–155.

Worm M, Hompes S, Fiedler EM, Illner AK, Zuberbier T, Vieths S. Impact of native, heat-processed and encapsulated hazelnuts on the allergic response in hazelnut-allergic patients. *Clin Exp Allergy.* 2009 Jan;39(1):159-66.

Xiao P, Kubo H, Ohsawa M, Higashiyama K, Nagase H, Yan YN, Li JS, Kamei J, Ohmiya S. kappa-Opioid receptor-mediated antinociceptive effects of stereoisomers and derivatives of (+)-matrine in mice. *Planta Med.* 1999 Apr;65(3):230-3.

Xu X, Zhang D, Zhang H, Wolters PJ, Killeen NP, Sullivan BM, Locksley RM, Lowell CA, Caughey GH. Neutrophil histamine contributes to inflammation in mycoplasma pneumonia. *J Exp Med.* 2006 Dec 25;203(13):2907-17.

Yadav VS, Mishra KP, Singh DP, Mehrotra S, Singh VK. Immunomodulatory effects of curcumin. *Immunopharmacol Immunotoxicol.* 2005;27(3):485-97.

Yadzir ZH, Misnan R, Abdullah N, Bakhtiar F, Arip M, Murad S. Identification of Ige-binding proteins of raw and cooked extracts of Loligo edulis (white squid). *Southeast Asian J Trop Med Public Health.* 2010 May;41(3):653-9.

Yang Z. Are peanut allergies a concern for using peanut-based formulated foods in developing countries? *Food Nutr Bull.* 2010 Jun;31(2 Suppl):S147-53.

Yarnell E. Botanical medicines for the urinary tract. *World J Urol.* 2002 Nov;20(5):285-93.

Yeager S. *The Doctor's Book of Food Remedies.* Emmaus, PA: Rodale Press, 1998.

Yu LC. The epithelial gatekeeper against food allergy. *Pediatr Neonatol.* 2009 Dec;50(6):247-54.

Yusoff NA, Hampton SM, Dickerson JW, Morgan JB. The effects of exclusion of dietary egg and milk in the management of asthmatic children: a pilot study. *J R Soc Promot Health.* 2004 Mar;124(2):74-80.

Zanjanian MH. The intestine in allergic diseases. *Ann Allergy.* 1976 Sep;37(3):208-18.

Zarkadas M, Scott FW, Salminen J, Ham Pong A. Common Allergenic Foods and Their Labelling in Canada. *Can J Allergy Clin Immun.* 1999; 4:118-141.

Zeiger RS, Heller S. The development and prediction of atopy in high-risk children: follow-up at age seven years in a prospective randomized study of combined maternal and infant food allergen avoidance. *J Allergy Clin Immunol.* 1995 Jun;95(6):1179-90.

Zeng J, Li YQ, Zuo XL, Zhen YB, Yang J, Liu CH. Clinical trial: effect of active lactic acid bacteria on mucosal barrier function in patients with diarrhoea-predominant irritable bowel syndrome. *Aliment Pharmacol Ther.* 2008 Oct 15;28(8):994-1002.

Zhang J, Yuan C, Hua G, Tong R, Luo X, Ying Z. Early gut barrier dysfunction in patients with severe acute pancreatitis: attenuated by continuous blood purification treatment. *Int J Artif Organs.* 2010 Oct;33(10):706-15.

Zhang J, Zhang X, Lei G, Li B, Chen J, Zhou T. A new phenolic glycoside from the aerial parts of Solidago canadensis. *Fitoterapia.* 2007 Jan;78(1):69-71.

Zhang JB, Du XG, Zhang H, Li ML, Xiao G, Wu J, Gan H. Breakdown of the gut barrier in patients with multiple organ dysfunction syndrome is attenuated by continuous blood purification: effects on tight junction structural proteins. *Int J Artif Organs.* 2010 Jan;33(1):5-14.

Zheng M. Experimental study of 472 herbs with antiviral action against the herpes simplex virus. *Zhong Xi Yi Jie He Za Zhi.* 1990 Jan;10(1):39-41, 6.

Zhou Q, Zhang B, Verne GN. Intestinal membrane permeability and hypersensitivity in the irritable bowel syndrome. *Pain.* 2009 Nov;146(1-2):41-6.

Ziemniak W. Efficacy of Helicobacter pylori eradication taking into account its resistance to antibiotics. *J Physiol Pharmacol.* 2006 Sep;57 Suppl 3:123-41.

Zizza, C. The nutrient content of the Italian food supply 1961-1992. *Euro J Clin Nutr.* 1997;51: 259-265.

Zoccatelli G, Pokoj S, Foetisch K, Bartra J, Valero A, Del Mar San Miguel-Moncin M, Vieths S, Scheurer S. Identification and characterization of the major allergen of green bean (Phaseolus vulgaris) as a non-specific lipid transfer protein (Pha v 3). *Mol Immunol.* 2010 Apr;47(7-8):1561-8.

Zuidmeer L, Goldhahn K, Rona RJ, Gislason D, Madsen C, Summers C, Sodergren E, Dahlstrom J, Lindner T, Sigurdardottir ST, McBride D, Keil T. The prevalence of plant food allergies: a systematic review. *J Allergy Clin Immunol.* 2008 May;121(5):1210-1218.e4.

Zwolińska-Wcislo M, Brzozowski T, Mach T, Budak A, Trojanowska D, Konturek PC, Pajdo R, Drozdowicz D, Kwiecień S. Are probiotics effective in the treatment of fungal colonization of the gastrointestinal tract? Experimental and clinical studies. *J Physiol Pharmacol.* 2006 Nov;57 Suppl 9:35-49.

Index

(foods and herbs too numerous to index)

ulcerative colitis, 30, 94, 96,
    98, 100, 101, 102, 158, 170,
    177, 180
ulcers, 16, 96, 99, 100, 103,
    122, 125, 127, 131, 168,
    171, 172
urban areas, 37
uric acid, 126
urinary disorders, 16
urinary tract, 125

urine, 119
urticaria, 66, 86
vascular permeability, 32
vitamin D, 46, 68
vitamin U, 168
VOCs, 36
wheezing, 46, 53, 86
xylanase, 63, 136
yeast, 69, 83, 176, 180, 211
zonulin, 21, 22, 73, 106

Made in the USA
Columbia, SC
22 July 2021